ANGELS OF MERCY

After qualifying as a doctor in 1943, Eileen Crofton served for the remainder of the Second World War as a captain in the Royal Army Medical Corps. In 1945 she married John Crofton, who, as professor of respiratory diseases at Edinburgh University, went on to pioneer the successful multi-drug treatment for tuberculosis. After raising a family, Eileen Crofton returned full-time to her career, and in 1973 became the first medical director of Action on Smoking and Health in Scotland. Appointed to the WHO's expert committee on smoking, she worked throughout the world to raise awareness of the harm caused by smoking and campaigned for increased tobacco regulation. Lady Crofton was awarded the MBE in 1984 for services to public health. She died in 2010.

ANGELS OF MERCY

*A Women's Hospital on the
Western Front 1914–1918*

'And one patient, desperately ill, must surely have spoken
for many when he said: *"Il y a des choses qui ne s'oublient
pas"* – "There are things that are never forgotten." '
Chapter Eight, concluding words

Eileen Crofton

BIRLINN

This edition first published in 2013 by
Birlinn Limited
West Newington House
10 Newington Road
Edinburgh
EH9 1QS

www.birlinn.co.uk

Originally published in 1997 by Tuckwell Press as
The Women of Royaumont: A Scottish Women's Hospital on the Western Front

ISBN: 978 1 84341 063 8

British Library Cataloguing-in-Publication Data
A catalogue record for this book is available from the British Library

Typeset in Monotype Garamond by Iolaire Typesetting, Newtonmore
Printed and bound by Grafica Veneta
www.graficaveneta.com

Foreword

by Tam Dalyell

Back in the 1990s, the late Dr Eileen Crofton rescued an inspiring episode in the history of Scotland, and in the history of the women's movement, from oblivion. Without her efforts, the story of the heroic women who set up a military hospital in the old abbey of Royaumont in northern France during the darkest days of the First World War would have vanished for ever.

I should explain why Birlinn have invited me to pen a foreword. It has nothing to do with politics, or my being 'Father' of the House of Commons (2001–2005). It has everything to do with my mother's distant cousin and great friend, Dr Elsie Dalyell, one of the intrepid doctors who – along with nurses, orderlies and others – worked day and night in the abbey hospital. Her story, like the stories of so many of the women at Royaumont – is a remarkable one. Elsie came from a family that had left Scotland for Australia, as my mother put it with a chuckle, 'shortly after Botany Bay'. She grew up a tom-boy in Sydney, and went on to study medicine, graduating in 1909 with first-class honours. On the outbreak of war in 1914 she volunteered her services to the War Office, but her offer was declined. Instead, she joined the Serbian Relief Fund that went to Skopje in 1915 to help deal with a typhus epidemic. After Skopje was overrun by the Bulgarians, she joined (in 1916) the Scottish Women's Hospital at Royaumont, and her time there is well documented in Eileen Crofton's book. After the war, she travelled to poverty-stricken Vienna, where she established herself as an authority on rickets, which she showed was due to poor diet – an important leap forward in public health.

Eileen Crofton was also keenly interested in public health. She went up to Oxford in 1938 to study medicine, and after qualifying became a wartime captain in the Royal Army Medical Corps. It was while serving that she met her future husband, John Crofton, at that time a lieutenant-colonel in the RAMC. They married in 1945.

In 1952 they moved to Edinburgh, where John Crofton took up the post of professor of tuberculosis and lung disease, in which role he and his team were the first to develop a successful multi-drug treatment for tuberculosis. Eileen, meanwhile, had her hands full raising five children, but in the 1960s returned, part-time, to medicine, publishing a number of papers on the epidemiology of various respiratory diseases, including a study of the social effects of chronic bronchitis.

In 1973 she really found her metier, when she was appointed first medical director of Action on Smoking and Health in Scotland, in which role she proved her skills as a tireless campaigner and thorn in the flesh of the big tobacco companies. In recognition of her services to public health, Eileen was awarded an MBE on her 'retirement' in 1984. Of course she did not retire. Instead, she became convener of the nascent ASH women's committee, which became active in addressing smoking issues specifically among women, an area of health campaigning that had previously been largely ignored. She also became increasingly interested in women's issues more generally, and it was this interest that led her to research the stories of the pioneering women who ran the Scottish Women's Hospital at Royaumont. Her book was first published in 1997, but has been out of print for some years, and I am delighted that Birlinn have now brought out a new paperback edition. At the time of her death in 2010, at the age of 91, Eileen was still at work on another book, recording the experiences of the first generations of women medical students in Britain, in the later 19th century. Sadly, this work remains unfinished.

Preface to the Second Edition

Angels of Mercy is a revised edition of my mother's book *The Women of Royaumont: A Scottish Women's Hospital on the Western Front*, first published in 1997. When my mother was writing the book, a small handful of the women involved in the hospital at Royaumont during the First World War were still alive, and she told me how privileged she felt to be able to interview and correspond with some of those survivors. There is now no one left alive who served during that war; that generation is past. My mother too – who served as a captain in the Royal Army Medical Corps during the Second World War – has also now passed on. She died at the age of 91 on 8 October 2010, her mind still lively and her spirit vibrant to the end. Her generation in its turn is daily diminishing.

The year after my mother's death, Birlinn asked me, as her literary executor, whether they might bring out a revised paperback edition of *The Women of Royaumont*. We agreed that we needed a new title, one that would better communicate to a wider audience what the book is about. We also agreed that the book should be somewhat shorter, and more focused on the main story. To this end I have undertaken a certain amount of editing and rewriting, and have cut out quite a substantial amount of material that was somewhat tangential to the core narrative, and perhaps of more interest to historians and other researchers than to the general reader. In this task I was assisted by my sister Patricia Raemaekers, who made numerous useful suggestions, making my task much easier than it might otherwise have been.

For this second edition, I have preserved unaltered the original Dedication, Preface and Acknowledgements that my mother included in the book when it was first published.

Ian Crofton
October 2012

Contents

Foreword   v

Preface to the Second Edition   vii

List of Illustrations   xi

Dedication of the First Edition   xiii

Preface to the First Edition   xv

Acknowledgements   xix

Map of the Western Front 1915   xxii

1   The Story Begins   1

2   The Hospital That Went to France   13

3   The First Year   35

4   1916: The Year of Testing   65

5   The Patients   100

6   1917: Strange Interlude   117

7   1918: Their Finest Hour   149

8   Aftermath: From Armistice to Closure   203

Appendix I The Hospital: An Assessment   219

Appendix II The Women   233

Notes and References   287

Bibliography   305

Index   307

List of Illustrations

The Abbey of Royaumont.

Miss Francis Ivens, *médecin-chef* of Hôpital Auxiliaire 301.

The Scottish contingent leaving Waverley Station, Edinburgh, on 2 December 1914.

Les doctoresses in the abbey cloisters, 1915.

The hard-working ambulances were well cared for, but do not give the impression of great comfort.

Chauffeur Banks stands proudly in front of her ambulance.

An operation in the theatre on the first floor.

The job of the Vêtements Department at the top of the building was to sort through the filthy, tattered and bloodstained clothing of the injured.

Miss Ivens on a ward round.

Nurses dressing the wounds of French soldiers in the Blanche de Castille Ward on the first floor.

Another view of Blanche de Castille Ward.

Patients were nursed in the cloisters in the summer months.

Another view of the cloisters.

The kitchen.

A decoration ceremony taking place in the cloisters.

Sister Williams with one of her Senegalese patients.

Abdulla ben Ati looks down to the cloisters from the terrace.

Miss Ivens looks on as a *poilu* receives a decoration.

The arrival of the post at Villers-Cotterêts.

Orderly Proctor.

Miss Ivens, wearing her decorations, stands outside one of the wards at Villers-Cotterêts.

Miss Edith Stoney in her x-ray department in the Scottish Women's Hospital in Serbia.

Doctors awarded the Croix de Guerre, December 1918.

General Descoings and Professor Weinberg of the Pasteur Institute.

Dr Leila Henry, the youngest doctor, and Dr Elizabeth Courtauld, the oldest, on the terrace.

Dr Elsie Jean Dalyell, the bacteriologist.

Sawing wood for fuel at Villers-Cotterêts.

Staff enjoying a picnic in the grounds of Royaumont.

Two *blessés* ('wounded') in drag, performing a skit.

Staff with *blessés*.

A wheelbarrow race at Royaumont.

Soldiers about to leave Royaumont.

Departing from Royaumont.

The abbey at Christmas 1917.

Dr Courtauld as an old lady.

Miss Ivens in her office.

Preface to the First Edition

This book arose quite by chance – a perfect example of serendipity.

A last-minute decision to attend a conference of the European Medical Association on Smoking and Health in 1990 led me to a totally unexpected sequel: some years of growing discovery and excitement, numerous interesting contacts and some valued friendships as the story gradually unravelled.

The conference was held in the beautiful Cistercian Abbey of Royaumont about 30 miles north of Paris, now a delightful cultural centre and an important tourist attraction. Arriving in thick mist on a dark November day, its beauty was not immediately apparent, but on succeeding days a conducted tour in better weather revealed the glorious architecture of the 13th-century building in its lovely setting among trees still resplendent in their autumn colours, and the surrounding canals and waterways in the grounds. We were told the story of the abbey – and, as an aside to me, and because I came from Scotland – our guide pointed out the plaque in a dark corner that commemorated the fact that the abbey had been a military hospital during the First World War, and was a 'Scottish Women's Hospital'. This, however, was not considered sufficiently important to be conveyed to the rest of the international group.

I was so intrigued by this that on my return home I began to make enquiries and to read the early accounts, published in 1917 and 1919,[1] from which I learned the names of a few of the women who served there, and some basic facts – although seen through slightly suspect rose-coloured spectacles.

As a medical woman – and proud of what medical women have contributed to medicine – my first intention was to concentrate on this particular aspect of the story of the hospital. I had not gone far, however, when I discovered that the part played by women doctors – of crucial importance as it was – was only a part of the story. I became more and more involved with all the women who were engaged at Royaumont in a unique and extraordinarily successful enterprise. I decided then that it was the story of this community as it evolved over the years of war that was the story I wanted to tell. It also became clear to me that the story had been forgotten. In the abbey itself, only the bare fact of its existence seems to be known. To most people in this country, if they have heard of the Scottish Women's Hospitals at all, they recall the tremendous retreat from Serbia over the mountains in 1915, the gallantry of Dr Elsie Inglis, and her tragic death on landing in England in 1917 after the retreat of her hospital from Russia. This story has now been told,[2] but the story of Royaumont is a fascinating one on its own and deserves a fuller study. I have tried to do justice to it. The main part of the book focuses on the events in the hospital throughout the war, as well as the difficulties faced by the pioneers in setting up their hospital and the problems arising from an ever-increasing volume of patients as the war dragged on and the French medical service struggled to cope. The book then concludes with an account of the personalities and careers of some of the women involved, both medical and non-medical. As is often the case in wartime conditions, there were periods of intense pressure and periods of comparative quiet and inactivity. These two aspects of life called for adaptability and qualities of character in those who participated.

One of the outstanding features of this story is the gradual emergence of a strong and unique sense of community, which lasted not only throughout the period of active service, but which persisted for many years afterwards through the Royaumont and Villers-Cotterêts Association and through many lifelong friendships. It must be almost unique that a wartime association should persist as theirs did, with regular newsletters and meetings, until as recently as 1973.

The strong sense of community – not always to be seen in an all-woman setting – was remarkable. It must have owed much to the quality of their 'Chief', Miss Ivens. It must also owe something to the fact they knew, and were proud, that they were doing a worthwhile job, one that was recognized and highly valued by the French authorities and in all the villages around who benefited from the presence of 'Les Dames Anglaises'. To be a 'Royaumontite', to be the recipient of the medal of the Scottish Women's Hospitals, and, for some of them also, medals from the French government, was a distinction and source of pride in their later lives.

The hospital was what they made it. Its success – and it *was* a success – was theirs and belonged to them all. They were dependent on their own resources and could not summon outside help in times of crisis. The success of the hospital depended on all the different departments. Efficiency in the kitchen and the clerical department was no less important than in the departments concerned with the direct care of the patients. There was mutual respect, which existed despite occasional misunderstandings, some of which are recorded in the story. That there should also be some misunderstandings with the committee at home is not surprising, but it was a tribute to the members of the committee who visited from time to time that a fuller appreciation of the difficulties faced by the unit working in what was in fact a totally unsuitable building led in most cases to their resolution.

The history of these women illustrates the changing role of women in the early part of the 20th century and, in particular, the impact of the war. For many, probably all of them, their experiences at Royaumont formed a watershed in their personal lives. For some it opened new windows of opportunity; for others their return to civilian life brought less change than they might have expected and perhaps hoped for.

Acknowledgements

I am sometimes overwhelmed by the number of people who have helped me in the writing of this book. I am grateful to all of them and only hope that I have not betrayed their trust in me.

I owe a big debt of gratitude to Miss Helen Lowe who generously placed at my disposal her register of the Royaumont staff, her collection of newsletters of the Royaumont and Villers-Cotterêts Association, and other material and whose unfailing interest has greatly encouraged me.

Dr Leah Leneman shared with me much material arising from her own researches on the Scottish Women's Hospitals that was relevant to Royaumont. Although we shared information, I am conscious that the debt was very much on my side.

I would also like to thank Dr Harold Swan, honorary archivist of the University of Sheffield, for his continuing interest and listening ear, and Professor Alexander Fenton, director of the European Ethnological Research Centre, for reading my text, encouraging me, and making many useful suggestions.

I acknowledge with gratitude the enormous help of my publisher, John Tuckwell, who has shown unending patience in guiding a tyro through the mysteries of publishing. Any deficiencies that remain are mine, certainly not his.

Finally I am grateful to Professor Ruth Bowden for much useful advice.

Among the individuals I acknowledge the help of: Mrs Audrey Acland, daughter of Orderly Starr; M. l'Abbé Bigo, Presbytère de Viarmes; Mrs Mona Calder, daughter of Orderly Watt; Dr Hilda Cantrell and Dr James Carmichael for memories of Miss Ivens and

Miss Nicholson; Mr Samuel Courtauld, great-nephew of Dr
Courtauld; Dr Betty Cowan, for information on Dr Guest at
Christian Medical College, Ludhiana; Mrs M. Crowther, daughter
of Dr Hamilton; Mr Tam Dalyell, Mr Wm Dalyell and Dr Martin
Davey for information on Dr Elsie Dalyell; Mme Marie-Christine
Daudy, daughter of M. Henry Goüin, and granddaughter of M.
Edouard Goüin for a tour of the abbey and making it possible to
examine the visitors' book; Sir Alastair Denny, for information on
Orderly Denny; Mr Harold Francis FRCS and the late Professor
Sir Norman Jeffcoate for information on Miss Ivens; Mrs Morag
Fairlie, niece of Chauffeur Smeal; Mr William Garrett, son of Dr
Lillie; Mr James Gray and Mrs Gray, formerly Cook Simpson; Dr
Jean Guy for information on Edith Stoney; Miss Rachel Hedder-
wick, daughter of Cook Littlejohn; Mrs M. Kappagoda, for
information on Dr Hendrick; Miss Heather Mackay, niece of
Auxiliary Nurse Chapman; the late Dr Grace Macrae, formerly
Orderly Summerhayes; Mrs Amy Maddox and Mrs Sue Morris,
nieces of the three Inglis sisters; Mlle Maloum-Gerzo, of the
Abbey of Royaumont; Mrs Anne Murdoch, daughter of Dr Henry;
Mrs Margaret Nisbet, daughter of Orderly Manson; Mrs Margaret
Oddy, daughter of Sister Dunderdale; Mr David Proctor, nephew
of Orderly Proctor; Miss Mary Pym for information on Miss Ivens;
Dr Elizabeth Rees, for information on Miss Ivens and Miss
Nicholson; Ms Margaret Randall, niece of Orderly Davidson;
Mr G.D. Richardson for information on the Dalyell family; Mrs
Catriona Reynolds, niece of Orderly Neilson-Gray; Dr Ann Shep-
herd, niece of Dr MacDougall; Mrs Ailsa Tanner, granddaughter of
Mrs Robertson; Dr J.F. Tessier for advice on French writing on the
First World War; Dr Christopher Silver, for a photograph of Miss
Ivens; Dr I. Simmonds, son of Chauffeur Banks; and Miss M.P.
Simms, niece of Orderly Simms.

I acknowledge also the help of many institutions, libraries and
museums: Mr Adrian Allen, assistant archivist, University of
Liverpool; Mr Michael Barfoot, Edinburgh Medical Archives
Centre, University of Edinburgh; Mme Thérèse Blondet-Busch,
Musée d'Histoire Contemporaine, Photothèque de l'Hôtel Nation-
al des Invalides, Paris; Mr Peter Carnell, library archivist, University

of Sheffield; Mr D.M. Cook, librarian, Liverpool Medical Institute; Mr David Dougan, librarian, Fawcett Library, London Guildhall University; Miss Joan Ferguson, former librarian and Mr Ian Mills, librarian, and his staff, Royal College of Physicians of Edinburgh; Miss A. Fletcher, medical librarian, Royal Free Hospital School of Medicine; Dr Leslie Hall and Miss S.M. Dixon, Contemporary Medical Archives Centre and Mr William Schupbach of the Iconographic Collection, Wellcome Institute for the History of Medicine; Mr Graham Hopper, Dumbarton District Library; Dr Elizabeth van Houts, archivist, Newnham College, Cambridge; Mr Peter Liddle, keeper of the Liddle Collection of First World War Archive Material, Leeds University; Mr Colin McLaren, head of special collections, university archivist, Aberdeen University; Mme Annick Perrot, conservateur du Musée Pasteur, Paris; Mrs Kate Perry, archivist, Girton College, Cambridge; Mr Simon Roberts, Department of Documents and Mrs Hilary Roberts, Department of Photographs, Imperial War Museum; Ms Margaret Robins, archivist, Women's College Hospital, Toronto; Mr M.A.M. Smallman, sub-librarian, Queen's University, Belfast; Mr K.E. Smith, archivist, University of Sydney; Mr Robert Smith, keeper of muniments, University of St Andrews; Mr Alastair Tough, archivist, Greater Glasgow Health Board, University of Glasgow; Dr Ian White, honorary archivist, St John's Hospital for Diseases of the Skin, St Thomas's Hospital, London; Miss Hazel Wright and her staff, Department of Rare Books and Manuscripts, Mitchell Library, Glasgow; and to the staff at the National Library of Scotland, the Edinburgh Central Library and the French Institute, Edinburgh.

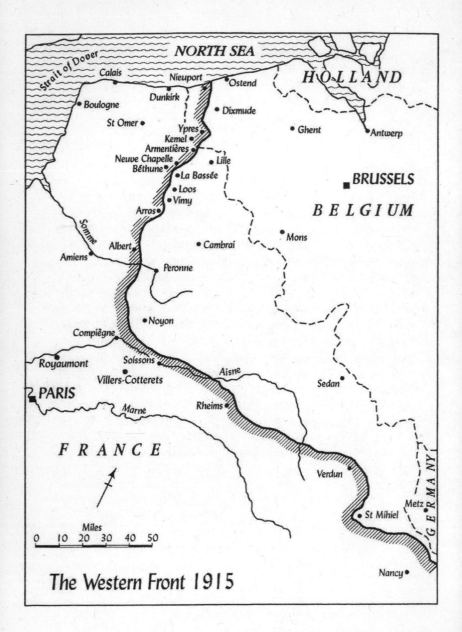

The Western Front 1915

CHAPTER ONE

৵

The Story Begins

This story concerns an abbey, a hospital, some women and the war.

It all took place in the Abbey of Royaumont, one of the most beautiful of all the lovely Cistercian abbeys of France. Set in gently rolling wooded country some 30 miles to the north of Paris, it is still in a relatively unspoilt area. The continual expansion of Paris has not yet engulfed it, though the nearby villages are gradually losing their local character. The roads are now of a quality that would have aroused the envy of those women ambulance drivers who, dodging potholes, tried to protect their wounded passengers from the jolts and bumps of the 12-mile journey on atrocious roads from the railhead at Creil.

The train service nowadays is perhaps not very much better than the one they knew. But for those travelling to and from Paris in the First World War it must have been a very much more beautiful journey than it is now, especially in spring when the orchards were in flower.

The journey from England now is, however, very different. A rapid and comfortable flight to Charles de Gaulle airport bears no comparison with the crowded cross-Channel steamers with the ever-present danger of U-boat attack, and the slow, and often devious, journeys by train to Paris and on to Viarmes.

Today from the air you can look down on a crossroads, where you can see, clearly visible, the Royaumont Monument, marking the limit of the German offensive in 1914 and commemorating those who died in the hospital. And if you are quick enough you might also catch a glimpse of the Abbey of Royaumont itself, among its trees and its landmark spire.

The forests where the women loved to wander and picnic are still there, but the trenches they sometimes explored are gone. There are possibly fewer of the wild flowers that so delighted them. Did they, perhaps, gather too many of the lilies-of-the-valley? We know that the *poilus** were allowed to do so, and that they delighted in offering great bunches to the sisters and orderlies. The beauty of the unspoilt countryside in those days made an unforgettable impression. In spring and summer they remembered:

> The fields blue with cornflowers and scarlet with poppies – the woods carpeted with cowslips, lilies of the valley, dwarf daffodils, and all made gayer and more exciting by gorgeous butterflies, dragon flies and moths.[1]

And in November:

> I have no words to tell of the beauty of that autumn forest [the forest of Beaumont]. The hush of St Luke's peace was over all the forest, that dream beauty which comes with a still November, a kind of hushed period of farewell when the tattered banners of scarlet and gold hang on the edge of the winds. A perfect sunset lit the forest aisles with subtle light ... and the misty blue distances between the tree vistas had the spell of moonlight on them. The names too of these forest alleys were a perpetual delight to me – imagine such a light shining along the 'Route de la Pierre Turquoise'. In these woods Blanche de Castille used to ride on her white palfrey. When we emerged from the wood a new beauty awaited us, a great copper moon rising on the loops of the Oise – Seen through the straight poplars it was like a Japanese painting ... That ride home through the little village of Beaumont and by the Oise in the last lingering purple twilight and glorious moonlight was unforgettable.[2]

* The informal name given to French private soldiers in the First World War, the equivalent of the English 'Tommy'. *Poilu* literally means 'hairy'.

The trees in front of the abbey – in their spring or autumn foliage, shrouded in snow, or sparkling with frost – are the same ones that grew there all those years ago; and the canals and waterways around the abbey, where convalescent *poilus* so hopefully went fishing, are there still.

The buildings themselves struck every newcomer then – as they still do today – with their beauty. The cloister court is unchanged, though the rose garden has disappeared. In imagination the visitor can picture the cloister court filled with beds, and patients lying there enjoying the healing power of the sunshine and the lovely surroundings and the nights of peace and quiet. 'On moonlit evenings,' Antonio de Navarro tells us in his 1917 account of the hospital, 'the scene was one of indescribable beauty. The old grey masonry, assuming then a ghostly pallor, shone like marble in the dark, shimmering sky.'[3] The terrace above the cloisters, where they used to sit and rest and chat, has now been removed – it had been a 19th-century addition. Behind the present buildings there is a field where a crater remains from a shell that landed in 1918.

The interior of the buildings is now much changed. The entrance hall, so large and impressive in the hospital era, has been divided, but happily concessions to modern ideas of comfort have not gone so far as to install a lift. The visitor must still climb 71 steps to the second floor, and is thankful not to be burdened with a heavy patient on a stretcher. Nor, with modern heating and plumbing, must fuel and water still be carried up all those stairs.

The hospital wards are recognizable from their beautiful vaulting and ornamental pillars. How impossible it must have been to black out those tall Gothic windows when the Zeppelins and Gothas were overhead.

The present well-heated bedrooms with their ensuite bathrooms are a far cry from the primitive conditions of wartime, and would have seemed an unbelievable luxury to the women who strove to keep themselves warm and clean in those early days. Perhaps also they might have envied the sanitary arrangements enjoyed by the monks of the 13th century, who were provided, in what is now known as the *Maison des Latrines*, with no fewer than 60 seats placed back to back and draining into a canal. A generous allowance, it would seem, for 180 monks. How useful these would have been for the patients in the wartime hospital, where the sanitary arrangements were pretty primitive and the graceful lectern in the refectory was used as a convenient depository for bedpans.[4]

All those coal-burning stoves seen in the archive photographs, with the flues finding their way out through the old stone walls, are gone without a trace. Gone also is the monstrous stove in the kitchen on which Michelet, the renowned chef, used to dance, and gone also is the sink. Instead there are priceless mediaeval tapestries, and a superb 15th-century statue of the Virgin and Child.

Standing in the great refectory, or perhaps enjoying one of the concerts that frequently take place there, the visitor requires a keen imagination to picture it when it was a ward of wounded – often desperately wounded – men: beds on each side and a row down the middle – 100 in all; brilliant scarlet bed covers against the soft grey of the Gothic pillars; and a giant Canadian flag reminding us that this was 'Canada Ward'. It must have looked even more colourful at Christmas time when it was decorated with great branches and bunches of mistletoe, and how beautiful it must have been when the old Curé celebrated Mass in the candlelight.

One member of that wartime community tells us what it was like to be a part of this great endeavour:

> I dreamed dreams of a grey, dusty austere Royaumont, where eager grey, blue and white figures hurried about, intent and tight-lipped, or enthusiastic and laughing; rows of red-blanketed beds in the quiet nights and the soft pad of feet and the long shadows moving on the high stone walls; of a purpose and unity of mind; of life and of death and of memories too deep for words ... something of which nobody left in the whole building knows.[5]

On their tour of the abbey the observant visitor might notice a rather worn and inconspicuous plaque, which translates as follows:

> Here from 1915 to 1919 Miss Frances Ivens CBE MS Lond was Head Physician of the Scottish Women's Hospital estab-

lished in the Abbey of Royaumont by the good grace of its owner, M. Edouard Goüin, and the generosity of British and Allied donors.

Ten thousand eight hundred and sixty-one wounded French soldiers received from an exclusively feminine staff the benefits of a devotion without limits.

What was this hospital? And who were these women?

ᥣ⃰

Before we answer those questions, let us first unravel a little of the broader history of the abbey,[6] which was founded by Louis IX of France (later known as Saint Louis) in 1229. His father, Louis VIII, had had the ambition to endow a monastery. When he died, his 12-year-old son lost no time in carrying out his wishes, with the help of his redoubtable mother, Blanche de Castille.

The little boy took his duties seriously. The abbey was to be under the Cistercians, a relatively new order that called for greater simplicity than that practised by the longer-established Cluniac foundations. However, as this was to be a royal foundation, simplicity was somewhat modified. It was to be known as Royaumont, or Mons Regalis ('royal mount', although there is little evidence of a mount). It was well-endowed – in fact its subsequent history showed that it was too well-endowed.

According to tradition, the boy-king would ride over to the abbey from his nearby castle at Asnières, mingle with the lay brothers engaged in the construction work, and encourage them to greater efforts by pushing a stone-laden wheelbarrow himself. He would rebuke those who made too much noise, or rested from their labours, telling them 'Monks keep silence, and so should you. Monks don't rest, and neither should you.'

With or without this encouragement, the abbey church was ready for dedication on Sunday 19 October 1235 (an event which the hospital staff commemorated in 1915, almost 700 years later). The church was dedicated to the Holy Cross, Our Lady and All the

Saints, and King Louis donated a piece of the True Cross, a fragment of the Crown of Thorns, some relics of St Thomas of Canterbury, and some relics of St Agnes.

Many stories are told of Louis' piety. He took part in the Cistercian custom of washing the feet of the poor (just as in a later chapter Orderly Starr records how she washed the feet of the wounded *poilus*). Louis, in an excess of zeal, wanted to go further to demonstrate his humility by washing the feet of the monks. He was restrained, however, by the abbot, who suggested some people might speak ill of it – in other words he might be accused of showing off.

Louis used to visit the infirmary, and with his own hands prepare food and place it carefully in the mouth of a leper, removing any grains of salt that might cause pain – just as, centuries later, Orderly Starr would feed her patient with the wounded mouth so patiently and so carefully. Like the orderlies 700 years later, St Louis swept the floors, and at mealtimes carried his plates to the hatch into the kitchen – the very same hatch through which meals passed when the monks' refectory was used as the staff dining area. Sometimes Louis would read to the monks from the pulpit where, on Christmas Eve 1917, Orderly Don (a trained opera singer) sang to delight her listeners.

King Louis died at Tunis on the Second Crusade, but his endowments to the abbey were continued and even increased. Consequently, the initial period of devotion and austerity gave way to an era of laxity and indulgence.

In 1516 King Francis I gained the right to appoint 'commendators'. These appointments, being highly profitable, were much sought after, and were a useful source of royal income. Religious duties were not required, and commendators could be responsible for the worldly affairs of a number of abbeys. One such commendator was Cardinal Mazarin, who added Royaumont to his list. For reasons best known to himself he handed Royaumont over to the ten-year-old Prince of Lorraine, in whose family it remained, becoming a beautifully furnished *maison de plaisance* ('pleasure palace'). A later abbot was not content with the abbey as it stood and built a palace (later known as the 'chateau') alongside. However, he was not to enjoy this. The French Revolution broke out, and the abbot fled to Austria, where he was reported to have died in misery.

In 1790, when there were only ten monks remaining, the National Assembly decreed the destruction of the abbey church. This was duly carried out in 1792 – but the northeast tower was too strong for them and still stands today as the *flèche* ('spire'), the emblem of Royaumont.

The abbey was sold, its contents scattered and a cotton mill installed, and in the 19th century pavilions in the grounds became popular holiday resorts for fashionable Parisians. In 1864 the abbey was sold again, to the Oblate Fathers, and then in 1869 to the Sisters of the Holy Family. It was a religious building once more. Much preparatory work was done after the damage caused by the industrial installations, but the return to a religious use was not to last. In 1905 a law was passed against religious orders and the sisters had to leave for Belgium. The property was bought by Monsieur Jules Goüin (who already owned the nearby chateau). It lay empty until the advent of the First World War, when Goüin's son Edouard offered it to the French Red Cross. This in turn led to its occupation by the Scottish Women's Hospital for four and a half years.

❦

The Scottish Women's Hospitals of the First World War were the inspiration of one remarkable woman. On the outbreak of war Dr Elsie Inglis conceived the idea of setting up hospitals that would be run exclusively by women, as a means of supporting the war effort. She carried through her project until her own tragic death in 1917, but she had laid such firm foundations that Scottish Women's Hospitals continued in active service up to and beyond the end of the war.

It was a magnificent achievement, especially in the face of society's attitudes towards women – particularly medical women – in the early years of the 20th century.

The 19th century had seen many struggles by women to raise

their standards of education, to widen the their opportunities in employment, and to correct at least some of the injustices they suffered regarding property and other rights. By the end of the century women had gained access to universities. After a long and sometimes bitter struggle, they were able to qualify in medicine and, by having their names on the Medical Register, could be legally entitled to practise medicine. When Elizabeth Garrett Anderson gained admission to the Medical Register in 1865, she was only the second woman to do so. The medical profession were perturbed: they closed ranks and denied women access for the next 12 years. But others – among them Elsie Inglis – were pressing hard on the closed door.

In Edinburgh Sophia Jex-Blake, having won her own personal battle for registration in 1877, was struggling with the Edinburgh medical establishment to get instruction, practical experience and access to examinations for women students. Elsie Inglis was one of her students. At an early age Elsie showed the stuff of which she was made when she, with others of her fellow-students, rebelled against Jex-Blake's autocratic ways and, with outside help, set up a rival – and successful – Medical College for Women in Edinburgh. She herself qualified in 1892, and set up practice. She went on to carry out pioneering social and medical work with poor women in the slums of Edinburgh.

Elsie Inglis soon became involved in the campaign for votes for women, and in due course became the honorary secretary of the Scottish Federation of Women's Suffrage Societies. The Scottish Federation was allied to the National Union of Women's Suffrage Societies (NUWSS), whose president was Mrs Millicent Fawcett, a younger sister of the pioneer Dr Elizabeth Garrett Anderson. The policy of both these organizations was to pursue their aims through peaceful and constitutional means. These were the 'suffragists'. For some women these methods were too slow. Mrs Emmeline Pankhurst and her daughters founded the Women's Social and Political Union (WSPU), which adopted militant tactics and whose members became known as 'suffragettes'. These women became increasingly active in the years before the war, and gained considerable notoriety. They actively sought imprisonment and caused the government of the day more than a little embarrassment through their policy of going on hunger strike when they were imprisoned.

In the mood of patriotic fervour that accompanied the outbreak of war, most suffragists and suffragettes resolved to lay aside their campaigns for the vote, and devote themselves to the war effort. To Dr Elsie Inglis the war provided a golden opportunity to demonstrate what medical women could achieve, particularly in a very different field from the traditional one of caring for women and children. Dr Anderson – now aged 80 – had no doubts either. 'My dears,' she told the volunteers, 'if you are successful over this work, you will have carried women's profession forward by a hundred years.'[7]

Elsie Inglis was an achiever. She had determination, and she knew how to be ruthless when she thought it necessary. She had a remarkable gift of persuading others to do what she wanted; she could gain support from influential people; and she could attract devoted followers. In addition she never spared herself.

Even before the war she was involved in the training of young women for Voluntary Aid Detachments, but on the outbreak of war she envisaged something much more ambitious. On 12 August 1914, at a meeting of the Scottish Federation of Women's Suffrage Societies in Edinburgh, Dr Inglis proposed 'that the Federation should give organized help to Red Cross work'. Miss Mair, the president, then proposed that the empty St George's School in Melville Street (the school for girls which she had helped to found, and which had moved to new premises) should be applied for and equipped as a hospital. One can almost feel Dr Inglis's mind leaping ahead as she then proposed 'that Melville Street should be equipped as a hospital staffed entirely by women – and if not required at home should be sent abroad'.[8]

Finding that the school building in Edinburgh was not available, Dr Inglis then proposed, with the backing of the committee, to offer the proposed unit of 100 beds to the War Office or to the Red Cross. Both offers were summarily turned down ('Go home and sit still' was the oft-quoted phrase). There was no interest in a hospital staffed by women.

Undaunted, on 15 October Dr Inglis wrote to the French ambassador in London:

> I am directed by the Executive of the Scottish Federation of Women's Suffrage Societies to ask Your Excellency's consideration of our scheme for organizing medical aid for the help of our Allies in the field.
>
> The Federation proposes to send out hospital units, officered by women doctors, and staffed by fully trained nurses and properly qualified dressers. The Units will be sent out fully equipped to nurse 100 beds. Should Your Excellency's Government desire such aid as we are proud to offer, it will be very willingly placed at the service of the French Red Cross. Our Units will be prepared to move from place to place as the exigencies of war may require, and to utilize such buildings as may be placed at our disposal.[9]

A similar letter went to the Serbian authorities. Both countries recognized that their own medical services were very inadequate, and both countries accepted the offer. The Serbian story is a fascinating one, but is not the subject of the present book.[10] Dr Inglis now had the enthusiastic support of the NUWSS, and they agreed on an appeal for 'Scottish Women's Hospitals for Foreign Service'. Meetings were arranged, including a very large one in London on 20 October, where Dr Inglis outlined her plans to a big audience.

Back in Scotland a specially convened 'Scottish Women's Hospitals Committee' was organized to receive donations and offers from volunteers. Sub-committees were set up to deal with hospitals, personnel, equipment, uniforms and cars. Premises were obtained in St Andrew's Square, Edinburgh, gifted by the Prudential Insurance Society.

Excitement was mounting, and money was flowing in; by 30 October *Common Cause* (the journal of the NUWSS) announced: 'Dr Inglis has got her first £1000! One hospital is secure and will go to Serbia.' There were plenty of volunteers – 'surgeons, nurses, medical students and members of Voluntary Aid Detachments ... but many more are needed'.

The press work in the NUWSS offices in London was co-ordinated and masterminded by V.C.C. (Vera) Collum, who was to play a major role in the subsequent history of Royaumont.

By 6 November £2800 had been collected; they now hoped to fund three hospital units, at an estimated cost of £1000 (later raised to £1500) to equip each 100-bed unit. By 13 November two units were ready.

By 20 November *Common Cause* reported that Madame de la Panouse, president of the French Red Cross, was actively seeking a building that would accommodate the unit of these '*Dames très sérieuses*', and by 27 November the decision had been taken that it should go to the Abbey of Royaumont. By the end of November the link between the abbey and the Scottish Women's Hospital was firmly in place, a link that was to last longer than anyone conceived at the time.

※

From the military point of view, the fighting in northern France between August 1914 and the arrival of the hospital in January 1915 represented one of the most dramatic periods of the war. It was in essence a war of movement, not to be repeated until the German onslaughts of 1918 and their subsequent repulse.

The so-called 'Battle of the Frontiers' began on 14 August. The Germans advanced rapidly, taking Amiens, Soissons, Laon and Reims; British and French forces were in retreat and Paris itself was threatened. What had seemed to be an inexorable onslaught was eventually halted at the River Marne, where the German advance was checked, signalling the end of the war of movement and initiating the horrors of trench warfare. In the first five months of the war the French lost 300,000 men killed, including 5000 officers; 600,000 men were captured, wounded or missing.

In September the Germans made a great effort to reduce Antwerp (in which they succeeded in October), and to destroy the Belgian army. The German cavalry, the Uhlans, swept across to the Belgian coast. With the Allies in full retreat, the Uhlans ranged at will over northwest France. It must have been at this time that they bivouacked in the abbey – and left behind quantities of straw and other debris for the first orderlies to clear. The German advance had in fact drawn very close to Royaumont. On 4 September 1914 they reached the crossroads only a mile from the abbey. It was here that the dearly loved Curé had stood for several days ready, if it should prove necessary, to plead with the German commanders for the safety of his village of Asnières (see Chapter Five).

By the end of 1914 stalemate had been reached; both sides were beginning to dig in, and it was not until February 1915 that fighting was renewed. By this time Royaumont was just beginning to get organized.

The story of the abbey, the hospital, the women and the war had begun.

❧

CHAPTER TWO

The Hospital That Went to France

By the middle of November 1914 the selection of volunteers destined for Royaumont was complete. In the first instance the unit was to consist of seven doctors, ten nurses, seven orderlies, two cooks, a clerk, an administrator, two maids and four chauffeurs (two of them men, as there was initially some doubt as to whether the French authorities would permit women to drive in the war zone).

The great experiment began.

What were the motives that led these women to volunteer? Some were looking for adventure, some were swept up by patriotism, some sought to wave the banner for women's suffrage. One of the volunteers, Dorothy Littlejohn, a highly trained cook from the Edinburgh College of Domestic Science, was not among this last group. Not only did she actively oppose women's suffrage, she entirely disapproved of women doctors. This was strange, as her father was the great Sir Henry Littlejohn, the first medical officer of health for Edinburgh. After initial hesitation about female doctors he had become a strong supporter of Sophia Jex-Blake in her prolonged and traumatic campaign to obtain medical education for women. But his daughter clearly had very different ideas. Indeed she was furious that on arrival in London the party was 'paraded' before Mrs Millicent Fawcett in the offices of the NUWSS. She wanted no part of that.[1]

Who were these seven doctors who were about to pioneer totally new fields of activity, fields that they had probably never even imagined a few short months before?

The appointment of Miss Francis Ivens* as chief medical officer (*médecin-chef*) was almost certainly the most crucial one in effecting the transformation of a small medical unit into a hospital of 600 beds, later described as 'the crack hospital of the war'. At the age of 44 she had an established position as consultant obstetrician and gynaecologist in Liverpool. She had been a brilliant student at the London School of Medicine for Women, and a gold medallist of London University. In addition she was only the third woman in the UK to obtain the degree of master of surgery. She had been keenly interested in the suffrage movement (the non-militant wing) for a number of years, and on the outbreak of war had volunteered her services to the women's unit in Belgium under the leadership of Mrs Stobart. However, the German advance had led to the withdrawal of the unit before Miss Ivens could join it. She was then free to volunteer for the Royaumont unit.

Miss Ruth Nicholson, a graduate of Durham University, had worked in the mission field in Palestine, where she had gained wide surgical experience. She later became second-in-command at Royaumont and served continuously until the hospital closed in 1919.

Dr Agnes Savill, one of Glasgow University's most distinguished women graduates, was a consultant in London with a high reputation in dermatology and electro-therapeutics. This involved radiological work, and it was in that capacity that her expertise was so valuable at Royaumont. Her connection with Royaumont was maintained throughout the war, though not on a continuous basis. She had played a notable role in the women's suffrage movement, having worked alongside two distinguished male surgeons in an inquiry into the appalling treatment of women hunger-strikers in prison (see Appendix Two).

Dr Winifred Ross had been resident surgeon in Paisley Parochial Hospital after her graduation from Glasgow University. Her surgical experience included the treatment of male patients, an area which some regarded at that time as too indelicate for women.

Dr Berry (née Augusta Lewin) had been a fellow-student of

* The title 'Miss' is used here for the chief surgeons (Ivens and Nicholson) in accordance with British custom. All others are referred to as 'Dr'.

Miss Ivens, and had experience in the field of public health. She served right through to the summer of 1918.

Dr Hancock had been resident medical officer at the Hospice in Edinburgh, an institution located in an appallingly poor and over-crowded area of the city. It had been founded by Dr Elsie Inglis (whom she would have known well) as a surgical and gynaecological service for women, and a centre for district midwifery.

Dr Heyworth had only recently qualified, and it was intended she would work in a junior capacity as a 'dresser'.

Such was the initial medical team; most of them will become familiar as the story unfolds.

Although not a medical person, another key figure from the outset was Cicely Hamilton, who was clerk of the unit from December 1914 to May 1917. On the outbreak of war she had already achieved fame as an actress and playwright, and had played a prominent role in the women's suffrage movement.

.⁂

The Edinburgh contingent joined up with members coming from other parts of the country and proceeded to Folkestone accom-panied by Dr Inglis herself, who had come to see them off, and who followed them a few days later. There was, on that Friday, a terrific gale blowing. The army decided that it was too rough to embark the troops, but Dr Inglis was insistent that her women would sail, come what may. She was not one with whom new recruits were prepared to argue, so on they went. Hatches were battened down and the wise ones took their seasick pills. After a 'simply terrible crossing' lasting three hours longer than scheduled, they landed at Boulogne and began the struggle with customs and red tape. Dorothy Littlejohn was in better shape than most, and also spoke some French, so it was left to her to negotiate with the authorities. This done, they proceeded to Paris.[2]

The following morning Sister Martha Aitken in Boulogne (who had no connection with the SWH) wrote an account of that fierce storm in her diary:

All night long it has blown a gale and the big windows in the casino shook very much. Every minute I expected to see them blown in. Rain, thunder and lightning accompanied the wind. The sea is lashed into a white fury and below the casino one can see the spray dashing the sea wall. The hospital ship had taken refuge in Boulogne Harbour. During a flash of lightning one can see the white cliffs of Dover. Towards morning we hear several guns being fired and two rockets sent up. I expect it is some poor ship in distress. Poor souls on a night like this.[3]

Cicely Hamilton, travelling a few days earlier than the main unit to take up her duties as clerk, also had a rough crossing. Looking back in 1946, she remembered

... the tumbling steamer as it neared the harbour, making wide circles to avoid the mines. The unfamiliar faces of Indian soldiers looking down from a familiar Boulogne quay, the slow devious journey to Paris – devious because mainline bridges had been blown. And finally Royaumont – picturesque, impressive and most abominably chilly.[4]

Meanwhile in Paris, Miss Ivens and a few others who had travelled with her had learned that their equipment had not arrived, and that its whereabouts were unknown. Furthermore, they heard from Monsieur Goüin, the owner of the abbey, that he had accommodated Cicely Hamilton, the clerk, and Mrs Owen, the administrator, in his own part of the abbey as a temporary measure, but that he could offer no further accommodation. He strongly urged them not to come. This was not in accordance with the ideas of Miss Ivens, who elected to proceed regardless of the warnings. She was as determined as Dr Inglis herself to get on with the tasks ahead, and it was no part of her plan to idle in Paris while work was waiting to be done. If there were no beds for her staff, she could buy mattresses, stuff them with straw, carry them by train, and lay them on the floor. So this is exactly what they did.

On 11 December Dorothy Littlejohn wrote home to her fiancé:

This Abbaye is 1½ miles from Viarmes, such a nice little country town, with quite good shops. The Abbaye itself is charming with lovely old cloisters and a real old-fashioned garden with a little fountain in the middle. The inside rather appals one at first, it's so very large and so many odd staircases etc; in fact it is very eerie, especially as there is no light anywhere at the moment, and, as you know, a candle doesn't give much. ... The room I had felt very musty and in the morning my dress felt so damp I was afraid to get into it so what the uninhabited portion will be like I dread to think.[5]

They had set out from home under the impression that the Abbey of Royaumont was 'a fine house with ample accommodation, good drainage and water supply, and electric lighting'.[6] This description was correct in only one respect: the abbey did have ample accommodation.

Apart from the deficiencies of water, heating and lighting, the abbey was in a deplorable condition. Dirt had accumulated everywhere over the years, and the vast rooms were cluttered with masses of heavy masonry, and with straw and rubbish left behind by the Uhlans who had bivouacked there during the Battle of the Marne.

On 17 December Cicely Hamilton reported:

Those first few days at Royaumont I shall always look back on as an experience worth having. In surroundings of mediaeval grandeur – amid vaulted corridors, gothic refectories and cloisters – we proceeded to camp out with what we carried. The Abbey, in all its magnificence, was ours; but during those first few days it did not offer us very much more besides magnificence and shelter. It had not been lived in for years and its water supply had been practically cut off when the nuns left for Belgium. Hence we carried water in buckets up imposing staircases and along equally imposing corridors. Our only available stove – a mighty erection in the kitchen which had not been lit for a decade – was naturally short-tempered at first, and the supply of hot water was very limited. So, in consequence, was our first washing; at times very limited indeed. Our equipment, after the fashion of baggage in these times of war, was in no great hurry to arrive; until it arrived we did without sheets and blankets, wrapped ourselves in rugs and overcoats at night, and did not do much undressing.[7]

Dorothy Littlejohn, working as cook in the kitchen, also left an account of the initial privations:

I had an awful morning trying to get food ready, with a plumber every now and then putting my fire out. We have got a huge chef's range, in fact some of the parts are so heavy it is quite difficult for women to shift them. You see, in this place, there is really nothing to work with until our things arrive from Edinburgh, so, for 25 people, we are cooking with two small pans, some rather wee bowls of the country, a kettle and that's all. The dishes are equally scarce, so it's a case of eternally washing up and also double meals and really by the time we have cooked and fed all that lot we are almost past food, but don't think I am grumbling; it will be better later on. ... This kitchen is a huge place with lovely arches and a nice door into the garden. At present we have nothing but candles, so it looks very gloomy, but they are going to put in a certain amount of electric light and also putting in a kind of hot water system which will be a comfort as at present every drop of hot water has to be specially boiled and also the kitchen is the only place you can get any at all.[8]

Cicely Hamilton had more to say about the difficulties:

We borrowed teacups from the village ironmonger, and passed the one knife around at meals for everyone to have a chop with it. We are as short of lamps as we are of knives – shorter; and we wandered about our majestic pile with candle-ends, stuck in bottles; little twinkling candle-ends that struggled with the shadows under the groined roofs ... we are getting electric light in now, and already I find it in my heart to regret those bottled candles with their Rembrandtesque effects. Two of them, faintly dispersing the gloom at one end of the vaulted kitchen – while the pillars climbed to lose themselves in the blackness ... I try to console myself for their loss by reflecting that the staring electric bulbs are more practicable for hospital purposes. But I am glad that I saw the kitchen before the bulbs were put in.

We did not easily get our staring electric bulbs; nor did we easily get our water laid on, our drains attended to, or broken windows mended. We live, you see, in the land of compulsory military service – where the plumber, the glazier, the electrician can only attend to your wants when he has not been ordered to the colours ... Our preparations have been slow – but if they have been slow they have been sure. Drains, water, heating, lighting – everything in spite of the difficulties, is finally getting itself done. A few days ago our equipment condescended to arrive – and now we have knives all round and blankets and towels.[9]

Looking back in 1955 Norah Mackay (clerk from January 1915 to July 1917) remembered when 'we scrubbed the floors by candle-light, the candle moving along as the scrubbers progressed'.[10]

These were the conditions with which Miss Ivens, who had the ultimate responsibility, had to cope. With her characteristic under-statement she reported on 6 December to the Scottish Women's Hospital Committee in Edinburgh that Royaumont looked lovely, but was 'rather uncomfortable owing to lack of household implements'.[11]

Miss Ivens had much to do. She made a tour of inspection with Monsieur Goüin, the owner, and his architect, Monsieur Pichon (who became a very good friend to the hospital). They discussed the best way to heat such an impossibly large and draughty building, and concluded that anthracite stoves provided the best solution, combined with a hot-water system. Top priority was to be given to the operating theatre.

They also reviewed sanitary arrangements. The discovery of a bylaw whereby no sewage could be discharged into the river was a near disaster (Goüin himself was unaware of this) and threatened the very existence of the hospital. Luckily, they discovered that there were cesspits underneath the abbey, and arrangements were made to adapt the plumbing accordingly. Sanitary facilities were never more than barely adequate at Royaumont. At one point Miss Ivens was even contemplating military-style earth closets, but this desperate measure seems to have been avoided. It was all a far cry from the original 13th-century arrangements, whereby 180 monks had the choice of 60 seats.

Miss Ivens made a number of visits to see how the French ran their own hospitals, and negotiated a written contract with Monsieur Goüin by which it was agreed that they could have the use of the abbey for a year or 'as long as the war lasts'. No one expected this would be another four and a half years.

It became apparent that permits would be required from the military authorities before patients could be collected from the railhead at Creil, and there were doubts whether women drivers would be acceptable. In addition, Miss Ivens found that doctors had to provide evidence that they were properly qualified. This would have been easy if they had known of this condition beforehand, and it was only after an extensive search that a copy of the British Medical Register was found in Paris.[12]

On 11 December the missing equipment – such as it was – arrived, but not surprisingly there were gaps. The committee had done its best, but they had a formidable task and no model to follow. The staff became skilled at improvising:

> Until a fire shovel appears Miss Hamilton replenishes it [the stove] with morsels of slack (stolen from the kitchen) with an ancient soup ladle.[13]

When the x-ray room was fitted up, a fish kettle served as a cistern for the development of the films, an operation carried out in a cupboard where a forgotten cold-water tap was discovered.[14]

Dr Inglis visited the hospital and did her best to speed up the supply of certain items, particularly cars, for which she had left instructions before she left Edinburgh. She scolded the committee for the delay: 'There is a perfectly magnificent opportunity before us if we can seize it ... we have made a really good start ... Royaumont is *perfect* and if we can get enough motors it will be one of the finest hospitals in France.'[15]

Miss Ivens had to decide the allocation of the various rooms. There was plenty of scope for choice as, in the first instance, they were only planning 100 beds. However, a 13th-century building did provide problems with damp, dirt and general decrepitude, combined with an extremely complex layout. Eventually Miss Ivens found space for the beds on the dry upper floors and in one room on the first floor. The rooms were fitted with stoves, electric light and primitive bathrooms (though they did not actually contain baths). They were scrubbed, scrubbed and scrubbed again. When the equipment arrived it was carried up the stairs by the women. They were proud of their work and what they had achieved in such a short time. The wards, they thought, looked most welcoming with the scarlet coverlets on the beds, and with the bedside tables, dressing trolleys and screens in place.

But there was still one hurdle still to cross. The hospital had to be inspected by the Service de Santé of the French Red Cross before being permitted to receive patients. The inspection took place on 24 December, and the outcome was gravely disappointing: only the ward on the first floor, Blanche de Castille (named after the mother of St Louis) was passed. The inspectors from the Sanitary Department of the Military Government of Paris couched their report in no uncertain terms. They wrote that apart from the beds in the wards, the installation was incomplete. The bottles in the pharmacy were still lying on the floor. The fittings of lavatories and bathrooms were rudimentary; the x-ray apparatus was still to be fixed up. They criticized the reception arrangements as too far from the entrance. The second-floor wards, aired and lit by skylights in their sloping roofs, provided insufficient ventilation for patients. The inspectors dismissed them as 'cowsheds'. Other smaller rooms designed for isolation were found to be quite unacceptable, unfavourable for either hygiene or health. 'It is a pity,' the inspectors declared, 'that by too much haste in the very praiseworthy intention of rapidly forming an auxiliary hospital the organizers did not think of grouping the rooms and to keep them close to the service rooms.' They disliked the slow-combustion stoves – 'most troublesome from the point of view of health, dangerous and should be forbidden'. They wanted porcelain wood-burning stoves and porcelain sanitary fittings.[16]

It was a bitter blow. Dorothy Littlejohn, from her kitchen, wrote home indignantly:

> The top wards we considered ideal were condemned. Simply disgusting, after all the hard work the nurses have had with them, and stoves and electric light put in and bathrooms made – one ward passed and now they have to make some very large and damp rooms on the ground floor turned into wards.[17]

The feminist Vera Collum was more outspoken: 'Brass-hatted inspectordom', she fumed, and 'Blame the women.'[18]

Miss Ivens herself, while not accepting every point, realized there was some sense in the inspectors' report. It was disappointing, but 'we are not taking official snubs too much to heart,' she wrote to Dr Inglis on 2 January. 'I am determined to carry the thing through against all obstacles.' She admitted that she had made a mistake in her initial allocation of rooms, and regretted that 'the change to downstairs was not done at once'.[19]

The women were all extremely tired, and not surprisingly there was a slump in morale. Dorothy Littlejohn reflected the general mood:

> Both Miss Swanston and I feel utterly disgusted with it all and that we are being of no use but to feed a lot of quarrelling women ... If we don't get wounded soon Miss S and I think we might look for something else ... I wouldn't mind slaving away all day if the place were full of soldiers, but these women, no![20]

The cooks were somewhat cheered by a gift from a local woman in the form of mistletoe decorated with flags and ribbons. In spite of her grumbles, Dorothy Littlejohn was much appreciated by the orderlies, and when she left to get married after the expiry of her six-month contract they presented her with a travelling clock inscribed 'To the hand that fed us, Orderlies, Royaumont 1915'. This remains a treasured possession in her family.[21]

At this point the magnificent leadership qualities of Cicely Hamilton and Miss Ivens came to the fore. The unit was to have the most superb Christmas festivities that could possibly be organized, and the disgruntled cooks rose to the occasion and excelled themselves with traditional Christmas fare. Cicely Hamilton brought all her experience of acting, playwriting and producing to design a pageant of the history of the abbey through the ages.

It was a turning point. Now the women felt more able to face the tremendous task of preparing the groundfloor wards, as required by the inspectors. All the clearing, cleaning and scrubbing was still to be done.

Two large rooms to the left of the entrance were prepared as the 'Marguerite d'Ecosse' and 'Jeanne d'Arc' wards, and a smaller room separated off from the entrance by a red curtain was for the reception of the patients. Beyond were the rather primitive bathrooms. The entrance hall was designed to impress visitors with the beauty of the inside of the building. The Goüins sent some of their beautiful furniture, and suggested the installation of potted palms. There were now 96 beds ready for use.

Things were now moving in the right direction. The operating theatre, sterilizing room, dispensary and x-ray room were complete, and the second inspection was awaited with some anxiety. On 31 December Miss Ivens recorded that the workmen were just about finished, but there was still no coal, anthracite or wood, and washing was 'a problem'.[22] Dorothy Littlejohn confirmed this:

> The great excitement today [20.12.14] was I had a bath for the first time for a fortnight ... I have set a fashion, everybody is clamouring for a loan of my bathroom.[23]

She wrote again on 26 December:

Yes, I have to use my canvas bath and find it very nice indeed, it's nearly always out on loan as I and one of the doctors are the only ones to have baths.[24]

Sister Jeffrey spoke later of 'the monthly bath in Paris'.[25]

Miss Ivens and Dr Savill took their difficulties to Dr Robinson, president of the British Red Cross in Paris. He explained there was constant antagonism between the civil and the military authorities: 'Dr Savill and I are both quite jolly for we realize we are not the only sufferers.'[26]

On 7 January Monsieur and Madame Goüin made their final inspection and declared themselves highly delighted. Mme. Goüin was reported to have said, 'You English are so practical', and M. Goüin found the sterilizers for the instruments '*le dernier cri*'. Miss Ivens herself felt 'the despised bathrooms were much cleaner already'.[27]

Things were looking up. Coal arrived, and on 6 January the second inspection took place, this time without a hitch – 'how nice he was, such a contrast to General Février – delighted with everything'.[28] Formal permission to admit patients arrived on 10 January. The unit could now call itself Hôpital Auxiliare 301 (HA 301).

They had to face yet another inspection – this time from Dr Coussergues, the head doctor from the *gare régulatrice* (clearing station) at Creil, who would be responsible for the allocation of patients. The director – or '*gestionnaire*' – at Royaumont (the official appointed by the French Red Cross to look after military documentation etc.) had advised Miss Ivens, 'It is more important to be on good terms with this man than the President of the French Republic.' Fortunately, when he came 'the stoves did not smoke and the x-rays worked beautifully'. Dr Coussergues was fully satisfied with all he saw, and was specially delighted with the x-ray installation – the only one in the neighbourhood.[29]

Meanwhile Miss Ivens and the *gestionnaire* travelled round the neighbouring villages in the Goüins' pony-carriage. They visited the mayors and the curés, introducing the hospital. Miss Ivens was well-received and was touched when she was presented with one franc from a French workman – the first French donation.

Miss Ivens also visited the evacuating hospital in Creil where patients were held until a decision was made as to their destination. 'Very rough and ready,' was her verdict. There were a lot of sick men, but some of the hospitals in the area were refusing to take them. 'Isn't it horrible of them?' she wrote. At one French hospital she watched some operations, recording that 'Their methods do not appeal to me.' Another hospital – at Senlis – was, she considered, 'appalling'. Royaumont was looked upon as a 'palace' in comparison.[30]

Miss Ivens had a heavy responsibility. Other members of the unit – nurses, orderlies, doctors and cooks – had the hard physical work. There were no great comforts for the staff. The kitchen floor was awash with water from the sink, which tended to drain on to the floor. Clogs brought in from the village solved that particular problem until more definitive arrangements could be made. On the domestic front two old women were employed to wash clothes and linen in the river. They were known as Mesdames Frotter as they used the time-honoured method of rubbing the clothes to clean them. Water remained a problem. Even some months later members of the unit 'were requested to avoid all waste of water: it is not suggested that they should cease to wash, but they must wash with discretion and economy'.[31] Drainage was a particular worry for Dr Berry with her background in public health. She was remembered afterwards for cleaning out the drains herself – she was always ready to turn her hand to any task that needed doing.

In January a new orderly (unidentified) was writing home:

Such a lovely old place, but Mon Dieu, the cold. We three sleep in an enormous room with a window at one end ... Last night we slept with all our worldly goods on top of us ... our mattresses are made of straw and smell of the stable ... the cooks, Miss Swanston and Miss Littlejohn make their orderlies work like slaves.[32]

For her part, Dorothy Littlejohn complained they had to give up the help of a French woman in the kitchen when the new orderlies arrived – 'most willing and know nothing so it's been a hard week for us'.[33]

In the early days – and indeed for a long time afterwards – staff recalled using the same enamel plate for meat and pudding, and having to help with the washing up – a greasy and a not very salubrious business. Doctors, nurses and orderlies, with much ingenuity, 'furnished' their respective sitting rooms and sleeping quarters. Packing cases were much in demand, and valuable bits and pieces were 'acquired' from various rooms containing un-wanted items from the neighbouring chateau.

The accounts were the responsibility of Cicely Hamilton, who proved to have a flair for bookkeeping. One of her more enjoyable duties was her monthly trip into Paris to have her accounts audited.

Fuel was a major problem. The Germans were occupying France's coalmining areas, and it was a notably cold winter. Some hospitals in Paris were even closing down as a result. Coal had to be brought from England, and transport was difficult until a motor lorry was acquired, and the chauffeurs had to add this to their long list of duties. In one 'coal crisis' the chauffeurs loaded 15 one-hundred-weight (50 kg) sacks of coal onto the lorry at a time, drove to the abbey, unloaded the sacks, then returned to the depot for more until as much as 40 tons had been carried, and the emergency – for a while – overcome.[34]

The lorry in question was acquired after the chauffeurs objected strongly – and very reasonably – to carrying heavy goods in their ambulances, which were in fact their own cars, bought with their own money, converted to carry four stretchers each. (Later on, the unit acquired its own purpose-built ambulances.) One chauffeur, Edith Prance, tells the story of how they persuaded their *médecin-chef* to write to the committee and request a lorry:

An ambulance was ordered to take Miss Ivens to Clichy Hospital, go on to the vegetable market while she was at the operations, and pick her up on the way home. That vile road, all cobbles and pot-holes … The chauffeur [it was Prance herself] bent down to the clock on the dashboard, put it forward ten minutes, and smeared its face with an oily rag. With a cheery 'Good morning' the Chief took her uneasy seat on the unsprung, thinly cushioned board next to the driver. Pleasant conversation beguiled the way along the Paris road till the turn was reached down that shocking street through Clichy, a 2-mile martyrdom, 'How are we for time?' Hastily polishing the clock face with a driving glove – 'Good gracious! – We shall be late – I mustn't on any account keep those doctors waiting – AS FAST AS YOU CAN!' Followed a furious drive, at express speed, twisting this way and that in a vain endeavour to avoid potholes, but succeeding only in plunging into the worst ones, to right and left we swung. Our poor Chief was hurled against the wooden side, flung up to the roof, hell for leather we went, and presently arrived bruised and breathless at the hospital. The Chief straightened her hat and entered the hospital … The chauffeur put the clock back. … On the return journey, the Chief – 'I don't think we should drive so fast now, there is no hurry really.' Then, as we turned into the Royaumont road: 'I see what you chauffeurs mean, this road is terrible, we must not use ambulances for this work (the marketing) – a lorry is a necessity – I shall go in to Creil with one of you anyhow and cable straight away for a LORRY!'[35]

The chauffeurs (they preferred this term to 'chauffeuses') were in a way a breed apart. They were required to be at least 24 years of age (Prance was almost 40). They were recruited from a class well-enough off to be accustomed to driving; many of them had their own cars. However, the British War Office refused passes to the women to drive their own vehicles in the French Military Zone. Yes, they could *ride* in their own cars, but men must drive them. As Vera Collum reported – 'Dr Inglis only grinned! "It will be alright," she assured them, and it was.'[36] Once in France, the owner-drivers were able to snap their fingers at London – and could also hold their own with the French military authorities. One of these independent-minded women was Marjorie Young, who on one occasion was instructed by a French soldier that it was not possible for her to go along a certain road. *'Pour moi tout est possible,'* she said, as she let in her gear and drove off.[37] Their independence was fostered by the fact that, at least for most of the time, they had their own quarters in the abbey stables. There were good reasons for this: casualties usually arrived at the railway station at Creil, 12 miles away, late at night or in the early hours, and patients who were to be evacuated left in the early evening. So meals were eaten separately, and there was little mixing with other members of staff.

Some of the orderlies, perhaps brought up with rather traditional views, looked a little askance at these 'modern' women, one of whom was even seen smoking a pipe. 'Could they be suffragettes?' they wondered.[38] The chauffeurs were certainly highly competent: not only were they accomplished drivers, they were also responsible for the maintenance of their vehicles and for minor repairs. The uncertainties about the use of women drivers had led to the initial employment of two men as chauffeur-mechanics, waiving the all-woman principle. But as the women drivers proved their ability to do anything the men could do, the presence of the latter became an embarrassment to Miss Ivens, who in August 1915 wrote to the committee to say how it placed her in an awkward position with the French authorities to have 'useless men hanging about' when the French already felt 'that England is not doing its utmost and it is most humiliating – not only that, but it does not look well to pose as a woman's hospital and yet have men here … it exposes us to criticism'.[39]

❧

Perhaps it is not surprising that the issue of uniform was one that aroused many grumbles, opposing viewpoints, offended sensibilities and general ill-feeling between those in the field and the committee at home. After all, the women at Royaumont were volunteers, and not subject to military discipline – especially as far as dress was concerned.

The uniform that was selected by the committee (and which was to be made by Edinburgh tailors) consisted, for the doctors, of a formal grey coat and skirt with facings of Gordon tartan. This was one bone of contention, as Miss Ivens herself registered a personal objection to wearing tartan. Dr Inglis herself complained to the committee about the quality of the tailoring:

> The stuff is shoddy and the sewing coming undone. Not a single collar fits – in fact – as Dr Ivens has said 'It is a mercy Royaumont is in the country – for we could not go out of doors in Paris.' ... Imagine coats and skirts that are not fit to be seen after a month's wear.[40]

Miss Ivens voiced her concerns to Dr Inglis on 31 December 1914:

> I think if the doctors had a well-cut grey tunic each nearly tight to the throat, with a belt, it would add to their comfort very much, for one is really ashamed to appear before the outside world in our present garments ... I don't think there is much wrong with the nurses. The chauffeurs have had to get hold of khaki overcoats. [This was a requirement of the military authorities.][41]

Later the chauffeurs also had to get rubber boots and heavy goatskin overcoats to protect them from the cold during their night work in freezing winters. And in 1918 when they were driving under bombardment they were issued with steel helmets.

Miss Ivens, always elegantly dressed herself, was still unforgiving about the committee's choice of uniform when, in July 1917, she told Dr Henry that she had no need to apologize for wearing mufti when she first reported for duty. Dr Henry had explained that she felt self-conscious in the drab cotton uniform issued in London. Miss Ivens reassured her:

> I'm glad you did. I have told the Edinburgh Committee that we are too near Paris to be dressed like nannies! Tomorrow Nicol in Paris will take your measurements.

The result, Dr Henry reported, was a 'coat and skirt of light grey twill with red velvet *caduceés* [a recognized medical emblem including serpents and wings] in the lapel and a heavy dark blue for winter'.[42]

When they learned about it, this blue uniform greatly displeased the committee. A telegram was sent: 'blue uniform unauthorized we are sending out grey material'. Miss Ivens responded that the doctors were already wearing blue. The uniform committee said they would not pay. The hospital committee then stepped into the fray – the uniform committee gave in and the doctors were satisfied and continued to wear their blue uniforms.[43]

There was worse to come, however, from the committee in London in 1916:

I have just seen in all its horrible details the uniform in which we send out our hospital nursing staff. It made me almost cry with rage and shame – shame for the poor girls who have to wear it, shame that members of our hospital should be seen in it, shame that foreigners should think such a rigout is the Englishwoman's idea of working and workman-like clothes, and rage that Edinburgh after more than two years' practical experience should be sending out something so ill-cut and ill-made, so unsuitable to the occasion.[44]

And this was at the height of the Somme battles! It seems that those who had to wear it had more urgent things on their minds – at least there is no record of the nurses having such violent views.

However, Millicent Armstrong, who was a clerk in 1917, thought:

Perhaps the Committee chose the design with a view to our protection among the licentious soldiery. [It seems that it was the outdoor uniform which made the hackles rise.] It was lucky, wasn't it, that our indoor uniforms were a lovely shade of blue.[45]

In September 1915, Miss Loudon, the administrator, was writing back to Miss Mair:

Please don't send out hats. We can get grey hats in Paris to match our costumes. We will have them very simple. The memory of the first doctor's hats is still green.[46]

French visitors were more tolerant:

The doctors have ... a very simple tailored costume in a grey that is soft on the eye, and which the chief doctor wears with grace, without any special badge ... All the doctors wear, as insignia, the *caduceés* of surgeon-majors in silver on grey velour. Sisters and orderlies are dressed in grey-blue, the former wearing the traditional headgear, the latter wearing sweet little mob-caps the same colour as the dress (or white for the cooks), which graciously frame their alert expressions.[47]

We leave the last word on uniform with an orderly, Marjorie Starr, going on leave and donning her mufti:

One gets thoroughly sick of going about like a Scotswoman in those hideous grey coats, so I feel like a lady again.[48]

❧

One of the greatest challenges for the women of Royaumont was the fact that very few of the hundreds of men for whom they would be caring would have any knowledge of English. The French Service de Santé wanted all the doctors and nurses to make a declaration that they could speak French. This was a little idealistic, and the requirement does not seem to have been taken very seriously.

Possibly the weakest members of the team in terms of language proficiency were the sisters. Some of them had absolutely no knowledge of French when they arrived, but they nevertheless proved successful, in varying degrees, in communicating with their patients. When Madame Fox, a local French lady, came to live in the hospital in 1917 after the death of her husband, Miss Ivens welcomed her for a variety of reasons, not least that the sisters would have an opportunity to improve their language skills.

The story is told of one newly arrived sister who was very puzzled and upset by the great distress of a patient on his return from the theatre: 'I'm sure I said nothing to upset him,' she said, as she had only one French word, and that was *'oui'*. The patient's distress was explained by the man in the next bed – *'Mon camarade a demandé à la sistaire: "Est-ce que je vais mourir?"* [My comrade has asked the sister, "Am I going to die?"]' She used the limit of her vocabulary in her reply: *'Oui, oui.'*[49]

One orderly, Yvonne Barclay, recalled a sister dressing a boy's foot. 'An' noo, *c'est fini*, bonnie laddie.' *'Qu'est ce que "bonnie laddie", Sistaire?'* 'Och. *C'est le* Scotch for Antret [his name].' They understood each other.

Many of the sisters devised their own system of communication. Sister Jessie McGregor apparently had her own inimitable way: 'Conversation was always carried on in a series of staccato monosyllables, half French, half English; yet every man understood what she meant.'[50]

Sister Janet Williams was remarkable. She had charge of the Senegalese ward. They knew very little French and no English at all, and Sister Williams knew even less French than they did. In spite of that they developed an extraordinary degree of understanding. She even discovered a great deal of their family history and the numbers of their wives.[51]

The orderlies came from privileged family backgrounds. Many had had a good education and knew a certain amount of French. Nevertheless, Miss Ivens declared herself shocked that the majority of girls were so badly educated.[52] Dorothy Littlejohn was able to deal with the local tradespeople from the beginning, and there were others who could manage quite well. A few took lessons in the village, though their fluency did not always improve as much as it might. One story was told of an orderly receiving a telephone call from the army authorities in Creil during the hectic summer of 1918, and being asked, *'Combien de lits disponibles?* [How many available beds?]' She could not say as they were already required to collect from *'une caniche toute pleine de blessés* [a toy poodle completely full of wounded]'. For weeks afterwards every passing officer was enquiring tenderly about the *caniche* and the fate of her large family.[53]

Another orderly, Florence Simms, writing to her old governess, bemoaned the fact that 'I'm afraid I shall never learn to speak properly, however hard I try. You see, I never know what people are talking about, they talk at such a terrific rate.'[54] Her friend, Grace Summerhayes, was much more confident. She reckoned she had two kinds of French – her correct schoolgirl French, and the French the *poilus* spoke: 'My French in the end was either very up or very down.'[55] Ella Figgis, a dispenser, was probably not the only one who 'spoke French rather correctly but slowly, conceding nothing to Gallic vivacity'.[56]

One of the greatest successes of the early appointments was that of Cicely Hamilton, who went as a clerk but rapidly became more and more indispensable to the smooth running of the whole organization. She was of enormous value to Miss Ivens in the early days with her facility in French, both written and spoken. Miss Ivens relied on her greatly to assist her in all the delicate negotiations with the French authorities. Miss Ivens herself, though she became completely fluent in French as the war progressed, had some difficulty in the early days. Her standard question to a newly admitted *poilu* was '*Êtes vous blessé ou malade, Monsieur?*' It became complicated for her to follow when the man replied that he was both wounded *and* sick, and then went on to supply a wealth of corroborating detail.[57] But, as with everything she undertook, Miss Ivens set herself to learn. She told one story against herself (which contradicts the assertion that she lacked a sense of humour) that after a ward concert given by some of the patients she rose and made a little speech, only to realize later that she had thanked 'ourselves for giving the men such a delightful concert'.[58]

Some of the doctors probably had more knowledge of German than of French, as a number who had qualified in the early years of the century had, in the face of obstacles back home, pursued postgraduate education in German-speaking centres such as Vienna, Freiburg and Zürich. In contrast, their proficiency in French was probably no greater than when they had left school. The outstanding exception to this was Dr Wilson, who arrived in November 1915 and who was an outstanding linguist. However, by the end of the war there appears to have been a general raising of the standard of French-speaking, as by Christmas 1918 the unit could put on a pantomime *Cinderella* with dialogue and songs all in French.

From the other side of the linguistic barrier some of the patients attempted to learn the language of their carers. One said goodnight to his sister every evening by singing 'Sleep, my little one, dream my pretty one,'[59] and they all became proficient in singing 'It's a Long Way to Tipperary' 'in excellent English and most tunefully'.[60]

One way or another, with mutual help, determination and sheer necessity, the question of language proved to be no insuperable barrier to communication or good relations in general, or to the maintenance of discipline.

CHAPTER THREE

❧

The First Year

Royaumont received its first patients in January 1915. From the military perspective, stalemate on the Western Front had been reached by the end of 1914, when both sides had dug in, and long lines of trenches ran from Verdun in the east, westwards through Reims, Soissons and Noyon, then turned northwards to Albert, Vimy Ridge, Loos, Neuve-Chapelle, Armentières, Ypres and to the coast south of Ostend.

It was not until February 1915 that fighting was renewed. Throughout that year much of the Allied war effort on the Western Front was concentrated on the eastern end where the Germans were straining to capture Verdun. However, in February and March the French made repeated attacks in Champagne, trying to penetrate the German defences. French losses were appalling – 50,000 men in these two months alone. Then in April they lost 64,000 men in a disastrous attack on St Mihiel, further to the east, towards Verdun.

Between 9 May and 18 June the French were attacking further north between Lens and Arras – losing 102,000 men in the process. Between 15 May and 27 May the British were engaged in attacks on Festubert, south of Neuve-Chapelle.

This enormous loss of life produced little change in the military situation. There was something of a lull until 15 September, when the French renewed their attacks in Champagne, and the French and British together attacked in Artois. Allied losses in these September campaigns amounted to 242,000 (nearly twice the German losses of 141,000).

In the later months of 1915 there was again stalemate and,

thanks to the onset of winter, a period of relief for the soldiers in the trenches and the hardpressed hospitals behind the lines.

Royaumont was particularly well-suited to take casualties from the Reims–Soissons–Noyon sector. All these areas fed by rail into the *gare régulatrice* (clearing station) at Creil, 12 miles from the hospital. It was at Creil that patients were distributed to the various hospitals in the sector; one of these was Royaumont. Apart from a short period in 1918 when the rapid German advance put Creil temporarily out of action, it remained a critically important centre throughout the war. It was convenient for the military authorities to have Royaumont where it was, but the 12 miles of bad roads between the abbey and Creil represented something of an endurance test for the hard-pressed chauffeurs, particularly during the 'rushes'.

Nevertheless, as Vera Collum commented, 'Chance or destiny flung our little emergency Unit of women into the one spot in the whole of France where it could prove of greatest value.'[1] The degree of activity at Royaumont fluctuated with the intensity of the fighting, and their greatest 'rushes' – or 'flaps' as they called them – came in April, May and September.

❧

On 10 January 1915 the hospital was recognized as a military hospital, to be known as Hôpital Auxiliaire 301 (HA 301).[2] The very next day the first six patients arrived – all sick. The authorities were not yet ready to trust them with wounded soldiers. These patients were brought in by French army ambulances, which had taken four hours to cover the 12 miles from Creil, and as a result the men were completely exhausted. After this example of gross inefficiency Miss Ivens was able to obtain permission for her women drivers to collect the patients in future. The unit was delighted to have patients at last – they were beginning the work for which they had volunteered.[3]

By the end of the month the unit was receiving a handful of wounded soldiers, and by 5 February there were 55 patients, half of them sick, half wounded. By the end of February the hospital was almost full, with 95 beds occupied.

The unit was being closely watched by the French medical authorities. Miss Ivens reported that she had to do a number of abdominal operations under their critical supervision – 'fortunately all went well'.[4] It was not surprising that the French were anxious – they had no experience of women working as doctors in hospitals, let alone as surgeons. Could these women really cope? However, Cicely Hamilton was delighted when she overheard the men telling a visiting colonel that they had a 'marked preference for the service of women doctors'.[5]

Towards the end of February, Miss Ivens was invited to staff a hospital at Mont-à-Terre, near Creil, to deal with a typhoid epidemic. Never one to turn down a challenge, Miss Ivens welcomed this as an indication that the French authorities were beginning to overcome their suspicion and mistrust. However, the epidemic abated rather rapidly and the whole exercise was cancelled.[6] This may have been fortunate in the light of the demands soon to be made on the hospital at Royaumont.

Further marks of confidence followed. The army authorized the unit to collect causalties direct from the train at Creil rather than from the Creil Hospital.[7] This saved the wounded men much unnecessary and painful movement. The women were also asked to provide another 100 beds. To accommodate these the former chapter house of the abbey on the ground floor became the 'Millicent Fawcett Ward', the guest refectory of the monks became the 'Queen Mary Ward', and the 'cowsheds' on the second floor became the 'Elsie Inglis Ward'.

The French army was now prepared to pay 2 francs a day for each patient and to supply petrol, tyres and other necessities for the vehicles, even though they were desperately short of vehicles at that time. The equivalent of £1000 was provided for the new beds – the beds themselves were to be returned 'after the war'. ('Very poor quality,' commented Miss Ivens.)

It had been agreed with the committee and with the French authorities that, provided the care of soldiers received top priority, any slack could be used to treat the civilian population. This was immensely popular with the local communities as there was a great scarcity of medical facilities of any kind. Miss Ivens reported on

19 March that the outpatient department was growing to an embarrassing degree. Women naturally predominated. No charge was made, but a box was provided for contributions.

Patients were increasing in numbers – on 22 March there were 137. But where was the equipment? Miss Ivens was more than a little concerned:

> We are in a dire need of equipment, no beds, sheets or blankets ... cutlery and utensils for patients dreadfully short. I shall have to stop taking patients today unless the equipment comes.[8]

And again she vented her anger on the committee:

> Patients have poured in daily, and as the equipment was painfully inadequate and meagre for 100 beds it reached vanishing point with 158 patients. In addition constantly increasing staff whose requirements were entirely unprovided for. Weeks ago I wired for more sheets and pyjamas but I got no response ... It is most discouraging for nurses to see their beds covered with stained, dirty sheets ... soldiers wandering to and fro to the x-ray room half-clad for lack of dressing gowns and pyjamas ... Dressings are practically exhausted and none have come ... The loyalty of the staff has been strained to the breaking point by the unnecessary discomforts ... We have had to borrow sheets and blankets from the poor of Asnières. The staff have given up their bedsteads and replaced them with borrowed horrors ... do try and get some constant supplies out. Otherwise we might just collapse.[9]

Vera Collum tells an endearing story that goes some way to account for the love her staff had for Miss Ivens:

> As usual the new equipment went astray and there was a raid on staff beds. It used to be uncommonly cold sleeping on the floor. If beds were not forthcoming at the first hint of their need, the Médecin-Chef had a way of giving up hers to start

with. I remember passing my bed on to her the first time. She sent this also to the new ward. Meanwhile I had commandeered another. Of course I had to offer it again – we could not have our M-C sleeping on the floor. Next time I got a broken bed which I patched up. It served the purpose fairly well; but again the M-C handed over her bed, and I was on the floor once more. So, with a sigh, I took along my broken bed, which she retained, I believe, as it was too 'groggy' for a wounded man. I had now given up a bed as a bad job, and till the missing equipment had come I slept resignedly on the floor.[10]

The patients always came first with Miss Ivens. On 6 April the equipment had still not arrived – but in spite of that they had a great bed-moving day. 'All the French horrors are banished to our rooms and the patients are nearly comfortable on our nice straw mattresses.'[11]

On behalf of the committee, Dr Inglis remonstrated with Miss Ivens: 'We thought we had sent you everything you asked for, and you evidently felt that you had asked for many things that you did not get.'[12] And on 30 March Dr Inglis wrote to the treasurer: 'There seems to have been a glorious muddle at Royaumont over everything just now.'[13] However, the situation was saved when large quantities of invaluable stores arrived from a hospital at Cherbourg that was closing down, and soon after that the long-awaited equipment from home arrived. The crisis was over.

Dr Inglis visited the hospital once more at the end of April on her way to Serbia, where she was to command one of the Scottish Women's Hospitals. She wrote a reassuring letter to Miss Mair, the president of the Scottish Federation:

I am more than ever delighted with the place. The wards are beautiful. The operating theatre is as perfect as any I have ever seen, and the whole place is in perfect order. The patients – 178 were in today – seemed most contented, and everyone on the staff seemed well and keen. There is no doubt that the hospital is a great success, and that the credit belongs to Dr Ivens. The staff has worked splendidly. So that, in my opinion the thing to do is to support Dr Ivens in her 'plans' – of course insisting on estimates, for *that* is her weak point![14]

And to the treasurer she wrote of 'Dr Ivens's management of the place, and her patience and persistence in the face of really extraordinary difficulties in the way of red tape etc has made our work there really something to be proud of.'[15]

Dr Inglis was also delighted to open and name the 'Elsie Inglis Wards' on the second floor. These were the same that had been so roundly condemned only three months earlier.

The extra 100 beds had to be inspected again, but this time the inspection went without a hitch, and the beds were passed as fit for use. The inspector actually apologized for his earlier 'boorish behaviour'. Miss Ivens wondered if his change of heart might be because he was 'obviously bowled over by the "petit bonnet bleu" of Miss Inglis [Etta Inglis, Dr Elsie's niece] who is a very charming person'. Much to Miss Ivens's relief he didn't ask about the lavatories – 'the one thing that is weighing on my mind and which I see no means of improving'.[16]

Miss Ivens had been very angry with the committee over the delays in sending equipment. She had been sensitive to the criticisms of Monsieur Goüin, the owner of Royaumont, who did not like to see patients wandering around without proper clothing, and she was also troubled by the suggestion that the patients were not getting enough food. It must have been humiliating for her to borrow from poor villagers, even though they were pleased to help the hospital that was already doing so much for them. It was possibly for her the most unhappy period of the entire war – she had a dread of falling down on any job. Later in August she wrote:

> Our experience in the Spring in trying to provide for the extra patients while we waited weeks for equipment ... would not encourage me to repeat such a nightmare of worry and anxiety.

Inevitably, there were a few misjudgements in the selection of personnel. The committee were inexperienced and were ignorant of what the work would entail, and equally ignorant of the qualities that would be needed. Some of their appointments were brilliant – or particularly fortunate. Among these were Cicely Hamilton, the first clerk (later administrator), and Vera Collum, who came as an orderly, but later became a highly skilled radiographer. The two problem appointments were actually made by Dr Inglis herself. Mrs Owen, the first administrator, was, it seems, totally out of her depth. She spoke no French and had no idea how to handle the difficult conditions she found. It was a relief when she resigned. Her replacement was Mrs Harley – who could not understand why Mrs Owen 'could not get on with Miss Ivens except that she had too difficult a task and got thoroughly worried'.[17]

Mrs Harley, who was then in her sixties, had been prominent in the suffrage movement, and was the sister of Sir John French, the commander-in-chief of the British Expeditionary Force. After three months at Royaumont she transferred to the tented hospital that the SWH opened at Troyes under Dr Louise McIllroy. When that hospital in due course was sent out to Salonika, Mrs Harley went with it. Her subsequent history until her death from an exploding shell in 1916 is part of the Serbian story and has been told elsewhere.[18] She seems to have been a difficult and autocratic character, although this was more manifest in her later career than at Royaumont. Probably her posting spared Royaumont some of the problems other units experienced.

Miss Tod, the first matron, who took up her post in February, was elderly, already retired, and had been accustomed to traditional nursing in traditional settings in Scotland. She, like Mrs Owen, found conditions at Royaumont more than she could cope with. Neither was she at all in sympathy with the 'modern women' who were so well represented at Royaumont. She was particularly suspicious of Cicely Hamilton, who would go about her business in a workman's smock. Was it true that she had been an actress? And what could have brought her to this? Recalling the incident later, Cicely thought she might have answered that it was 'the drink' – at least, that is what she would have answered if Mrs Tod 'had not been so kindly, so serious and so Scotch!'[19]

Another personality who came under Miss Tod's disapproving gaze was Mrs Williams, an administrator whose expert knowledge of French made her a very valuable acquisition. However, Miss Tod was unhappy that Mrs Williams powdered her nose and scented her bath, and considered her silk underwear positively demi-mondaine.[20]

Miss Tod was not even sure that any woman should be a doctor in the first place, and reportedly told one sick orderly, 'Don't you think you should send into Paris for a man?'[21] Miss Ivens found her 'not loyal' to women doctors, and 'too old and unadaptable for the hand to mouth existence we have here'.[22] Mrs Harley reported that Miss Tod grumbled, found fault and discouraged the orderlies, and concluded that she would have to go. It is to the credit of Dr Inglis that she was at pains to spare Miss Tod from humiliation and to allow her to return home 'with honour'. 'She is too old for the post and we oughtn't to have asked her. But we did put her in, and so we must not hurt her in getting her out ... Don't let her know that I told you she cried. She is so proud she would hate that.' When Miss Tod died in 1929 there were some in the unit who remembered her with affection, 'perhaps having forgiven us all for turning out to be adventurous ducklings so very different from the sedate chicks she had expected to hatch'.[23]

With the increasing number of patients, tasks multiplied. For Cicely Hamilton there were the forms required by the military authorities:

> The number and docketing of French military patients is not a job to be trifled with. Four documents for every man entering and the same for leaving, and seventeen for a death. Reca-pitulatory reports, telling everything all over again – every five days.[24]

According to Miss Ivens it was as bad or even worse for her. She and the French *gestionnaire* (administrator) had 27 military forms to sign as soldiers arrived.

Another unforeseen task was dealing with the soldiers' clothing. Vera Collum takes up the story:

> On arrival I was confronted with seventy piles of filthy tattered clothing, most of it in sacks, ranged in some semblance of order round and across the room, each sack with a number, from one upwards, corresponding to rough pencil entries in a penny notebook, giving the owner's name, and the ward he was in, and the date of his admission ... The cowsheds with their stinking, crawling burden, became a nightmare. I remember our great field day with the soiled clothes, when we had prevailed upon a village washer-woman of the pre-Marne days to get her fires and boilers going again. The pile was higher than my own head: we packed the clothes into half a dozen ticking mattress cases and took them by motor to the village: the reek of them penetrated into the inhabited wing of the hospital and brought a horrified CMO [chief medical officer] to the scene, who at once acquiesced in our scheme cost what it might.[25]

The *vêtements* (clothing) department, having started in the 'cowsheds', was moved up to the very top of the building – 'One could have set a row of cottages with their back yards inside it.'[26] An enterprising orderly devised a pulley to haul up the heavy sacks, thus saving the weary orderlies at least one of their heavy chores. The French army were not renowned for looking after the welfare of their troops, and were unable to provide replacement clothing. So, whatever the condition of clothing, it had to be repaired.

A routine was established, basically unchanged throughout the life of the hospital:

> The clothes are fumigated in great cupboards, and next day the sacks are sorted, soiled linen is sent to the wash, and outdoor clothing hung from the rafters in a good courant d'air. The mending is undertaken by a wonderful Frenchwoman, Madame Fox, the wife of an English resident in our village.[27]

Most of her helpers were volunteers, but the owner of a local factory, Monsieur Delacoste, loaned two of his workers every afternoon:

> We ourselves tackle the uniforms with the noble assistance of Mrs Hacon, a prominent member of the Shetland Branch of the National Union of Women's Suffrage Societies, through whose ingenuity I have seen the 'veste' of an artillery man, minus half a sleeve, made into a wondrous garment with warm woollen cuffs – all because there was nothing in the world to mend it with but a pair of navy blue bedsocks – and an old scarlet sock repair a breach made by shrapnel in a pair of infantry trousers![28]

(This was before the French army were clad in *horizon bleu*, their version of khaki.)

The women were proud of their *vêtements* department. Cicely Hamilton reported that

> ... rumour has it that the Royaumont men turn up at Creil depot considerably smarter than the majority of the other 'évacués' of the District, and that Mme Fox is to go to Creil one evening in order to compare the results of her handiwork with less successful efforts in the mending and cleaning line. She has been granted the honorary rank of 'directrice-adjointe du bureau de vêtements de l'hôpital auxiliaire 301 de Royaumont'. I invented the title myself and she deserves every single word of it.[29]

Hospital routines evolved by degrees for staff and patients. These included the arrangements for the arrival and departure of the wounded. Dr Henry, who arrived in 1917 when the routine was well-established, describes how the hall porter, having been alerted from the distributing centre in Creil, listened for the sound of the ambulances. She then blew her horn, summoning the orderlies to rush to the entrance, leaving only one on duty in charge of the ward. 'Each', she said, 'had her station as on board ship.' The orderlies unloaded the ambulances, and the stretchers were

> ... laid on the flagged floor of the inner hall. Tags attached to the uniforms were checked. These gave indication of the type of wound, whether from bullet or shrapnel. Those who had haemorrhaged or were already suffering from infection were quickly discovered by the stench. Clothing was cut off; swabs taken and sent to the laboratory ... hot drinks were available to all, then they would be borne up the wide stairs to the next floor where the x-ray and operating theatres were ready for them.

Some were taken straight to the wards – for those headed for the second floor there were 71 steps to climb. 'There were no men orderlies and no elevators. The girl orderlies undertook all these heavy tasks.' Dr Henry remembered how the *poilus* in the wards greeted the newcomers. They would:

> Introduce him, sit beside him and calm his fears. I have seen such gentleness between the veterans and the young recruits. You'd hear a new patient being questioned 'Can you sing? – What kind of music do you like? – Well, we all sing here, but it's comme il faut, some verses we leave out. These are all English ladies.'[30]

Miss Ivens was quite aware that some of these verses were not fit for the ears of the young orderlies in her care. She deputed one of the auxiliary nurses, Marjorie Miller, who had good French, to ensure that nothing *pas convenables* (inappropriate or indecent) was heard.[31]

The chauffeurs drove entirely alone along those bumpy 12 miles from Creil. One of them remembers opening the door on arrival wondering if her casualties were alive or dead.[32]

Discharges also followed a certain routine. They usually took place about 6 p.m., and the discharged men were given a good send-off by their fellow-patients and by the staff who had looked after them. Miss Ivens herself made a point of being present whenever possible. Some of the discharged men went on leave, others for further treatment in another hospital. Some unfortunate ones were sent straight back to the Front. Feelings were very mixed when they left, but the staff tried to make it as easy as they could:

> Practically every evening and punctually at six, we, to use the French term, 'evacuate' a certain number of patients, and their departure is usually the liveliest moment of the day. It looks, sometimes, as if everyone who is able to walk had come to cheer them on the road. Variety of costume is always charming, and the crowd round our front door, in so far as it consists of patients, is clad chiefly in pyjamas of different hues, and wears what headgear it fancies, chiefly 'kepis' and Zulu straws. Miss Ivens reads over the men's papers – a necessary precaution this, as any warrior without the correct documents is liable to be returned on our hands. We have never yet fathomed what would happen if anyone's papers were absolutely and irretrievably lost, but we imagine that in such an eventuality he would have no legal existence, and that the only way out of the difficulty would be to exterminate him and bury him secretly. The evacuated ones, having been duly identified, there is much hand shaking, much thanking of doctors and nurses. It takes some time till everyone and everyone's bundles are hoisted in and the car is off.[33]

With routines established and with the accompanying growth in confidence, the hospital was now on the way to becoming a 'unit'. After certain disagreements and incompatibilities in the early days, and the departure of one or two misfits, it does seem that a very positive esprit de corps developed – a striking feature of the hospital throughout its life, and one that was maintained for years after the war through the Royaumont Association. This esprit de corps was undoubtedly fostered by the appreciation of the *poilus*, the admiration of the neighbouring villagers, and the increasing value set on the unit's services by the military and medical authorities.

Dr Ross, on a visit back to headquarters in June 1915, was asked by the committee if there was much discontent among themselves? She replied that 'it was a "perfect paradise" compared to similar institutions in this country'.[34] And in September Dr Boissières, inspecting on behalf of the French authorities, said Royaumont was 'one of the few Hôpitals Etrangères [foreign hospitals] which had not given them "unspeakable ennuis"'.[35]

In May Miss Ivens began an experiment in which sunshine was used to treat wounds. Beds were wheeled out into the cloisters, at first by day only, later by day and night. Wounds were exposed, protected by gauze soaked in saline solution. This treatment, combined with the peace and beauty of the cloisters, produced good results. In his contemporary account of the unit, Antonio de Navarro wrote:

> The beautiful Gothic cloisters and box-bordered court offered a habitation that for picturesque repose was unobtainable even by millionaire sanatoria: by day, a harbour of unaccustomed novelty and enchantment; and when evening was come, a night of silence and stars – the soothing babble of the fountain lulling the nerve-racked sufferers to peaceful sleep.[36]

The hospital continued to develop. In May a laboratory was prepared on the top floor, under the direction of Dr Elizabeth Butler. Royaumont was fortunate to obtain her services. She had graduated from Glasgow University with honours in 1890, and took her MD degree with 'the highest honours the University could bestow'. In due course she was awarded a Beit research fellowship from the Lister Institute. (Dr Elsie Dalyell, an Australian, who worked later at Royaumont, had also been a Beit fellow. These were two of the most eminent women scientists of the time and contributed in no small measure to the high reputation that Royaumont came to hold.)

For Dr Butler the opportunity to work at Royaumont came at a very appropriate time. She had been working on a cancer research project in Lemberg, Austria, but when hostilities broke out she resigned her fellowship, concealed her papers (hoping to recover them after the war), and returned home. She and her husband were then without any means of livelihood. Being fluent in French and German, she wrote to the secretary of the Lister Institute, 'I shall be glad to help as a doctor, dresser or nurse, at home or abroad.'[37] This led to the Royaumont appointment. One must assume that Miss Ivens did not know of Dr Butler's willingness to work as a nurse, as she always insisted that women doctors should work as doctors and have the same conditions of service and pay as men. Dr Butler's husband worked for a short time at the unit as a chauffeur, so the Butlers' employment problems were resolved for the time being.

On 25 June the new laboratory was opened, and a 'deluge of generals' descended to inspect it.[38] Whether the generals had any qualifications to judge its quality was a moot point, but there was still intense interest in what the women were doing, and, besides, visitors always enjoyed the Royaumont teas.

The prestige of the laboratory was further increased by the interest taken by Professor Weinberg of the Pasteur Institute in Paris. Weinberg was the leading expert on gas gangrene (see Appendix One), and his confidence was such that he conducted many of the trials of his new gas-gangrene sera at Royaumont. Lecturing in Glasgow in March 1916, Weinberg expressed his admiration for the way that each case at Royaumont was treated, and said he could not imagine any activity on the part of women that would so effectively further the cause of the women's movement as the work of the Scottish Women's Hospitals.[39]

In addition to Dr Butler, a number of other new doctors arrived in 1915. Dr Jean Meiklejohn was a pathologist who had been a Carnegie research fellow, a rare distinction for a woman. Dr M.E. Wilson was an experienced missionary doctor from Palestine. Dr L. Hawthorne took on the supervision of the x-ray department in the absence of Dr Savill. (Dr Savill divided her time between Royaumont and her consultant work in London.) It was Dr Hawthorne who trained Vera Collum in radiography. Collum's talent for photography had been noticed by Miss Ivens, who was always on the alert to spot the potential of her orderlies. Collum later distinguished herself in the great 'rushes' resulting from the Somme battles of 1916, and again in the last desperate struggles of 1918.

With a new administrator (Miss Kate Loudon) to replace Mrs Harley and a new matron (Miss Isabella Duncan) to replace Miss Tod, Miss Ivens was relieved of some of the work that had fallen so heavily on her shoulders. Miss Loudon probably did not fully realize the extent of the problems she was to face in the next 18 months, but her delightful personality and concern for the welfare of the whole unit won her many friends, some of them lifelong, and the affectionate nickname 'the Robin'. She fell in love with Royaumont and wrote enthusiastically of her first impressions:

> I am very happy here, and the staff are so nice and what is really delightful is they all have Royaumont first in their minds and are determined that it shall be second to none. You would be amused at the quite friendly – but quite obvious desire to keep well ahead of Troyes! [the second SWH hospital in France]. It's like rival schools. Of course we [observe the 'we' after a fortnight] are extraordinarily fortunate in having a Chief like Miss Ivens.[40]

As the laboratory opened, the number of admissions increased – a nightly average of 28 compared to the previous 4 to 12 – mostly coming from the shelling in the Albert–Arras sector. 'Still, though the staff is distinctly pressed just now, it likes it. It likes to feel that Royaumont is known as the hospital where a man gets his full 100% of chances.'[41] The appreciation of the patients was the greatest encouragement. 'One patient badly wounded in the arm assured me that he should [sic] take away with him a very substantial souvenir of Royaumont – his arm!'[42] The surgeons at Royaumont took great pains to preserve limbs, in contrast to many other hospitals, where amputation, often regarded as the easiest option, was all too readily performed.

Some slackening of pressure in July enabled the women to celebrate Bastille Day on the 14th with a concert in the refectory organized entirely by the patients. Cicely Hamilton described the colourful scene:

Rows of beds with their vivid scarlet coverlets on one side, long cane chairs on the other – benches in the centre – groups of nurses, orderlies, chauffeurs and kitchen staff. Gay red of coverlets and soldiers' bed-jackets, beautiful blue of orderlies' dresses, sprinkling of military uniforms and snowy veils, with the sober grey of the little knot of doctors made a magnificent colour scheme in the old Gothic building with its stained glass windows filtering the afternoon sunlight on the parquet floor, and the stone pillars, the blankets and the uniforms.[43]

At this time the patients were in the throes of a craze for making *bagues boches* – rings fashioned from fragments of shells or other pieces of military debris – which they would present to wives, sweethearts and every nurse and orderly within sight. The search was on for unringed fingers, and great was the competition to adorn them.[44]

Athletic competitions were organized in which patients, orderlies, sisters and doctors all took part. Events included stretcher races, tugs of war, potato races and so on – a novelty to the patients, who were delighted with this example of British eccentricity.[45] Another diversion came in August, when the unit marked the founding of the abbey by Saint Louis – celebrating the occasion, not entirely appropriately, with modern music and a tombola.[46]

Domestic problems interrupted the smooth running of the hospital. Money had to be found to improve the hot-water supply. The kitchen orderlies were now too busy to wash the floors themselves, so French women were recruited. The solution was more trouble than it was worth, however, as they flooded the floor with copious buckets of water and conditions were worse than before. An SOS went back for eight or nine strong, healthy, 'Scotch' servants.[47]

There were endless problems with coal and electricity. The dynamo for generating electricity simply ate coal; they tried coal dust but this was inadequate. Some of the underground electrical wires were damaged, and the whole installation was totally insufficient for the work it was required to do. Electric light had to be limited to the theatre and the x-ray room; a dynamo was hired from Paris at considerable expense – but even with this the supply of light for the theatre could not be guaranteed. They were reduced once more to candles in bottles, and Miss Loudon found that 'penny Chinese lanterns do very well for candle-sticks'. Poor Miss Loudon was torn between the need to heat and light the hospital and the need to keep expenses down.

> I have come to the conclusion that the most necessary qualification for an Administrator is a knowledge of plumbing and engineering, of both of which I am entirely ignorant.[48]

There was not enough electricity for sterilizers, and now even alcohol for spirit lamps was running short. There was a shortage of blankets – the staff were passing theirs to the patients. Miss Loudon begged the committee for 5000 yards of gauze and one hundredweight of cotton wool every month. Couldn't we use more moss for dressings? she wondered. (Sphagnum moss, collected by volunteers in the boggy areas of Scotland and elsewhere, was sterilized, dried and packed, and its absorbency and softness proved very useful for the copiously discharging wounds of modern warfare.)

In September the women were cheered by the arrival of a beautiful new x-ray car, gifted by the London Society and fitted out with the very latest equipment. The car had its own dark room, an independent water supply, and facilities for developing films in transit. It was to be used for the benefit of other patients in neighbouring hospitals, none of which at that time had even the most rudimentary x-ray machine. Patients would now be saved unnecessary and painful journeys. Madam Curie herself had advised on the equipment, and took a great interest in the adaptation of x-rays to serve the war effort and the needs of humanity. However, there was a drawback in having such a very wonderful machine, and putting it on show in London before taking it over to France. It may have encouraged contributions to the Scottish Women's Hospitals, but – it was seen by the War Office! Cicely Hamilton reported to Dr Savill in London on 28 August:

A new and dreadful hitch to the x-ray car – The War Office commandeered the engine, then they refused to release the car from the works until Austins had delivered a specified number of cars to them. Yesterday we heard that at last our car was released and could start; but now they refuse to give Captain Humphries leave to come out [he was to help in getting it operating] and Major Barrett doesn't want to go without him ... Most satisfactory if you [Savill] would come over for a day or two and let them go through everything with you ... if possible Butt [the manufacturers] will agree to send out one of their own men ... I am so afraid that if we are not quick at getting it out of the country the War Office will think of some new hitch.[49]

Dr Savill did come out, and the x-ray staff were trained. The War Office was foiled.

On 24 September the hospital was alerted that a rush was imminent. They were ordered to evacuate as many patients as possible. 'I think we have evacuated every man who could crawl,' Miss Loudon reported. The rush materialized over the next five days and nights. Wounded poured in from the Arras and Souchez sections of the French Front, and later from the heavy fighting round Hébuterne. They were all, Miss Ivens reported, 'horribly infected. I have never seen such wounds, gangrenous and offensive to a degree. We amputated three limbs, and there are several on the verge.' Even her Downs forceps were worn out with heavy use.[50] On one day they performed 22 operations, and 18 on the following day.

A young Canadian orderly, Marjorie Starr, who had recently arrived at the abbey, recorded her impressions of the tough conditions: 'A little fountain plays perpetually ... water just tantalizes me, no bath now for two weeks and none in view for another fortnight.'[51] Starr found her first flea – 'We scrub and clean so much there isn't a corner for them to live in (must have come from the trenches at Arras).' Starr, however, was 'not tired at all, just dirty'. She seems to have been flung in at the deep end. On 15 September she wrote: '15 beds to make myself, perfect stream of bedpans, 3 horrid dressings to prepare and then bandage up and clear away – and when the other sister came back if she didn't get me to scrub lockers and I jolly well had to smile and do it.'

Cleaning feet and nails was a 'smelly job'. They were 'very particular about nails here on account of the microbes'. She saw her first operation:

> ... all tendons and nerves mixed up – agony of dressings so great they gave him chloroform, and it took 6 of us to hold him while he was going under – got all sprinkled with blood and pus as he was very septic.

By 18 September she was 'never so tired in all my life'. They were short-staffed, there were painful dressings, the new cases were 'simply filthy'. 'Then, when they were all cleaned up, the chimney sweep arrived – there was soot everywhere even on the patients' bandages, a man came down from operation, the patients' suppers had to be served – and all at once.' On 24 September:

> ... everyone worked to death ... in our cleansing room pipe burst and flooded ... the kitchen boiler went wrong and kitchen fires had to be put out, so no hot water ... and the electric light engine got cranky and light so dim.

Through the next three days they were in the thick of the rush. 'Spent the day cleaning dirty people.'

She described the reception of the patients:

> When the Hall Porter hears motors coming she blows a horn and we all flock to the entrance except one in the wards, lift stretchers and lay on floor ... if stretchers go to out-patients' room where we blanket bath ... clothes into sack. Walking cases to cleansing room – bath there behind curtains and one of not badly wounded [patients] ... bath them. Then we finish them up and get them to bed. I never saw such filth ... straight from the trenches – all gory. Still they come, the wounded. Every hour as soon as one lot is cleaned and put to

bed the next ambulance arrives, and the worst of it is that in the middle of the excitement the meals for the others have to go on. Also ... in the middle of dressing a horrible wound, have to run to someone else with a bedpan.

And again, on the 28th:

How we all groan when we hear that blast[ed] horn and then we stampede for the entrance with all the blue dresses and caps of the sisters lifting the stretchers out of the ambulance, and really today each one seems worse than the last: one arm will simply have to be amputated, he had poison gas as well, and the smell was enough to knock me down, bits of bone sticking through and all gangrene. It will be marvellous if Miss Ivens saves it, but she is going to try it appears, as it is his right arm. He went to x-ray, then to theatre, and I believe the op was rather wonderful, but I had no time to stop and see as I had to help and carry the stretchers. They come right from the trenches, with only temporary dressings, and we operate, and as soon as possible move them on. No poky little wounds now, they are all serious. I mind the smell, or should I say stink, of the wounds more than anything. I can't seem to get away from it. I get to bed about 9.30, and after a good wash [her own rubber bath had arrived by this time] sprinkle my bed with perfume so as to get it out of my nostrils as my clothes even smell of it. We have so little disinfectant, not enough to drown the odour of it all. The operating theatre is a horrible hell these days.

They were fitting up a second operating theatre in one of the ward kitchens.

As all the ambulant patients had been discharged in anticipation of the rush, the orderlies no longer had their help with the chores, and to add to their heavy work in the wards they had to carry all the coal, and the stretchers themselves. 'It is the stretcher cases that wear us out, carrying heavy men up those stairs is much too heavy for girls, even four of us.' The orderlies were getting up at 4.30

a.m.: '40 beds to be made, 30 helpless – all beds to be changed as
dressings soaked through. High nervous pressure while dressings
are being done 8–12.30. Everyone worn out and nerves all on
edge.'

Starr's difficulties were increased by the sister who was supposed
to be training her:

> And really I never knew whether I was standing on my head
> or my heels, and I never seemed to get through, as she never
> let me finish anything in peace, always fly away to get this or
> that, then why wasn't it done? I suffered in silence, but I
> would just come up here when I was off and cry from pure
> wrought-up nerves.

Her stress was noticed and she was placed under a different sister –
'And now it is just heaven in comparison – she is from the Royal in
Glasgow. [This was probably Sister Lindsay.] Everyone was pitying
me and I evidently won Matron's favour by never complaining.'
How thankful she was later on to have this change of sister:

> It rather sent my heart to the bottom of my boots when I lifted
> the stretcher out and saw what I had, or rather smelt it . . . all his
> lower jaw was blown away, and it was fearfully sceptic [sic] and
> his clothes and body were in the last word in dirt and goriness. I
> am sure he had been lying sometime in mud unattended to
> before being picked up. [This was highly likely as at that period
> the collection of wounded from the battlefield was very
> inefficient, particularly in the French lines.]

This patient became very important to her. Her knowledge of
French enabled her to help him through, and the sight of his
gradual improvement, in which she played an important part, must
also have helped her through her own period of stress.
Next day:

> . . . the man with the awful mouth seems a little better. I had
> to try and get an egg down his throat but it was no use, he

couldn't swallow: his tongue seems half gone. They always have to call me to him as I seem to be the only one who can understand what he wants to say.

On 1 October she found herself in charge of a ward all alone (with a sister nearby to call if needed), responsible for serving supper to 16 men, four of whom had to be fed. 'The man with the wounded mouth was to have liquid food poured down his throat through a tube: it isn't a pleasant job but anything to help the miserable man.' By 4 October 'my poor man with the wounded mouth is getting on. I feed him on milk every time I have a minute to spare, through a rubber tube.' On 8 October 'my smelly friend with the mouth is doing well and he is a little more wholesome to go near'. On 18 October, after a spell away from the wards, she saw him again – 'I got a shock when I saw the man with the mouth. He had been shaved and walked into the refectory himself, he can eat soft food quite well and his mouth is nearly healed and he can talk quite well.' And on 4 November: 'I think the man with the mouth will soon be away now, and as he is quite cured and very little disfigured and he talks quite well and eats enough to make up for lost time.' Finally, on 28 November: 'my "smelly friend" as I call him (the one with the shattered jaw) is so well that they operated to get a stray bit of shrapnel out of his neck . . . it was a great success and he is doing well'.

Starr was beginning to feel the strain. There was some relief for her when she went on night duty – no longer getting up at 4.30 a.m., and spared the ordeal of the daily dressings. She described her new work:

> . . . such an eerie existence in the old Abbaye at night with only a lantern, and I had four fires to stoke, and if they went out I jolly well had to light them and fish for sticks and nothing to chop them with if you do find any, but I managed to find the lid of a box and chopped it with a shovel.

Miss Loudon, the administrator, arranged for her to have a few days' rest in Paris and then a month in the kitchen 'till my nerves get better':

It will not be so interesting of course, but I am not thinking of seeing things now, I just want to rest my mind and get away from the horrors for a little. Several of the girls have given up completely under the strain, but I hope this change will just pull me up in time, and I won't mind the hard work if I have no responsibility.

Starr's experience shows that as far as the demands of the work allowed the staff did consider the needs of the young orderlies. In Starr's case they relieved her in time, as her subsequent career showed. Her spirits rose and she found she was enjoying life again:

We work in the quaintest old place, all stone arches: it must have been where wine was served to the monks in the old days, and then later was the scullery of the convent. Three girls usually run it and the other two here are awfully nice and we have lots of fun over our dish slinging. You ought to see us throwing those tin plates about, they go like lightning.

After this short spell in the kitchen she began work as a store-keeper: 'I am sure I shall feel a perfect lady, no more dirt for a few days anyway.'

She described the procedure on the death of a patient:

The night orderly, [Marjorie] Miller, had to help carry the body to the chapel – she says it was rather a gruesome sight. Miss Duncan, the Matron, went first down three flights of steps and through the moonlit cloisters carrying a lantern and these three girls carrying the stretcher, draped in a sheet and a piece of paper pinned on his chest with his name, age 19, and then the name of the witnesses who were there when he died, Miss Ivens, the surgeon, a sister and Richmond. [Miss Susan Eleanor Richmond, later Mrs Haydon, was an actress and subsequently had a very successful career on the London stage.]

On another occasion she witnessed a funeral at Asnières and left this account:

First a line of choirboys followed by the coffin, then the priest, after that the old mother of one and the relations of the other, then their comrades from the wards ... Then crutches, slings and bandaged heads followed each other two by two, then two of our lady doctors in uniform and a band of village women all in black who go to all the funerals so that the poor souls have plenty of mourners. It seems strange that they don't have a military funeral still this is war in grim earnest and there is no time nor men to be spared for show. The wounded who followed had their uniforms on, as in the hospital they wear blue trousers and red flannel coats belonging to us, that is when there is enough to go round: now we have 204 patients so there is a variety of costumes given out, but nothing like the variety of the French soldiers at the funeral, some were Zouaves, some even had black faces [probably Senegalese], some in blue trousers, some in red, but none ever so clean in all their soldier lives as they do [sic] when they leave here with all the uniforms cleaned and disinfected and mended. [At this time there was indeed a great variety of uniforms in the French army. It was only in 1916 that the army was provided with steel helmets and 'French blue' uniforms – not as good camouflage as the British khaki or the German *feldgrau* but much the same when covered in mud.]

Starr's interest in the medical work continued. On 4 November she recorded:

There are several very bad cases of gas gangrene, which is nasty and smelly and, of course, very dangerous. I was very glad I wasn't the poor VAD* yesterday who got a leg to burn as the theatre sisters were too busy to attend to it. [An incinerator was provided for the disposal of limbs, dressings and other rubbish.] It is bad enough to hold the stump for dressings without having to handle the lifeless limb.

* A member of the Voluntary Aid Detachment, which provided field nursing services in both world wars.

On 20 November she was reporting a lull – for the time being the rush was virtually over. Back to nursing in the wards again, she was called on by the doctor to translate a patient's story. The man described the terrible mud, and how the shells made holes in the bottom of the trenches. With mud up to his knees it was impossible to see where the holes were, and he fell in up to his chest. He struggled for five hours to get out until, responding to his whistle, rescuers got ropes and hauled him out. He was one of the lucky ones – on the same day three men had been drowned in the mud.

Throughout Starr's account one can sense her pride in the hospital and her admiration for the work of the surgeons. Of two badly wounded patients she wrote: 'Their legs are really awful, and in a French military hospital would have been amputated long ago, but Miss Ivens is doing her best to save the limbs.'

The sense of strain betrayed by Starr was shared by others. While she was nursing the matron during a short illness, Starr remarked on what a difficult time the matron had with so many squabbling sisters. Miss Ivens herself had a problem with one of the doctors. Dr Rutherford had arrived at Royaumont in June 1915, and resigned suddenly on 23 October. She wrote to Mrs (Dr) Russell of the committee:

During the greater part of the time the hospital has been established the cases have been chiefly of a light nature, but recently more serious cases have been received. Unfortunately during the past few months two patients have been trephined with grave results. On the 20th inst another cerebral case occurred in which surgical interference seemed imperative, and owing to the unfortunate result in the former cases I ventured to suggest to Miss Ivens, for her own sake and that of the hospital, the advisability of obtaining a second opinion. She received my suggestion in bad part, and afterwards, in public, asked me to leave the theatre. After the operation I reiterated to her that my suggestion was a friendly one and not in the nature of a criticism, but offered to resign immediately as she had resented my action. Accordingly I left Royaumont the following day. I regret if this slip has caused inconvenience either in the Hospital or to the Committee, but in the circumstances no other course was possible.[52]

Mrs Hunter, the chairman of the hospital committee, said that she had received a number of complaints about Dr Ivens's surgery on a recent visit. The committee also received a letter from Miss Ivens stating that 'she had just become aware of disloyalty in the medical staff', and she wanted the committee to recall one member. Mrs Hunter felt she could not continue in her office unless these complaints were thoroughly investigated.

Mrs Russell, a member of the committee who was medically qualified, went out to Royaumont with the specific remit to 'explore the situation'. In other words, was Miss Ivens up to it? It was a delicate task for Mrs Russell, but she reported back after her visit that she had 'investigated thoroughly, studied the medical statistics and interviewed affected members. The French authorities were abundantly satisfied – they were still sending cases after these reports had reached them, Dr Coussergues [*médecin-chef* of the army zone in which Royaumont was placed, and therefore representing the highest medical authority] frequently brought visiting doctors to visit and invited Miss Ivens to inspect work at other hospitals and the hospital was thoroughly inspected at regular intervals.' Mrs Russell went on to reassure the committee that 'they had no cause for anxiety whatever, but on the contrary had cause to be proud of the work being done by Miss Ivens and her assistants'. The committee resolved unanimously that they send a vote of confidence to Miss Ivens.[53]

Most surgeons would agree that Miss Ivens had some justification in requesting an assistant to leave the theatre if she had been criticized – publicly – for her handling of a very difficult operation. Most surgeons would also agree that in the conditions prevailing at that time there would inevitably be some cases that would go wrong. All surgeons were learning on the job how to deal with war wounds. Miss Ivens was no exception. She had, in her usual thorough way, taken great trouble to equip herself in her new tasks. Looking back from a knowledge of the achievements and the results obtained at Royaumont by the end of the war, it seems Mrs

Russell's report was justified and no mere whitewashing exercise.

To be fair to Dr Rutherford, though she was not as wise as she might have been in the way she acted, she had been genuinely worried when she saw a case 'going wrong'. After leaving Royaumont she went on to serve with the Royal Army Medical Corps (RAMC) in Malta and Salonika, and after the Second World War worked as a medical officer in UNRRA (United Nations Relief and Reconstruction Administration).

Dr Rutherford's departure on 23 October must have left a problem for the remaining staff – Miss Loudon reported the week from 24 to 30 October was 'rather dreadful':

> The doctors and nurses and theatre orderlies work from morning to night and from night to morning; if there is another advance I don't know what will happen. The wet weather means much mud in the trenches, and mud on wounds means dirt and that usually means poison and gas gangrene and all sorts of horrors.

She reserved a room at the hotel in Creil for the use of the chauffeurs, who often had to wait for long periods in the cold and wet for the arrival of the hospital trains. And just then the cesspits had to be cleared out. 'You can imagine the odours,' she moaned – and this was in addition to the smell of gas gangrene. And those damaged electric cables were not yet repaired.[54]

❧

The progress and achievements of the hospital were followed with great interest by many of the leading women doctors of the time, who recognized that the reputation of women in the medical profession depended in part on their performance in difficult wartime conditions. If they could perform well in those circumstances it would be difficult for the sceptics to maintain that women were not strong enough or able enough to be regarded as the equals of men. It was already recognized that women could give valuable service in looking after women and children and in filling unpopular but necessary positions in the local authority 'workhouse' infirmaries, but could they really be proficient in general surgery, and, even more doubtfully, in military surgery? Were they, in short, tough enough? And what if they should fail?

Miss Louisa Aldrich-Blake (later Dame Louisa, only the second women to receive that honour) had no doubts on the subject. She was herself a distinguished surgeon – she was the first woman to obtain the degree of master of surgery (Miss Ivens was the third). From 1914, in addition to her surgical work, she was dean of the London (Royal Free Hospital) School of Medicine for Women. Her heavy workload prevented her from volunteering for service overseas, but she used her vacations to work at Royaumont in 1915 and again in 1916. She turned her hand to many kinds of activities, from making toast to major surgery. Orderly Starr, looking at her from afar, decided she was a 'charming person'. The patients, who referred to Miss Ivens as *la Colonelle*, decided Aldrich-Blake was *Madame la Générale*.

It was a happy arrangement, and after Dame Louisa's death in 1925 Miss Ivens recalled her visit to Royaumont in 1915:

> The greater part of her time was spent in the theatre, looking for elusive bullets or bits of shells in inaccessible positions. Her patience and pertinacity impressed both theatre staff and x-ray departments. I can only remember one failure, but there were many brilliant successes.

And in 1916, when 400 beds were in use:

> Cases of gas gangrene had poured in, and the work had been strenuous and exhausting. With her characteristic energy Miss Aldrich-Blake dressed in the wards, did re-amputations, or anything else that was needed. She was much interested in the sera treatment of gas gangrene, which we were then success-fully trying in some of the worst infections. ... She was most sympathetic with our difficulties, and I do not remember hearing a word of criticism though she must have noticed a great deal that could have been improved upon.[55]

Another prominent medical woman to pay a working visit to Royaumont in 1915 was Dr Louisa Martindale. Travelling in her first-class carriage from Paris, she was recognized by a member of the unit and was introduced to the economical ways of the staff of the Scottish Women's Hospitals, who were all, including Miss Ivens, travelling third class. When she arrived at the abbey, Dr Martindale found that her 'cell' had a bed, a chair, a packing case and a basin, but no bathroom. At mealtimes she had a single enamel plate that had to serve for two courses, and a single enamel mug which did duty for wine and coffee. (Later, the staff had to do without the wine, though for the patients it was always a part of their rations.) But the food was splendid – Michelet, the famous chef, was then in the kitchen on a temporary basis. Knives were in very short supply, and the first thing Dr Martindale did when she got home was to send out a dozen or so for the doctors. She spent her time dressing wounds, operating, filling in forms, writing reports, and doing other necessary chores. She was

> Tremendously impressed ... There were no men to help carry the heavy patients. Women, some of whom had never before done any housework, worked all day at washing up in that huge, badly equipped, ancient kitchen, or helped to clean, mend and repair, each soldier's kit ready for departure. Most of all I was lost in admiration of the splendid organizing and administrative powers of the CMO [chief medical officer], Miss Ivens – of her endurance, courage and above all her surgical skill.[56]

Various other women doctors also spent their holidays working at Royaumont, showing the enormous interest and pride felt by medical women in the work being done by the unit.

❦

Towards the end of the year there was another worry for the hospital committee at home – this time financial. Royaumont was proving very expensive. It now cost £1000 a month in addition to the 2 francs a day per patient that they received from the French government. (Dr Inglis had originally calculated £500 per month.) Did they really need 72 pairs of rubber gloves per month? The demands for gauze seemed to the committee to be exorbitant.

They really must try and use less than one ton of coal per day. And did they really need a staff of 90?

Miss Kemp and Mrs Russell went into this very thoroughly on their visit of inspection. They said clearly and definitely that there was 'no extravagance at Royaumont'. It would be quite impossible to work the hospital with a smaller number of staff. The size and inconvenience of the building and the serious nature of the cases necessitated keeping the staff at the present level.[57] Right through to the end of November the hospital was particularly full – there had been an influx of bad cases since the advance at Loos.

With the slackening of the work as winter approached, Marjorie Starr spent some of her spare time exploring the trenches nearby (these were never actually used, but had been prepared after the Battle of the Marne). There were other new activities:

A lot of doctors and orderlies and even some of the nurses have organized a hockey team, but yours truly won't join, the suffragettes would be too much for me . . . The hockey team is getting on – I wouldn't care to play with them, they are a burly lot, a good many of them suffragettes. I say they are keeping in training for after the war, but I must say they are a jolly lot just the same.

On 2 December there was a party to celebrate the opening of the hospital in 1914. Miss Ivens supplied champagne and 'gave us a spanking supper'. They put on fancy dress and danced till midnight. There was another party on 13 December, this time put on by the men. They had a gramophone, and those who were able danced. Poor Starr would 'quite like to have danced with them too, but it wouldn't do, we have to keep our dignity, or we wouldn't be able to keep order as we do and get respect from them'. The year ended with a splendid Christmas party, at which Cicely Hamilton produced a scene from her own play, *Diana of Dobson's*, which had been such a success on the London stage.

And so 1915 drew to a close. They had had their first baptism of fire. In later years Vera Collum looked back with nostalgia to 'the more leisured days of 1915'.[58]

ૐ

1916: The Year of Testing

The military situation in 1916, which formed the background to the work of the hospital, was influenced initially by the great struggles further east. As far as the French army was concerned, the winter lull ended on 21 February with the German push towards Verdun. On 25 February the Germans captured Fort Douaumont, one of the key strongholds, which the French had left, inexplicably, virtually unmanned. Had the Germans realized it at the time, the way to Verdun was wide open, but they missed the chance, and the opportunity never recurred. Instead, an increasingly grim war of attrition developed with repeated attacks by both sides, enormous losses, but barely any change in the front.

Then on 9 April the Germans launched a full-scale offensive along the whole of the Verdun front, on both banks of the Meuse. Fighting continued with little gained on either side through May and into June. Conditions in the trenches were appalling; there were periods of continuous rain and other periods of excessive heat. Suffering was intense.

On 7 June Fort Vaux, the second great fort supposedly guarding Verdun, fell to the Germans. On 11 June General Pétain, who was now (although only temporarily) in charge, pressed Joffre, the commander-in-chief, to bring forward the relief offensive that had been planned with the British on the Somme. On 20 June the situation became even more desperate with the first use of the new gas diphosgene, which paralysed the French artillery. On the 23rd the Germans made a significant advance.

The preliminary bombardment on the Somme by the British began on 24 June, and on 1 July both French and British infantry went 'over the top' and advanced towards the German lines. The preliminary bombardment proved to have been tragically ineffective and the casualty rate among the attackers was unbelievably high. On that one day the British lost 60,000 men, of whom 20,000 were killed. The French lost as many men as they had in the previous three months' fighting, which had, itself, been on an enormous scale. This was the terrible beginning of the 'Great Push'. It was followed by five months of pointless slaughter.

Now began the period of greatest stress that Royaumont had known so far, which was eclipsed only by its experience in the great battles of 1918. But it gave Royaumont the opportunity to prove what it was capable of.

❧

The New Year came in quietly enough. Surveying her staff, Miss Ivens was pleased. The *bouches inutiles* ('useless mouths'), as she called them, had left, and morale was high.

As 1916 opened, the women felt they were beginning to get to grips with the conditions in which they were working, and relations with the French authorities were becoming increasingly friendly and trusting. Dr Bossières, inspecting, had already expressed his confidence in the unit, while another visitor reported: 'Today it is known far and wide in the countryside as a refuge for the wounded under the care of the *dames écossaises*.'[1]

Royaumont did not confine itself to purely medical care. One day in early January, 180 men, exhausted, hungry and cold (but unwounded), arrived at the abbey. They had been on the road for several days – victims of the French army's lack of canteens and rest centres; and with pay a mere pittance of 20 sous a day they were in no position to help themselves. At the hospital hot meals were quickly provided, and straw was laid on the floor of the great refectory for the men to sleep on. Later, to the astonishment of the staff, the men roused themselves and gave them a concert by way of thanks.[2]

Beds were now increased to 250. Dr Coussergues, in charge of the *gare régulatrice*, begged the loan of two of the Royaumont sisters to direct a large new surgical ward at the Creil Hospital. Miss Ivens, with the blessing of the committee, agreed to send two or three sisters each month in rotation, provided always that the abbey's needs were met.[3]

Some improvements in the domestic arrangements were made. Monsieur Pichon, the architect, 'went over the drains most carefully',[4] though the later history of the abbey seems to suggest that, as the population increased and the years rolled on, the sanitary problems were never entirely resolved in spite of frequent emptying of cesspits. The washing now went to a military laundry instead of being farmed out to a number of individual women in the surrounding villages.[5]

Wine was obligatory for the *poilus*, as decreed by the army, and was now to be available at army rates, but the hospital still had to cover the cost. Miss Ivens, generous to a fault where the welfare of the hospital and the patients was concerned, asked the committee to use the £100 increase in salary they had offered her, and which she said she did not really require, to cover the cost of wine for the men.[6]

By early April, a new petrol-run electrical generator (costing 12,000 francs) was up and running.[7] The scullery still required a new sink and a new *marmite* (cauldron) for heating and storing water, and a second lorry was becoming essential. Intense cold and snow exacerbated the transport problems, and again the supply of coal was threatened. The military authorities proved helpful, and supplied the unit with a weekly truckload from Rouen, to be fetched in their hard-working lorry. Even the six and a half tons allowed was barely sufficient, and kitchen fires had to be ruthlessly cut.[8]

In January Royaumont experienced its first loss, when Sister Mary Gray died some days after an apparently successful operation for appendicitis. She was buried in the local churchyard with full military honours. One of her patients wrote of 'good, kind Miss Gray who has always something gently to do with us'.[9] She and her sister had been among the very first arrivals in November 1914, and her sister – who called herself 'Disorderly' (by all accounts a most inappropriate nickname) – gallantly returned after a short period at home. She then remained, a valued auxiliary nurse, throughout all the later tumultuous periods in the history of the hospital till the final closure in 1919.

In April the committee sent over two of its members to make a thorough inspection. Mrs Laurie and Mrs Robertson were impressed with the organization:

> Our impressions of the Abbaye de Royaumont are of the most pleasant, the work being carried on there appears to be excellent; the members of the staff are working most harmoniously together, there seems to be a tremendous feeling of esprit-de-corps among them all, and the patients speak in most appreciative terms of all that has been done for them by our noble women.
>
> The curés of Asnières and Viarmes as well as the municipal authorities of other little towns surrounding the hospital are all most grateful for the assistance we have been giving to the civil patients whom Dr Ivens has, – with the consent of the Committee, and, I consider, very wisely, – been taking in whilst the number of her soldier patients has been decreasing. We inspected very thoroughly the whole of the hospital, the orderlies' dormitories, Sisters' bedrooms, wards, kitchen, store and other departments. Mrs Hacon has now taken over the superintendence of the kitchen department ... an admirable arrangement as constant supervision is necessary, and this is the department where the greatest saving can take place, and where close attention to detail must be given to curtail waste as much as possible.
>
> There is no doubt that the patients are extremely well fed.[10]

Miss Ivens gave much thought to maintaining the morale of the patients: concerts were a regular feature, some given by staff, some by the men, and there was great rivalry between the wards. They were allowed into the woods to pick the lily of the valley, and they fished in the stream. The presentation of medals was an occasion for celebration for the whole hospital. Miss Ivens organized a competition for the men to write their personal war stories. For many this was not simply a way of passing the time, but a means of exorcizing some of the horrors they had undergone. Every entrant (and there were 64) received a prize – a photograph of the abbey. The best got a larger photograph, so everyone was pleased.[11] One entrant, Eugène Boutet, a farmer in civilian life, wrote of his experiences since the Battle of Loos (September 25–26, 1915):

> On the evening of the 26th, with several of my companions, we buried many of the unfortunates who had been killed on the 25th – they were all without arms or legs, or their chests torn open – it was frightful. This was my first experience of the labyrinth trenches. During the month of November we suffered many privations, bad weather (every day it poured), shells, mud and water up to our waists. At night we were frozen; it was, indeed, 'agréable'![12]

As the unit approached one of its peak periods during the Somme battles of 1916, some unknown person made accusations of waste and extravagance. Miss Ivens took these accusations seriously, and reviewed the administration. Mrs Hacon, now kitchen superintendent, was succeeding in 'feeding staff and patients as cheaply and efficiently as possible under difficult conditions'. She pointed out that 'a well-equipped store room does not mean that stores are given out lavishly. The most expensive times are when we have to live from hand to mouth, buying in Paris from day to day.'

But as regards dressings and drugs she was adamant. She pointed out to the committee:

> It is absolutely essential now to be ready for a heavy demand. The inspecting generals expect us to be prepared for all emergencies and any deficiency would be noted at once, and placed against us as a bad mark ... As I think I told you before, our standard has to be that of the Paris hospitals, in which zone we are placed geographically, while our preparations have to be of such a character as to enable us to meet any emergency at a moment's notice as we draw our wounded straight from the Front. To combine the two is by no means an easy task, and if I sometimes appear to make unreasonable

69

demands let me assure you they are well-considered. I am well aware that the hospital has cost a great deal of money, but I think that it has done its best to get good value, ... 1693 soldiers and 138 civilian patients have been treated, with only a mortality of 17. 1898 operations have been performed. Figures which I think speak for themselves.[13]

So Miss Ivens was consciously preparing for the testing time to come. The quieter times during the spring were, she explained, because the French army's main involvement was in the battle for Verdun, and the wounded from there went to Lyons, or Paris, not to them. But, she went on, 'we all anticipate a great offensive soon'.[14]

By 21 May Miss Ivens was reporting that she had been approached by Dr Coussergues on the feasibility of increasing capacity to 400 beds if needed. She was 'afraid we are to be in for a terrible time. All our *blessés* are to be evacuated Thursday.' She arranged a second temporary theatre in the Blanche receiving room – it had a stone floor and a good light. The organization for the reception of the wounded was reviewed and the staff prepared. Domestic arrangements were again overhauled:

It is now a pleasure to go into the kitchen and see the improvements that have been made in the direction of both cleanliness and order, and to feel that every item is scrutinized so that no leakage shall take place. Mrs Hacon works in conjunction with Tollitt and Grandage, the store and linen keepers, and I feel that they are all competent and conscientious.[15]

To ensure an adequate supply of orderlies, on whom the whole unit was crucially dependent, advertisements appeared in June: 'Ladies 24–35. Able to speak French or German fluently, and must have had some hospital experience or training in domestic science ... Lose no time in applying.'[16]

Miss Ivens was now happier with her nursing department. In April she had reported that it was 'in better control and efficiency' under Miss Duncan. She felt the selection of nurses by the committee was much improved. 'I like your nurse [Winstanley] very much. She is, as are also a number of newcomers, a much nicer type of nurse than we had some months ago.' (Miss Ivens did not mince her words.) 'There seems to be much less disagreeableness than there was amongst them,' she informed the committee. 'The better educated they are,' she continued, 'the more they like being here. The more ignorant and lower class ones miss the town, and have not sufficient resources in themselves to avoid being bored in their off time.'[17]

On the medical side Ruth Nicholson was now second-in-command (as she had been unofficially since the beginning), and the major surgical work was shared between her and Miss Ivens. Dr Courtauld was principal anaesthetist. The laboratory was now under Dr Elsie Dalyell, who had followed Dr Estcourt-Oswald in May. The x-ray department, under Dr Savill, now had three very well-trained radiographers: Vera Collum, Jean Berry and G.L. Buckley. The wards were looked after by Drs Berry, Ross and Wilson. They knew each other well by this time. It was a strong team and they worked well together. Apart from Dr Wilson, who died in 1917, lifelong friendships were forged between them.

Dr Courtauld had been a fellow-student of Miss Ivens at the London School of Medicine for Women, after which she had gone to a mission hospital in southern India, where she gained experience as an obstetrician and anaesthetist. Miss Ivens herself had invited her to apply, and she had joined the unit in January 1916. Although she was the oldest member of the unit, she stood up to the 'rushes' well. Dr Wilson came from the mission field in Palestine. Dr Dalyell was already distinguished in her field of bacteriology, and like Dr Butler before her she was a Beit research fellow of the Lister Institute in London. She was very successful in training selected orderlies to carry out the necessary laboratory procedures.

The hospital now had considerable expertise, and when the 'Big Push' came it was probably as well prepared as it was possible to be under wartime conditions.

Dr Savill pointed out that, as well as the organization of the hospital, 'experience of dealing with heavily infected wounds had been gradually built up throughout 1915 ... a course of action had been worked out'. Every case on admission was examined by one of the ward surgeons, and smears were taken from the wounds for bacteriological examination. In the minds of all was the horror of gas gangrene. It was this dread that dictated the order in which patients were sent to the theatre, as delay in operating could make the difference between life and death.

And so they waited. June passed, relatively quietly, but with growing anticipation. Miss Ivens, like the wise chief she was, tried to give everyone a period of rest.

❧

This quiet period was not to last. Just after it had started, Dr Savill described the long expected onset of the Big Push:

> We had received warning that the offensive was to begin about the end of June, and when we heard the guns thundering by day and by night from the 25th of June we realized that our share of the labour entailed by all military operations was about to commence. ... On July 2nd the anticipated rush began, and for 10 days, almost without intermission, it continued. ... Royaumont is situated only 25 miles behind the firing line, and cases reached us a few hours after being wounded when sent direct from the Front, and 2–3 days later when they had been detained for 'rest' in hospitals nearer the Front.[18] [This 'rest' was later realized to be a thoroughly bad idea – prompt operative treatment was essential to limit infections and in 1917 the whole system was changed to take account of this; see Appendix One.]

The most vivid description of 'The First Week of the First Great Push' was written by Vera Collum, then working in the x-ray department:

> On the first [of July] we waited, full of tense, suppressed excitement. The Great Push had begun – how were the Allies

faring? Our hospital had been evacuated almost to the last man. Our new emergency ward of 80 beds had been created in what had once been as big as an English parish church [*sic*; this was the refectory] – our theatre and our receiving rooms had been supplied with a huge reserve of bandages and swabs, of lint and gauze and wool; our new x-ray installation [a second machine] had been fitted up to the last connection; our ambulances were waiting ready to start at a moment's notice in the garage yard. The incessant thunder and boom of the great guns had never been silent for days. This day, at dawn, the thunder had swelled to an orgy of terrific sound that made the whole earth shiver; then, a few hours later, had ceased, and we could hear once more the isolated reports of individual cannon. Those of us who had been at the hospital through the attacks of June 1915, and the more serious push in Artois on September 25th, went early to bed. If the call came in the night we could always be summoned – meanwhile, we slept when we could. The later-comers marvelled at our lack – our apparent lack – of anticipation and excitement, and waited up long into the night. July 2nd dawned. The morning hours dragged on, placid in the hot sunshine of high Summer. Our ambulances were called out to await the first train of wounded at our clearing station. It was at noonday dinner that the telephone message came through that they were arriving shortly with very bad cases. The ward Sisters and their staffs went over their arrangements once more; the women orderlies stoked up their hot water *marmites* attached to each ward and to the operating theatre, and the Sister who presided there counted over again her reserve drums of sterilized cloths and swabs. We, in our department, once more tried our tubes to make sure they were regulated and working to a nicety, and the little group of women doctors collected by the window that opens above the entrance hall and watched for the cars to come.

Absolute readiness – and then – speed without haste. That was what we had to aim at; on that must depend the chances of many a human life. The long blast of a whistle from the entrance hall – how well we were to know it! – and almost to dread its insistent iteration during the next few days. This was the porter announcing the arrival of the first convoy from Cr[eil], sixteen stretcher cases. No sooner had the men been lifted out and carried to the various receiving rooms than the cars went back to the *gare régulatrice* for more. Trains were arriving from the Somme in one long stream. The drivers never ceased journeying backwards and forwards all that afternoon and all that night, and the three women and the man, who drove our four ambulances, carried over a hundred cases over the first 24 hours of that nightless week. They slept a little by turns, so that during the first twenty days of the great push there were always some of our cars at the clearing station, night and day, and the cases distributed to our hospital never had to wait there longer than was necessary.[19]

Collum described how, as the men were brought in more quickly than they could be dealt with, she was put in charge of the second x-ray machine, which had recently been installed in another room, and then the patients could be 'put through' more quickly:

Very soon, the surgeon-in-chief was hard at work, with the anaesthetist and the assistant in the operating theatre, each ward surgeon bringing up her own cases and assisting with them. It grew dark, and still the wounded came in. By ten o'clock we had a long line of stretchers lying in the corridor outside the x-ray rooms and the theatre, – at one end wounded men waiting to be examined by us; at the other, those who had already been examined, and who were waiting their turn for operation. The two storekeepers and the kitchen orderlies, who had gone off duty, organized themselves into a stretcher squad, and kept the x-ray couches and the operating theatre supplied. Down another corridor the other assistant radiographer had arranged her developed plates to dry – dozens of them. Some time after midnight our doctor [Dr Savill] had to retire to bed. She was not a strong woman and she had to be ready for the new day's work at 8 a.m. At four o'clock the other assistant, having developed 63 photographs since two o'clock in the afternoon, followed her. We knew the surgeons had more cases waiting for them than they could possibly operate on during the night. One or two of the ward surgeons dropped off, aware that they would have to begin work early in the morning. But the theatre went on, and the other surgeons who were waiting their turn to get their most urgent cases done, filled up the time by getting on with the list that was to be examined under the x-rays.

She went on:

Cases continued to come in all day, but as everyone was a stretcher case, and each car could only carry four, while the clearing station was 12 kilometres [actually 12 miles] distant, the hospital was able to absorb them as they came in, so that there was little if any delay in attending to the poor fellows.

Their wounds were terrible ... many of these men were wounded – dangerously – in two, three, four and five places. That great enemy of the surgeon who would conserve life and limb, gas gangrene, was already at work in 90% of cases. Hence the urgent need for immediate operation, often for immediate amputation. The surgeon did not stop to search for shrapnel and pieces of metal: their one aim was to open up and clean out the wounds, or to cut off the mortifying limb before the dread gangrene had tracked its way into the vital parts of the body. The stench was very bad. Most of the poor fellows were too far gone to say much.[20]

She remembers that they then

... had accommodation for 400, and for weeks we worked, once we were filled, with never a bed to spare. Our operating theatre was hardly ever left vacant long enough to be cleaned during the small hours and it became a problem how to air the x-ray rooms during the short hours of dawn that stretched between the ending of one day's work and the beginning of another's. We were fighting gas gangrene and time was the factor that counted most. We dared not stop work in the theatre until it became physically impossible to continue. For us who worked, and for those patient suffering men, lying along the corridor outside the x-ray rooms and the theatre, on stretchers, awaiting their turn, it was a nightmare of glaring lights, of appalling stenches of ether and chloroform, and violent sparking of tired x-ray tubes, of scores of wet negatives that were seized upon by their respective surgeons and taken into the hot theatre before they had even had time to be rinsed in the dark room. Beneath and beyond the anxiety of saving men's lives, there was the undercurrent of anxiety of the theatre staff as to whether the boiling of instruments and gloves could be kept level with the rapidity with which the cases were carried in and put on the table, as to whether the gauze and wool and swabs would last! – and with us it was anxiety for the life of the tubes, anxiety to get the gas gangrene plates developed first, to persuade them to dry, to keep the cases of the six surgeons separate, to see that they did not walk off with the wrong plates – for we had pictures that were almost identical, duplication of names, and such little complications. And it all had to be done in a tearing hurry, and at the end of a day that had already lasted anything from 10 to 18 hours, and no mistakes to be made. I do not think we lost a case from delay in locating the trouble and operating in all that first terrible week of July. The losses were due to delay in reaching the hospital.[21]

Collum tells of her personal work schedule over the first few days:

July 2nd 2 p.m. till July 3rd 7 a.m.
July 3rd 11 a.m. till supper time. Rest till 10 p.m.
Worked 10 p.m. till 6 a.m. on July 4th.
July 4th Slept 6 a.m. till noon. Dinner. Worked till supper. Rest till 10 p.m. Worked 10 p.m. till 4 a.m. July 5th.
July 5th Four hours sleep after 4 a.m. Worked till 11 p.m.
July 6th Sleep one hour, then wakened as a new convoy had come in and some of the cases needed immediate operation.

She describes how she felt:

> I do not think I have ever felt so sleepy and tired as I did when I got downstairs – it is so much easier to carry on than to be called up, when you are nearing the end of your powers of keeping awake. We worked as in a dream. My legs and hands did not seem to belong to me, and I heard my own voice far away as if it came from somebody else. It had become impossible to work quickly, and I found it necessary to make great efforts to remember little things and do them correctly. We got to bed again before dawn.
>
> On the last day of the week our x-ray staff had an addition, the chief assistant having come back hastily from leave in England.[22]

This was Buckley, a medical student who had interrupted her training to come to Royaumont as an orderly. She had gone home to sit a medical exam. Collum continues:

> Thenceforward we were able to tackle the work comfortably, each getting some time off during the day, and dividing the night's work among us in shifts of two. Further, since the hospital was full, we could not be rushed by any great influx of serious cases. We settled down to steady, hard work that continued through the rest of July, August and September, varied once or twice by emergencies, such as when we admitted 80 cases in one day (after having evacuated a good number to make room for them), and before nightfall had examined 40 of them under x-rays and operated on 20.[23]

There were other vivid recollections of that first desperate week. Dr Savill snatched a few moments on 4 July to write home:

> We have had a ghastly time of horrors since Sunday. Men badly wounded pouring in at the rate of 70 to 100 per day. We took 150 photos in x-ray rooms since Sunday noon, and many screenings and localizations in addition. . . . Our photos had to

dry all along the wall in the gallery. You can picture the scene
– surgeons demanding their photos and I chained to the x-ray
room. ... Miss Collum has worked singlehanded for the two
nights and afternoons. Miss Berry all day long in dark room
developing at post-haste, I alone in x-ray room ... When Miss
Berry was not developing she undertook singlehanded one of
the x-ray rooms. ... Miss Ivens had operated Sunday 1.0 p.m.
to 5.45 a.m. next day; then from 9 a.m. Monday to about 5
this morning; and again from 10 a.m. to-day, and is still hard
at it and likely to be so till tomorrow.[24]

Dr Dalyell, heading the bacteriological laboratory, also recalled
those first few days:

> ... there have been simply awful days and nights. I hear the poor
> people in the operating theatre cleaning up madly ... a swab of
> every wound is taken immediately after admission and sent
> instantly to the laboratory. I examine them on the instant – did
> 180 in three days – and a bacteriological report was despatched
> within about half an hour. All the gas gangrene cases were
> sorted out by this means and the incipient cases were spotted at
> once and operated according to the severity of the infection as
> notified by me. By that means we saved lots of limbs, as they
> were spotted early and opened up in time. So many of the cases
> where I insisted on immediate operation proved to have early
> gas formation at the bottom of a deep narrow shell wound that
> it would certainly be fatal to leave them; they would probably
> have lost a limb, if not life. So far we have had only 5 deaths and
> we did 112 bad cases of gas gangrene without stopping. As I did
> the bacteriological work in batches of 20, my excellent girl
> orderly did yeoman service in collecting the swabs and pre-
> paring of the specimens, I was able to take a hand in the theatre
> and plied between the lab and the operating table without
> ceasing day or night.[25]

For the surgeons there could be no system of shifts. The second
theatre was now in full operation. The junior surgeons were

admitting and classifying the wounded as they came in, applying the dressings of those who had been operated on, and watching the patients closely for signs of deterioration – which could occur with dramatic suddenness. They were also performing the smaller operations themselves, and assisting the chief surgeons.

That first night they were operating continuously till 7 a.m., and after only an hour or two of rest they were back in theatre. The urgent priority was to check the spread of gas gangrene. In some cases this involved immediate amputation; in others they had to open up the wounds and remove damaged tissue and pieces of tattered clothing, which would otherwise provide a potent breeding ground for the bacteria causing gas gangrene. Only these most urgent procedures were carried out in the first instance. Over the succeeding eight days several of the women had no more than 16 hours of sleep in total. 'Three hours consecutive sleep was an unbelievable luxury.'[26]

Miss Ivens was under pressure, not only from the constant inflow of patients, but also from the French medical authorities. On 3 July she telegraphed the committee: 'SERVICE DE SANTÉ DEMANDS WE ENLARGE HOSPITAL VERY URGENT WOUNDED ARRIVE CONSTANTLY IVENS.' The committee wired back: 'GLAD AGREE WHATEVER NECESSARY.'[27]

On 16 July Miss Ivens found a moment to write a letter, with an emphasis (typical of her) on practical considerations:

> We are hard at work. We have had in nearly three hundred cases during the last fortnight and they are nearly all *grands blessés* [seriously wounded] – cases they cannot send any further. As you know we were at once asked to double our beds – I was able to arrange this at once.

The army supplied the actual beds – she put 50 in the cloisters and nearly 100 in the refectory, which was then named the Canada Ward:

> Everyone is working very hard and I am hoping you will soon be able to send us the nurses and orderlies as soon as they can

possibly come with or without uniforms. It has been a case of day and night for many, and of course they cannot keep it up. There is every prospect this rush will last for several months. They seem to think that we can be of the greatest value to Creil as we take in heavy cases of gas gangrene to whom a few more hours means a fatal end. The wounds are dreadful. Last year was child's play to it, but so far we have got over the ground well. Refectory makes a lovely ward. M. Pichon has arranged a little stove and taps etc in adjoining store room, and three extra lavatories. We have got in two French helpers for cleaning temporarily. I must not stay for more. Every moment is precious.[28]

Vera Collum elaborated further on the work in the wards and how orderlies throughout the hospital rose to the occasion:

The wards were an unforgettable sight. Light dressings and gallows splints were the order of the day. Morning dressings were no sooner over than evening dressings had to begin. Stretchers were constantly coming and going from the receiving rooms, the theatre, the operating rooms. It must have been heart-breaking to nurses accustomed to the clockwork round and the neat rows of counterpaned beds in civil hospitals at home. To the girls who were serving as ward orderlies – and during this period of stress had to play the part of staff nurses – it must have been a long drawn-out period of dreadful strain and physical fatigue. The day staffs would work on till nearly midnight to help the night staffs; and the night staffs, instead of going off duty at 9 a.m. would work on in the wards till dinnertime to help the day people. In the same way the kitchen staff, the laboratory orderly, the store-keepers and Vestiaire clerk, would wait up every night till long after midnight, working as a volunteer stretcher squad to carry the stretchers backwards and forwards between the wards and the operating theatre. When they went to bed the cases were carried by the theatre Sister and her assistants; and if they were too busy swabbing up a too slippery floor, the surgeons would carry them themselves. Several of the poor fellows died, the only wonder was that they had lasted so long, wounded as they had been, after an exhausting struggle, and then sent on that long journey by ambulance and train from the Somme railheads to our clearing station.[29]

Cicely Hamilton records that 121 cases were admitted in the first 24 hours (2–3 July). During the first week over 200 were admitted, 231 bacteriological and 406 x-ray examinations were made, and 160 operations performed. 'The greater number of the cases have been exceedingly grave – some of the men have arrived actually dying. We are serving the Army of the Somme District where fighting is incessant and shows no sign of abatement. Every struggle and advance on the Somme means added work for the hospitals in the rear of the Somme line – of which Royaumont is among the largest.'[30]

It must have been with enormous relief that the unit welcomed the arrival of two more doctors in July. Dr Eleanor Hodson, who qualified in Edinburgh in 1900, had been in charge of some of the French Red Cross hospitals in France and was therefore able to transfer rapidly to Royaumont in the emergency. Dr Edith Martland was a young but brilliant graduate from the London School of Medicine for Women, and had been working in a children's hospital.

A third new arrival – but not until September – was Dr Helen MacDougall, a gold medallist from Edinburgh, who had been in Serbia with the Scottish Women's Hospital with Dr Elsie Inglis. She had been taken prisoner by the Germans, and after many adventures and much hardship she had eventually been repatriated via Zürich in February. She had had a grim time, but she seemed to be ready for more when she volunteered to come to Royaumont.

In addition to strenghening the medical staff, on 9 August a much-needed reinforcement of four nurses and three orderlies arrived from the Scottish Women's Hospital in Ajaccio in Corsica.[31]

Although the hospital remained very busy for the next three months, the most acute period was when they increased their occupied beds from five (for they had evacuated almost completely in preparation for the expected rush) to nearly 400 in less than three weeks. This was the period of greatest strain for the staff.

One more sharp peak of activity occurred on 30 August, when they were warned to evacuate as many as possible and to receive 80 seriously wounded men in one day. Miss Ivens was desperate for more pairs of hands and telegraphed the committee: 'WOUNDED ARRIVING ORDERLIES URGENTLY REQUIRED'.[32]

Miss Ivens herself was probably the most resilient of all the staff. On 13 August she was writing: 'I am quite fit, and ready for another rush.'[33] And to her stepsister, on a postcard: 'We have had a great time with 350 *grands blessés* from the Somme. Day and night for a bit. Everyone was splendid.'[34] Nevertheless she was aware that not everybody shared her phenomenal stamina:

> There was a good deal of illness in the staff ... with all those to nurse we are very short of orderlies, and while we can just get on with only 200 beds occupied another rush would be somehow disconcerting.

There was a tendency among some of the orderlies to express themselves in verse. Here is an example, from Geraldine Mackenzie:

IF –

(With apologies to Rudyard Kipling).

Dedicated to the night orderlies at Royaumont and particularly in memory of June, July, August and September, 1916.

> If you can make your walls of dusty sacking,
> And in an unswept barn by daylight sleep;
> If you can laugh when furniture is lacking,
> And keep your things in one ungainly heap;
> If you can smile when gramophones are braying,
> And Etienne shouts at Cardew till he's blue;
> If you can listen to the black boys laughing,
> And make allowance for their laughing too.
>
> If you can hear the staff who stamp and clatter
> When Buckley calls her fire-brigade to arms;
> If you can bear it when the sisters chatter
> To fetch the tea they find so full of charms;

If you can hear the victims in the theatre,
And only pity when they groan and scream;
If you can know the cars have just been sent for,
And weave it all into a blissful dream;

If you can rise though no one comes to call you,
And share one candle with five gloomy friends;
If you can eat cold porridge in the cloisters,
When in the darkness salt with sugar blends;
If you can feed your sister to her liking
On eggs or coffee, jam, or something roast;
If you can answer wisely when our Binkie
Offers a sausage on a piece of toast;

If, when the marmite fire sinks lower,
And, spite of all your efforts, goes quite dead,
You then can face St John in gusty moonlight
And calmly meet the ghost without a head;
If, when the men are restless, and the kitchen
Echoes with laughter and resounding fun,
You still can keep your temper mid the turmoil,
And whisper gently – 'Think of Blanche – or Jeanne?'

If you can carry stretchers by the dozen,
Polish the brasses, count three hundred sheets;
If you can work with all your heart, though knowing
The day staff always disbelieves your feats;
If you can crowd the unforgiving minute
With three hours' work and never feel the strain –

Yours is the world and everything that's in it,
But – though I seek you – it is still in vain.[35]

(Etienne was a former patient who stayed on to help with
mechanical problems. Mr Cardew was employed as a chauffeur
and mechanic. Buckley was the radiographer who was also study-
ing medicine. 'Binkie' was Constance Birks, an orderly. The 'black

boys' were the Senegalese, renowned for their cheerfulness. St John was presumably one of the Royaumont ghosts. Blanche and Jeanne were wards full of seriously wounded soldiers).

The following poem is by 'Anon', but must surely speak for all who were at Royaumont during the Somme Push:

> I wish I were a little rock
> A-sittin' on a hill,
> And doin' nothin' all day long
> But just a-sittin' still.
>
> I wouldn't eat, I wouldn't drink,
> I wouldn't even wash;
> But sit and sit a thousand years
> An' rest myself, by Gosh![36]

Miss Ivens was particularly appreciative of the work of the orderlies, and urged the committee to consider rewarding them appropriately:

Some of them have had a considerable amount of experience, and could be trusted to act as seconds in the wards ... they should be promoted to Auxiliary Nurses, be given a salary of £20 and wear Army Sisters' caps with ordinary uniform which would make a distinction. I am sure that some feel that they do not get promotion here, and really they do more work, and with more intelligence, than an inferior type of fully-trained nurse. In this way we should gradually replace some of the sisters (viz those who are sisters in name only) by some of our own training, and I do not think the work would suffer in any way. Miss Duncan [the matron] quite agrees.[37]

And of the chauffeurs Dr Erskine from the committee reported: 'Their work appeared to me quite excellent, and during the rush it must have been very hard.'[38] Miss Ivens now wanted them to have an allowance for their uniforms, and, as they were very much 'in the public eye' she did not want uniforms sent out from home 'which were badly cut and of poor material' – instead, they should visit a good military tailor in Paris. They were all volunteers, and as Mr Cardew, who got a salary of £60 per annum, was leaving, the three chauffeurs should have a salary of £20. Cardew 'was not as good as the girls who got nothing'.[39] Later, in 1917, this led to quite a major confrontation with the committee.

The welfare of the hospital and the fair treatment of staff was high on Miss Ivens's list of priorities. She was aware of the major fundraising efforts that were being made at home, and that when the SWH scheme was initiated no one expected the war to go on so long. She herself had a secure position behind her with her consultant practice in Liverpool, but many of the volunteers, working without pay, were beginning to have financial difficulties. When the committee offered to increase her honorarium, again she refused it, but asked them to increase Cicely Hamilton's salary to £200 from her present £50.[40] Hamilton had two old aunts particularly dependent on her, and was having problems. At the same time she was an absolutely key person in the hospital, and was in practice taking on more and more of the administration from Miss Loudon who, delightful person though she was, was finding the administration difficult. Hamilton duly received a raise.

Miss Ivens was also worried about the quality of the food. On 19 August she was writing to the committee:

> We shall only be paving the way for more serious trouble if sufficient palatable food is not supplied ... Bread and tea is a very poor preparation for a morning's hard work, and I know myself that I have felt quite faint in the middle of a morning after such a repast.[41]

This was reinforced by Dr Erskine in September:

> The margarine was uneatable ... and the bread was unpalatable, dark and sour. ... The staff were very badly fed – after the rush so run down that it was found necessary to have wine at the mid-day meal [though she hastened to add that it was used very sparingly].[42]

Dr Erskine warned the committee that they must be prepared for increased expenditure on food. Her other concern was the lack of washing facilities: 'The staff feel the lack of a bath very much ... They do not mind carrying up the water to fill it if there could be some mechanical means of emptying it.'[43] This must have touched the hearts of the committee, as a consignment of tin baths was despatched almost immediately. (The records do not say how they were in fact emptied, but there is a story that two orderlies narrowly missed the matron when they tipped their bath water out of the window.)

One or two practical problems arose during, or resulting from, the rush, both of which were solved with the help of Monsieur Delacoste, always a good friend to the hospital. The incinerator was proving unable to cope with the enormous quantity of used – and dangerously infected – dressings, and the all too numerous amputated limbs that had to be disposed of. Delacoste sent along a number of his workmen to build a new, large and efficient *déstructeur*. That problem was solved.[44] The second difficulty arose from the transformation of the refectory (formerly used as the staff dining room) into the Canada Ward. In the first instance the staff were able to eat outside in a corner of the cloisters not occupied by patients, and this arrangement continued until winter had pretty well set in – by which time those who had them were donning their fur coats for their meals. They must have been very grateful when Delacoste built a wooden hut adjoining the main building and fitted it with a stove.[45]

Mrs Robertson, a member of the committee, described the experience later in the year:

We are still [3 November] having all our meals out in the cloisters except the doctors' breakfast and tea, and on these moonlit nights it is a striking sight to see the trembling lights round the long white tables, and the moonlight striking on the grey arches and plashing fountain. We all wear fur coats for supper. Of course the blessés are never exposed like that, they get all their meals indoors, but now the refectory is Canada Ward so there is nowhere else for the staff to feed.[46]

And as late as 14 November:

> The doctors are still having dinner and supper in the cloisters, and though beautiful it is still very cold in the evening and we usually all sit in furs. If you are not very punctual the food is ice-cold. Everything is put on the side table by the door to the kitchen and you help yourself on an enamelled plate. When you've finished your soup you put aside the spoon and take your next course on the same plate. No matter who comes, Prof. Weinberg, Lord Esher or the Embassy chaplain – or the Comtesse de la Rochefoucauld – they all do the same – No one has seemed surprised.[47]

The morale of patients and staff was boosted, as Miss Ivens well knew, by ceremonies and visits, and some of these were particularly valuable. She arranged a formal opening of the new Canada Ward, so called because the money for equipping it was raised in Canada. Madame D'Haussonville represented the French Red Cross, and Mademoiselle Montizambert came from the Canadian Red Cross to perform the opening ceremony on 18 July, bringing with her a large Canadian flag to decorate the ward. Weak and ill as they were, some of the men managed to raise a cheer.

On 25 August Monsieur Doumergues, the French minister for colonial affairs, arrived to visit the colonial troops being treated in the hospital, chiefly Senegalese and North African. What this visit meant to these troops, who had very little idea of what the war was all about, why they were involved in it and why they were paying such a heavy price, must remain obscure; but perhaps they did appreciate in some way that important people were regarding them as important people too. Of more practical significance was that M. Doumergues had some funds to distribute, and 10,000 francs were passed over to be spent on their welfare.

Of even greater significance for the prestige of the hospital was the visit of the president of France, Raymond Poincaré, with Madame Poincaré, on 22 September. There were 330 patients at the time and both the president and his wife spoke to every man. In addition Mme. Poincaré gave each man a little bag of presents (history does not relate what was inside), and a message '*Jusqu'au bout*'.[48] This phrase could be, and no doubt was, interpreted in different ways ('all the way to the end' being the most likely contender), but it was certainly intended to be encouraging! The occasion was heightened by a band playing throughout, and by the crowd of local villagers and local VIPs who lined up to see their president.[49]

What more could be done to amuse and occupy the minds of the patients? On 27 August Miss Ivens asked if the committee would send out Mrs Robertson 'to organize raffia and basket work for the *blessés* and little entertainments to keep their minds off themselves'. Another reason, which Mrs Robertson indicated later, was to help settle certain 'diplomatic questions and difficulties'.[50]

Mrs Robertson arrived on 25 October in the motor lorry, driven by Mr Cardew, along with Mrs Hacon, an orderly and 'piles of cabbages, eggs, skinned rabbits etc etc'. With the tyres fragmenting, and in constant expectation of a burst, they finally arrived safely:

> Splashed and bumped up to the front entrance of the Abbaye in great style ... They were all at lunch in the cloisters, but came very soon to the hall as soon as ever the news spread – at least Dr Ivens and Miss Loudon did and also Miss Hamilton just behind ... Dr Ivens seemed genuinely glad to see me, and Miss Hamilton too; both have given me a great welcome – it's nice to feel that people like that want you with them.[51]

One of her tasks was compiling 'histories' of beds named after donors, which were to be published in the *Common Cause* (weekly journal of the NUWSS) and relayed back to the donors – so encouraging a continuing flow of contributions. With the great rush of patients this public-relations work had fallen behind, and it was time to take it up again. She described a session with Miss Hamilton in Canada Ward distributing name-plates to the beds. It was a happy occasion for them all:

All the blessés wanted 'des dames ou des demoiselles' over their beds – but there were not enough to go round and some had to take Colonels, Sirs – Mr and Mrs or even Railway Coys [companies]. When I had hung all round the walls and on the pillars there were still many beds in the centre, but these were for the time being unoccupied. I found at the end I had still two cards with ladies' names – So I went up the ward calling 'J'ai encore deux dames à placer, qui désire des dames?' ['I still have two ladies to place, who wants a lady?'] All the men who had colonels or CPR shouted and we had great fun exchanging them in the end ... It interested the men greatly as they had always felt jealous of the other wards having named beds and they not. So now there is great letter writing going on to the American donors.[52]

Mrs Robertson's good knowledge of French proved very useful, for example in helping Dr MacDougall to get items of x-ray equipment, and in purchasing materials for the laboratory, not to mention the continuing search for a good French cook. Mrs Robertson also took her turn with the *dévouements*. This was the rather unpopular duty of accompanying the seemingly endless stream of visitors around the hospital. The doctors shared this duty between them, and if one did an extra turn to help out she would expect to be repaid. Mrs Robertson had

... helped Miss Wilson with some bores of hers the other day, so was very much injured because the hockey match prevented her repaying her dévouement debt. However Mrs Hacon nobly invited us to the hockey tea which was also the opening of the new mess-hut in the yard ... Scotland won the hockey match, so great was the rejoicing and we had a very merry tea.[53]

(Hockey was a serious matter in the unit: one orderly was a hockey international.)

On All Saints' Day there was a ceremony and service at Asnières cemetery to which the convalescents and as many of the staff as possible were to go in military procession. An attack of bronchitis prevented Mrs Robertson from attending herself; in any case Miss Ivens wanted her to stay to cope with any visitors who might turn up. On this occasion the visitors were what she described as 'three specimens of the ancienne noblesse'. Two of them had the whole direction and arrangement of the female stretcher-bearers and infirmarians for all the military hospitals in Paris, where women were rapidly replacing men. They wanted to see how Royaumont coped. One positive benefit for Royaumont was that they managed to turn up an under-cook.

> I went to Marguerite [the Marguerite d'Ecosse Ward] among the men, after seeing the procession start off, first of all the blessés who c[oul]d with crutches and sticks, then the sisters in their veils, and orderlies in uniform, and lastly the doctors, Miss H[amilton] and Miss L[oudon]. I believe the little ceremony in the cemetery was most impressive. The maire [mayor] and the curé going to each grave of those who had died of wounds here and pronouncing a little oration, and Sisters laying wreaths on the graves. There was special mention made of Sister Gray who died here last year.

And then:

> When the party returned from the cemetery General Sieur from Paris arrived to confer the Médaille Militaire and Croix de Guerre on two men in Canada [Ward], and we had a very pretty little ceremony there. Miss Ivens loves a ceremony in which she is at one with the French people.[54]

Mrs Robertson found that she had arrived in time for the 'Gay Season'. After the stresses of the Somme rushes this must have been not only welcome but therapeutic. The first party was on Halloween, a new experience for the men. It was held in the beautiful Blanche de Castille Ward:

> The sisters and orderlies take no end of trouble in decorating their wards and getting up a little programme of entertain-

ment to which the men themselves contribute a large number of items. On Friday night we had Halloween potatoes with all sorts of things stirred in them, rings, buttons, badges, and even British threepenny bits – One poor chap got both a button and a thimble in his little lot and great was the fun and teasing when he was told that he would certainly never get married! 'Tant pis [too bad],' he said sadly – but was not at all consoled when I suggested that it might be that he was to have two wives – 'Oh, no, one is enough.' Another man was the proud possessor of two threepenny bits. A few of course got nothing, but we made it up to them otherwise. We had games too, hunt the slipper and musical chairs without the chairs, when you flop on the ground when the music stops and the last left standing goes out. It was so funny to see the 'niggers' at the games. [This word jars on the modern ear, but in 1916 it did not carry the same racist implications.] They love the parties better than anything and enter into the games with the greatest enthusiasm. Poor boys, they are so young, and have been fighting for a land which is of course alien to them. Little Sali Fon is 16, and has lost his right arm from the shoulder. He is a fine-looking boy as black as ebony, with dancing eyes and a splendid upright carriage. Another black man has lost his left arm. These two and several others go round to all the parties, they are charming guests, enjoying everything with much gusto. It was a young French sergeant who was the victor at the musical chairs after a tough tustle with an orderly who is an international hockey player. Hunt the slipper gave an opportunity to those of us who are better with their arms than their legs. Then we had a great sing-song, all the men's favourite trench songs 'Le Petit Chapeau', 'Tipperary' etc – and ended with the 'Marseillaise' and 'God Save the King'.[55]

A few days later it was the turn of Canada Ward:

This was a most gorgeous halloween party. When we arrived they were ducking for apples. Imagine the scene – the

Canadian Ward is the old refectory. It was most beautiful with
its lights shaded with red, and Chinese lanterns hanging from
the grey stone arches. A space had been cleared in the centre
between the pillars, and all round were the rows of beds with
their red coverlets; each containing a smiling blessé. In the
cleared space there was a motley gathering of blessés, convalescents in red jackets, sisters in flowing veils, Senegalis [*sic*]
with coal-black faces and flashing teeth and eyes. Doctoresses
in uniform, Zouaves, Arabs and orderlies in their pretty pale
blue uniforms and frilled caps, and a sprinkling of civilian
guests including young M. Goüin in full evening dress of the
beau monde. Many of the men were ducking for apples with
the greatest gusto in a big round shallow bath pan and
catching them in their teeth most cleverly – amid shouts
of laughter. Cigarettes, chocolates and biscuits were passed
round the beds and among the blessés at intervals. Songs were
sung and games were played. About a dozen of the convalescents were dressed up in fancy costumes and some were
very clever. A witch with high black peaked cap and red gown
with cabalistic signs struck terror into the hearts of the
blackies [again, such terms did not then have the racist
connotations that they do today]. There was a stalwart High-
lander in a kilt made from a travelling plaid and housemaid's
brush for a sporran. Uncle Sam in a wheel chair, a sailor, a
Mees (the patient's word for an orderly) and a Sistaire etc etc.
What delights the men most is to dress up in the sisters' and
orderlies' uniforms and play at being nurses.

Sir Roger de Coverley was a great sight danced here in this
wonderful setting and by this motley gathering. Surely quite
unique in the world's history and typical of the contrasts in
this world war. There was Miss Loudon tripping down the
middle with a huge negro from Martinique, demure little
orderlies and one-armed French poilus, Mr Ed Goüin and fat
Mrs Hacon, the kitchen superintendent – Dr Wilson with a
Senegali, Miss Courtauld with her white hair and gold eyeglasses and Sali-Fon Kanara with a red fez stuck jauntily on
his black wool, and his pink-striped pyjamas tucked into his

socks while one sleeve was pinned up over the missing arm. I
went up in the little musicians' gallery and looked down on
the wonderful scene. We all joined hands round the immense
ward, including the bed people when it was possible and sang
'Auld Lang Syne' – and surely it never was sung under
stranger circumstances. Of course all our parties end with
the Marseillaise and God Save the King.[56]

And the next day (truly this was the 'Gay Season'):

When I got back [she had been in Paris trying to find a cook]
the preparations for the Sisters' party were in full swing, and
there was also a party going on in Mary [Queen Mary Ward]! I
had to go and give prizes to the men as usual and then one of
the sisters dressed me up as an Arab lady from the Arabian
Nights with sheets and a gorgeous turban and veil and I
joined the party in the sisters' room. ... The costumes were
wonderful, but the 'clou' [star turn] of the evening was Miss
Hamilton as a tank. She had got inside her zinc bath wh[ich] is
a long oval and about 18 inches deep. She had big boots on
both hands and feet, and a tremendous noise and rattling
going on inside. She came in lolloping and crawling under it.
Another successful do was Dr Nicholson as the wolf from
Red Riding Hood all in grey woollen and with a big grey
wolf's head made out of cardboard. Dr McDougall was Red
Riding Hood. Miss Loudon Rose Red all in crinkled paper.
There were the three bears, Haroun al Raschid, the Babes in
the Wood, a Red Indian Squaw etc etc. We ducked for apples,
danced, and I told fortunes in my lair for a franc a head for
the blessés prizes or rather I read hands wh[ich] I know
nothing about, but I made some lucky hits.[57]

The next evening Marguerite Ward held its own party, the highlight of
which was a charade in which two or three orderlies and some patients
'embodied all the little hospital jokes and "took off" the Sisters and the
ward discipline and the objection of the men to fresh air, and their
amusing ways of getting round the meeses to perfection'.[58]

On 14 November it was the turn of Salle Elsie on the top floor, which held the Senegalese and the North Africans:

... I made a point of going up ... nothing would have induced me to disappoint Sister W[illiams] and Miss Courtauld their 'first Mammy' who always pretends she is not fond of them, and makes fun of Sister Williams' enthusiasm, but who was fussing over them all evening like a beneficent hen lest they should hurt or over-exert themselves with the games. One of the Mohammuds [*sic*] was capering about with a tube in his lung – a man whom she had insisted with wee McDougall two days previously was too ill to be taken down to the x-ray room! And grandpère with his just-healed thigh rushing about and dancing! These Arabs are so very live and graceful and so quick on their feet even with their wounds – The Senegalis are heavier and more deliberate, except of course the two young Sali Fons who have each lost an arm! All the Senegalese and Arabs had dressed up as they love to do. My big Kuli Bali as a 'soldat écossaise' copied from the picture postcard I gave him. Sali Fon was a girl of the period with a feathered hat and pink-cheeked mask. His black neck and hands below the mask and fine feathers was very funny. Naephle was a bear, a dancing bear, led by Abdulla who beat a cymbal in time to the gramophone and led the bear on a long chain as it danced about in a big fur coat and a bear's head. They played games, twos and threes and hunt the slipper, and danced 'Sir Roger' which is always very funny here. The proceedings ended by a distribution of prizes as usual. I had got something for each man in the ward, games, cards, briquets [cigarette lighters], little mirrors etc etc. Then there was three cheers for 'Maman Anglaise' (me), 3 cheers for Maman Camerade [possibly Miss Courtauld] – for Mees, for Sistaire Nuit and Mees Nuit, and finally for the chef who had made the cakes for the party. How this is done is as follows (the cheers not the cakes) the victim is hauled into the middle of an excited gesticulating dusky group and almost torn to pieces in their enthusiasm. We have no piano up in Elsie but the men love the gramophone and keep it going from 6 in the morning. They play cards, draughts and dominoes and love the cinema when it goes to their ward.[59]

On another occasion, Mrs Roberston describes taking some of the African patients for a walk:

Imagine about a dozen coal-black convalescents in pyjamas and blue overcoats most of them minus an arm with scarlet caps on their black wool and a varied assortment of injured Arabs, little Sister Williams and myself, tramping through the woods and over ploughed fields – marched to the orders of Sallifon [*sic*], Moussa or Couli Bali [*sic*] who being only privates in the ranks love ordering us to 'form fours' or 'right about face.' The funniest thing was when in the middle of a ploughed field we got the order to 'kneel'! We made each of them 'command' in turn. We had the two dogs with us – Smith and Jack the puppy, and dozens of pheasants rose whirring quite close to us – at wh. the blessés threw their sticks. Smith had a swim when we got to the Oise and shook himself all over us, and we returned bearing sheaves and great branches of Autumn leaves and scarlet berries for my room, wh. the Arabs loved getting and carrying.

Later she looked out of her window as she heard great shouts of laughter:

I found Sister Williams and one or two orderlies surrounded by the blacks and Arabs playing a kind of cricket with a big india-rubber ball I brought them the other day from Creil. The runs and the batting were the funniest things I have seen for a long time, and Sister in her flowing veil like a beneficent little dove darting about seeing that everyone of her black charges get a fair chance and fair play. Each day I am more lost in admiration and astonishment at the work she has done.[60]

Back in June 1915 a patient had been admitted who was to play a very important part in the life of the hospital. His wounds were not serious, and before long, as his condition improved, he was found to be disappearing from his ward and drifting towards the kitchen – a place that seemed to have an irresistible attraction for him. He was soon lending a hand, and gradually took a greater and greater share in the preparation of the meals. This was Michelet – who, before being called up, had been a renowned and brilliant chef in the service of a Paris millionaire. Miss Swanston, who was in charge of the kitchen at the time, wrote:

> He is now convalescent and helping in the kitchen, and we are charmed ... I feel confident indeed that this man is first class, and unlike most chefs, he will prepare the vegetables or do anything and the cooks are delighted to have his help with the staff cooking.[61]

Unfortunately for Royaumont, Michelet was rapidly returning to health. According to Navarro there were attempts to deceive the authorities that his state of health did not warrant discharge, but they were not so easily fooled. The sad day came in August 1915 when Michelet had to return to his unit. Miss Loudon reported to the committee: 'Michelet the chef left us on Monday to the great sorrow of the whole hospital. He wept, and we very nearly did.'[62] Miss Ivens, however, recognizing the enormous benefit such culinary skills could bring to the morale of the hospital, exercised her charm and not inconsiderable powers of persuasion in getting Michelet seconded to the hospital for the duration. Of course at that time no one expected the war to last so long. He returned in November 1916, as reported by Mrs Robertson:

> He was most delighted to return here, and was received with open arms by all the kitchen people. He will undertake all the catering and marketing, and has the experience and knowledge of the markets and prices necessary for this work ... There is a very happy and hopeful spirit prevailing in the kitchen just now with Michelet at the helm. [63]

Royaumont soon became known as the best-fed hospital in France. Michelet had a way with potatoes – he had a way with meat – and he knew how to rise to any occasion. Dr Henry tells us in her reminiscences:

> Once we were warned that 250 walking cases were en route, they had been on the road three days without food, going from one field dressing station to another. They sat on the stone benches all round the cloisters, were given water and towels, then Michelet our chef lived up to his reputation and provided a good meal before they moved on.[64]

Just before Christmas 1916 Mrs Robertson wrote:

> There are about 250 men in and Michelet is surpassing himself to give them the best Christmas fare available in war-time. Michelet is really splendid – he showed me with great pride last night his rows of turkeys all stuffed and ready.

And he colluded with all the little private parties the orderlies and sisters organized for themselves from time to time.

Sister Adams, who admitted that she had no great personal affection for Michelet, relented somewhat when he presented her with a plate of apple fritters when she passed through the kitchen. As an old lady she remembered how 'Michelet was a great source of entertainment ... He continually told me how he loved the "doctoresses, the Meeses and the Sistaires".'[65]

'Little Simpson' (head cook in 1918), visiting the old kitchen in 1961, recalled how Michelet used to

> ... spin the cocottes like curling stones across the stone floor to the sinks. Woe betide feet and ankles in their path! There I pictured him in the dusk, when all was quiet, as we awaited the night staff, cross-legged on the window sill playing his flute with the crickets for chorus, or again, in the darkness slipping furtively in from the park, with several pheasants tucked inside his coat – pour les docteurs, pour les misses! What wonderful suppers we all enjoyed.[66]

Grace Summerhayes (an orderly who later qualified in medicine) remembered him dancing on the enormous kitchen stove.[67]

It would be pointless to deny that friction did not arise from time to time as the weary war years rolled on. The question as to who was in charge in the kitchen was never completely resolved. Mrs Russell had pointed out that 'unless Miss Ivens went herself to the kitchen there is no one of any authority to administer between Michelet and the other people working there'.

The situation came to a head in June 1918 when Cook Simpson had repeated quarrels with Michelet following the departure of Miss McLeod, who had preceded her in the kitchen and who had also had problems with Michelet. The matter was brought before the committee, who asked Miss Ivens to consider very carefully the question of his employment 'as it seems rather hopeless to send out women cooks to work in the same kitchen with him'.[68] Miss Ivens spoke up for him: 'Michelet has his faults but cooks meat splendidly, and is devoted to the patients.' She resolved the issue – so far as it was resolvable – by turning a hut into a second kitchen for preparing meals for the hospital staff, with British personnel in charge, while Michelet remained responsible for cooking for the patients – at that time, in 1918, a very large commitment, with up to 600 beds occupied.[69]

※

As Christmas came round again in 1916, Royaumont received a large Christmas tree from the army bakery in Boran. The tree was erected in the great refectory, and the more able patients brought in armloads of evergreens from the forests to decorate it. Michelet's turkeys were consumed, and families invited from the nearby villages. There was singing of carols, Père Noel arrived on a sledge bearing gifts for every patient, and the day ended with a concert given by a group from Paris.[70]

For the unit the year 1916 had been one in which periods of intense activity had alternated with quieter times – as is so often the case in war. The records indicate that after the frantically busy time the rate of admissions dropped (the hospital being full to capacity) and normal routines were reestablished. The merry round of parties and entertainments suggests that there was still plenty of energy around. And there was certainly a degree of pride as the women reflected how well they had met the challenge. They had gained valuable experience in the 'rushes' in 1915, and this served them well during the greater demands of 1916. The volume of work carried out in a comparatively small hospital was certainly impressive. Miss Ivens gave some of the figures in a paper she published at the end of 1916.[71]

From January 1915 to October 13 1916:

Soldiers admitted 2267

Of these, Wounded 1694

Sick 229

Surgical, unwounded 229

Of the 1694 wounded cases 464 were infected with tetanus and gas gangrene. At the peak, 2 July, 127 cases were admitted in 24 hours. Gas gangrene was present almost without exception.

676 patients were examined under x-rays in the month of July, and in the second half of 1916, almost 3000.

As the year drew to a close many must have wondered what was in store for them in the year to come. In the words of Vera Collum:

During the Battle of the Somme the strain on us was terrific – physically, psychologically. We were stretched taut, and not a strand of the rope was frayed. We held![72]

ꝏ

The Patients

So far we have followed the story of the hospital up to the end of 1916, seen how the women dealt with problems of organization and treatment, and also learnt of the personal experiences of individual members of staff. But perhaps this is the appropriate place to examine more closely the background of the ordinary *poilus*, the men who made up the vast majority of the patients.

The nickname *poilu* ('hairy one'), applied in the First World War to a private in the French army, was said to have arisen from the fact that many recruits at the beginning of the war looked more like poachers than soldiers. Even though the amount of hair on the face of the average *poilu* reduced through the war, the name stuck. Many of the *poilus* were simple uneducated peasants, for whom life in the army must have been an extraordinary and bewildering experience.

It has to be said that the *poilu* had a pretty raw deal. Conditions for the ordinary French soldier were considerably worse than they were for his British or German counterparts – though some improvements did occur when General Pétain began to introduce measures to look after the welfare of the ordinary soldier, something that had been seriously neglected in the first two years of the war.

One of the most notable hardships was the extremely low pay: 20 sous a day (equivalent to two old pence), which compared badly with the British Tommy's (far from generous) shilling per day. This meant that the *poilu* was totally dependent on the services that the army provided for him – he had no means to help himself if the supply of food failed; he had no means of finding a bed if transport arrangements broke down (as happened all too frequently); and there was a woeful deficiency of canteens and rest centres. One instance has already been given where a large group of men, on foot, almost collapsed into the abbey after they had been on the road for several days. This was not an isolated occurrence – it was repeated in 1917 when Michelet fed another large contingent of 180 soldiers marching on foot from one posting to another.

One French account[1] describes the supply of food to the trenches. The *homme de soupe* carried the food from portable kitchens behind the lines. It arrived cold, if it arrived at all. If a shell exploded nearby the whole meal could be lost, or it could be mixed with generous supplies of soil and mud. The meal normally consisted of rubbery macaroni, solid rice and what they called *singe* (monkey). This was a stringy tinned beef in coagulated fat, greatly inferior to the British 'bully'. In 1916 during Lent the *poilus* were served with salt cod, which resulted in torments of thirst. The man detailed for fatigue duty was slung around with water bottles containing *jus* (black coffee, weak, but well sweetened). He also carried the *pinard*, the rough red wine, of which the regulation allowance was *un quart* per day. The *pinard* was the 'source of comfort, of happiness and endless chat'. Water was always in short supply in the trenches, though plentiful enough behind the lines. Discarded food ended up in the *feuillées* (latrines), whose upkeep, and even existence, depended on the sector being quiet.

On the march the *poilu* was exceptionally heavily laden. Alistair Horne[2] lists the articles he was supposed to carry – amounting to some 85 lbs (39 kg). His kit would consist of two blankets rolled in a ground sheet, extra boots, a sheepskin or quilted coat, a shovel or a pair of heavy scissors for cutting barbed wire, a mess tin, a large water bottle containing his ration of *pinard* (probably one of his more acceptable burdens), 200 cartridges, six hand grenades, a gas mask, and his personal belongings.

It seems that relations between officers and men were often poor, though officers did visit their men in Royaumont and the men were apparently glad to see them[3]. Junior officers in the British army were expected to be responsible for their men's wellbeing – inspecting their feet daily, for example, and always being ready to lend a sympathetic ear to personal problems. A similar attitude prevailed in the German army, but no such tradition existed in France. When *poilus* were out of the line, whatever accommodation was available was occupied by officers and NCOs, and the men had to fend for themselves. By 1916, Horne suggests,

> The division between officers and men was probably wider than it had ever been. Allied observers were often shocked at the way in which French commanders, after a successful attack, left their troops lying out on the destroyed enemy position for days and nights after they should have been relieved.

Class distinctions were upheld, even as far as sanitary arrangements were concerned: '*W.C. pour Mm les officiers, Cabinets pour les sous-officiers, Latrines pour la troupe.*'[4] One French colonel apparently declared: 'At the Front the soldier may be a hero; in the rear he is merely tiresome.'[5]

Leave periods (*permissions*) were few and irregular. Transport arrangements were often so muddled and unreliable that the unfortunate *permissionaire* might barely reach his home before it was time to return. The lack of canteens, which were generously provided to the British armed forces by the YMCA and other voluntary bodies, was a source of great hardship. It was not until 1917 that the French authorities realized their obligations, and called upon the SWH and other British voluntary organizations to help.

It was the appalling experience of trench warfare that formed the horrendous core of the *poilu*'s life. He might live for days and weeks at a time in the trenches. It was only after Pétain's reforms of 1917 that the men received regular periods of respite behind the lines, though this had long been routine procedure in both the British and the German armies. Apart from the actual fighting, the *poilus* had to suffer extremes of heat, cold and wet. The soil was more often than not waterlogged, their feet could be constantly in the mud, their boots always wet, and often their clothing as well. Deep shell holes filled up with water and turned to liquid mud in which men could actually drown (as Orderly Starr's patient related in 1915, this was not at all an isolated incident). Lice, rats, the smell of decomposing bodies (on which rats waxed fat and bold), the lack of sanitation (hygiene in the French trenches was particularly poor), the irregular supply of unpalatable food, the shortage of water, and – often during battles – the agonies of extreme thirst: this was the physical background to their lives.

A first-hand account from a French soldier paints a grim picture of entering a new trench:

A poisonous smell seizes our throats ... In torrential rain we find the walls stuffed with canvas. Next day at dawn we discover our trenches are in the middle of a charnel house. The canvas had hidden the corpses. Several days of burning sun brought flies. Appetite disappears. When the rations of beans and greasy rice appear we balance them on the parapet. Only the *pinard* and *gnole* [spirits] are welcome. The men's faces are waxy, their eyes hollow [author's translation].

Another describes the rats and flies that abounded among the unshaven, unwashed men; piles of straw with the indescribable acrid smell of urine; rubbish everywhere; the never-ending search for *totos* (lice); the constant torment of the rats when a man tried to sleep.[6]

A third French soldier wrote:

I've spent ghastly nights wrapped in my groundsheet and greatcoat – I feel these filthy beasts all over me. Sometimes there are 15 or 20 on each of us. After they have eaten our bread, butter and chocolate, they start on our clothes. It's impossible to sleep in these terrible conditions.

Others described the rats as 'enormous, fat with human flesh'.[7]

If he were wounded and unable to make his way to the nearest dressing station, the *poilu* depended on the stretcher-bearers.

Collection of the wounded from the battlefield was appallingly difficult – it was generally done under cover of darkness. The stretcher-bearers were a group of men of often outstanding courage who, together with the men who carried food and water into the trenches, were said to have the highest casualty rates of all. Once collected by the stretcher-bearers and field dressings applied to his wounds, the *blessé* (wounded man) was bumped painfully along in a two-man hand cart to the nearest casualty station. Here there was little chance of any real treatment being carried out, and the *blessé* was sent – if he survived that far – in a primitive ambulance (solid wooden tyres and unyielding springs) on a long and painful journey to the rail station. He would then be piled into a coach, often a cattle truck fitted with shelves. Sanitation was almost non-existent, and even water – for which the wounded men were desperate – was in short supply.[8]

Miss Ivens, writing a medical account of the hospital's experience of dealing with gas gangrene,[9] reported that out of 107 cases only 36 were admitted within 24 hours of being wounded. The remainder experienced much longer delays, even up to 12 days (though some of these might have had limited emergency surgery in a field ambulance). Only a few of her cases were in a 'tolerable' condition; some were collapsed and desperately ill; a few were near death.

The majority of wounds in the First World War resulted from shellfire. The shells were larger than any that had been used in previous wars. On explosion they shattered into ragged fragments of metal that caused horrific, usually multiple, injuries. In earlier wars bullets had caused the greatest number of casualties (after disease); they resulted in relatively clean wounds, usually single, and far simpler to treat. Horne comments:

It was only astonishing how much mutilation flesh could suffer and survive! To cope with these mutilations on so massive a scale, medical services were singularly ill-equipped. In this respect France was notably, and notoriously, behind both Britain and Germany. She remained so throughout the war. Her medical services had been prepared in 1914 for a short, sharp war and were hopelessly caught out ... Of the three Western powers France led with easily the highest rate of deaths to wounded: on top of a total of 895,000 killed in action, 420,000 had died of wounds or sickness.[10] [There is considerable uncertainty about casualty figures in the French services. Those quoted here may well be underestimates.]

It was no wonder that the men who had the good fortune to be admitted to Royaumont called it 'the Palace', or, as Private Breuil wrote, 'This charming Scottish hospital, that the *poilus* call Paradise.'[11] (This and the following quotations from French soldiers are only given in translation.) Corporal Mathieu wrote: 'If by chance black gloom lies in wait for us, the kind Misses soon take it away because here everyone has a happy heart.'[12] In 1917 one of the staff overheard the following exchange: 'Who is she?' 'She's one of the Scottish ladies, the happiness of the *poilu*.'[13] The records are full of such affectionate tributes; one man declared that he 'wouldn't mind being wounded again if it meant going back to Royaumont'.[14]

There was an easy friendliness between many of the French patients and their 'Meeses'. To the delight of the men, on 1 April 1917 Marjorie Chapman and two other orderlies disguised themselves as *blessés*. With heavily bandaged faces and wearing French *horizon bleu* uniform, they got themselves admitted into a ward and put to bed – and all before the inevitable discovery. The patients loved it – 'Oh, naughty Miss!' was their delighted comment.

The patients had their own sense of fun, and Chapman relates one memorable instance. It was the custom to surround *le cabinet* (the ward commode) in a discreet covering of bright red material. When a French general came on a visit of inspection, clad in the gloriously colourful uniform of his rank, a patient was heard to cry out, '*Ah, le cabinet, le grand cabinet!*' It was unlikely that the general caught the allusion.[15]

Naturally a large proportion of the patients were French, but there were also significant numbers of French colonial troops. These were largely Senegalese, and Arabs or Berbers from North Africa. There were a few from the West Indies, and soldiers from the French Foreign Legion included a number of nationalities, particularly Spanish; there was also an occasional Russian or Swiss serving in the French army. Later in the war there were British, Canadian and American patients at Royaumont, and a few German and Austrian prisoners of war. The monument in the Asnières cemetery commemorating some of those who died at Royaumont includes one 'unknown soldier'.

Vera Collum wrote glowingly of the courage of the French soldiers. It was her job to make thorough radiographic examinations, and this often involved positioning the patients – painfully – on a hard x-ray table to take the necessary pictures. She described one such patient:

> To endure all that after hours of tense waiting for the attack, more strenuous hours of fighting, the noisy hell of a modern bombardment; then with those two shattering wounds and the long wait, under fire, for succour; and after that the painful journey to the dressing station, and then the long journey by ambulance train and motor! He has the Médaille Militaire now and is doing well.[16]

There was one young French officer, Lucien Campora from Algeria, who caught the eye of Mary Peter, one of the orderlies, and so provided a Royaumont romance. In later years former staff remembered seeing Peter pushing Campora in his wheelchair in the furthest corners of the abbey grounds.[17] They married in 1920, then settled in Algeria where Campora built up a successful milling business. The last news the unit had of them was that they were celebrating their golden wedding in 1970.[18]

There were naturally a wide variety of types among the French troops: officers and men, scholars and simple peasants; élite troops like the Zouaves and Chasseurs-Alpin, and men from the punitive battalions (civilian convicts and military prisoners who were given an opportunity in the army to redeem themselves). Vera Collum, whose spectacles were inclined to be rosy, seems to have admired them all; towards the end of the war she wrote: 'They behaved always like the gentlemen they were – and the kind of gentleman a

French poilu can be is a very fine gentleman indeed.'[19] At the age of 98, Dr Grace MacRae, formerly Orderly Summerhayes, remembered: 'The poilus we liked very much indeed – not really the officers much – but the poilus – yes, they were nice chaps.'[20]

Dr Courtauld told Mrs Robertson of an unfortunate youth from Martinique:

> He was so badly smashed up when he arrived and gas gangrene had made such awful inroads that it was impossible to do anything; he was surely doomed. Still the impossible almost was done to relieve him, and Miss Courtauld sat with him herself by the bed away beside the window in Elsie. He lived for an hour after coming up from the operating table where his awful wounds had been cleaned. The details Miss C. gave me were sickening. And shortly before he died he turned to her and said with an expression of unutterable longing in his eyes: '*Dans mon pays, la bonne Guadaloupe, il n'y a pas de guerre!* [In my country, the good Guadaloupe, there is no war!]' There was sunshine without and the Oise was stealing in a silver thread through the lush meadows but France for him was a land of bloody battlefields and unutterable woe, and his thoughts were with papa, Maman and Babette his little fiancée of whom he babbled unceasingly.

We have already seen in the previous chapter how the Senegalese entered wholeheartedly into all the entertainments in the hospital, and the extraordinarily good relations they had with Sister Williams. Mrs Robertson expands on this:

> Now I want to tell you something about the dusky patients of Salle Elsie, who are the spoilt children of the whole hospital. Dr Courtauld is in charge there and they call her First Mammy. Little Sister Williams simply adores them and they reciprocate it. If she is 'pas contente' with them they weep and howl. She is about the size of tuppence, but they obey her lightest word. She has found out somehow a great deal about their family history – how many wives they had etc, which is

very astonishing as they speak little French and no English, and she speaks less French still, but they certainly do understand each other, and the discipline and fine feeling in that ward is very wonderful. When they came here the first time months ago they were absolute savages and their manners and habits were deplorable, but now they behave like gentlemen, have learnt self-control and nice manners and their attachment to the hospital, and everyone who has to do with them is quite pathetic. Of course they are having the time of their lives, and dread leaving Royaumont. And no wonder for there will be a poor welcome in Senegal for limbless heroes.

Vera Collum – who, like Mrs Robertson, shares the then-prevalent European tendency to patronize colonial subjects – describes how during the Somme rush they had a large influx of colonial troops:

These poor black fellows from Senegal, and the Arabs from Tunis and Algeria were very severely wounded: men with less iron constitutions must have died where they fell of such wounds. Yet the agony of their wounds was as nothing to the terror of their minds when they realized that a visit to the operating theatre often meant the loss of a mangled or gangrenous limb. They spoke only a few words of pigeon French, and the horrible legend spread among them that the first visit to the theatre meant incisions – mere senseless slashings of the surgeon's knife, to their unsophisticated intelligences; the second, amputation; and the third the slitting of their throats. It was days before their terror subsided, and weeks before their suspicious fear of the white women with sharp knives and wicked-looking forceps gave place to the dog-like devotion and gratitude that characterized their attitude to surgeons, nurses and orderlies, eventually. One broad-nosed woolly-headed giant, black as ebony, awakened from the anaesthetic on the operating table; he looked round in abject fear, though the instruments were all in the tray and the orderly had almost finished bandaging him: then his eyes lighted on the Chief Surgeon (divested of her gloves and gauze mask) who, as it happened, had dressed him in the ward and evidently gained his confidence. A black arm shot out towards her as she made towards the door, and clutched her hand, which he grasped and laid against his cheek, closing his eyes contentedly once more as he murmured, 'Moi connais toi' [I know you].[21]

One little fellow of 21, with a face like a child's golliwog had enough shrapnel in him to kill three men. His arm – both bones shattered beyond repair, and so full of metal that it would have been impossible to put a six-penny bit on any clear part of the x-ray photograph and not have covered a piece of shell – was amputated; but his thigh, from knee to buttock, equally full of bits of metal was left, since the buttock itself had been equally torn away. Yet five months later this black boy was tearing round the hospital park like a young deer, full of the wildest spirits, and reconciled apparently to his one-armed condition and his uneven gait by the fact that his French comrades regarded him as quite a little hero and that he was to receive the Croix de Guerre.[22]

Navarro describes the problem the Senegalese caused to those looking after them by the casual attitude they took towards their dressings, splints, drainage tubes and so on:

Among the Senegalese, the most curious and alarming experiences are the moments of recovered consciousness when the patient, curious as a child, tears off bandages, tubes and splints to see the effect of a missing limb or the result of a minor operation – the combined strength of surgeons and nurses ridiculously inadequate against the savage determination of the patient. One giant black who had three times in succession torn off his splints (six bad wounds in his two legs), murmured each time with satisfaction, '*Bon! très bon!*'[23]

Navarro tells the story of one particular Senegalese, reported to be a king,

... who was discovered one day seated on his bed, head bowed, weeping copiously. Beside him lay the body of a young Senegalese who had just breathed his last. Later, the king appeared suddenly within the screened enclosure (still weeping), explained that the deceased was one of his subjects, and expressed a wish that a ring on the young man's finger should be given to him as a memento. The nurses suggested showing him the face of the deceased. 'Non!' he answered, with arresting dignity, '*Non, laissez-le! C'est un grand guerrier!* [No, leave him. He is a great warrior!]'[24]

Less has been written about the North Africans, but Vera Collum writes:

The Arabs were very different patients: highly strung, nervous, complaining of their sufferings, they nevertheless bore them bravely enough when they became almost more than human nature could support. Their mental pain must have been acute when the strange foreign women, rather than let them die in possession of their shattered limbs, took them off, and thereby closed for ever the gates of Paradise against them should they succumb after all. If they recovered, the loss of a limb troubled them little; but when they came face to face with death, it must have been bitter for the orthodox to face eternal banishment from Paradise as well.[25]

On a lighter note Dr Henry remembers:

One Arab, enamoured of an orderly, used to follow her around with adoring eyes, and proclaimed that after the war was over if she'd come to Africa, he'd make sure that she would have potatoes every day. [Potatoes were always very popular with the troops.][26]

One of the auxiliary nurses recalled how the North Africans used to sit up in their beds, clap their hands and sing just like the bagpipes being tuned in.[27] They were a little confused when they met European-style sanitary arrangements for the first time. Ella Figgis, a dispenser, describés one such incident:

> A newly arrived blessé (I think he was an Arab) was told to go and have a bath, the salle de bains being indicated by a wave of the hand from the 'Seester'. A few moments after, on entering the salle de bains to see how he was getting on, we found him inside the marmite [cauldron] pacing up and down with all his might, the temperature of the water gradually increasing every minute! We hauled and got him out – and he was none the worse for which we were truly thankful.[28]

There are few specific comments about British patients – they were few in number and they did not represent sufficiently different cultures and values to arouse much interest. But one British patient – astonished to find himself in a hospital with a totally female staff – thought there could be only one explanation. 'SWH', he decided, with a sudden enlightenment, must mean 'Still Wanting Husbands!'[29]

As far as the American patients were concerned, the orderlies seem to have had mixed feelings. Evelyn Proctor wrote:

> We have some Americans too, some are nice but on the whole they are not half as nice to deal with as the French tommies. They expect a great deal and are inclined to grouse if we are simply through lack of staff and time unable to give them what they want. They are not considerate patients like the French.[30]

Orderly Summerhayes shared Proctor's reservations about the Americans: 'they thought they'd won the war and were swanking about' (this of course was in 1918). But it was their size that she really held against them: compared to the often underweight *poilus* they were so very heavy to carry.[31]

There were also some Germans in 1918. Dr Courtauld had two very badly wounded in her ward – 'quite decent youths' – but also a 'terror of a German officer'.[32] Dr Henry found her young German soldiers were 'happy, full of courage and adjusted well', but she had little respect for the Prussian captain in an adjoining room. When she told him about his German companions, he 'asked about their rank and explained that as he was a high-ranking officer he felt pain more'.[33] Vera Collum considered the German private soldier 'plucky enough', but was highly critical of a German officer who complained of everything and addressed his nurse as *Schwein* (pig).[34] Summerhayes recalls that only sisters were permitted to nurse the German officers, 'because they spat at us' (i.e. the orderlies).[35]

Of the civilian patients treated at Royaumont, mention should be made of a French girl called Madeleine who was badly injured in an explosion while working in a munitions factory in Compiègne. Mrs Robertson had a very soft spot for her, and enormously admired her courage. To quote Mrs Robertson:

> The poor girl was brought in in a dreadful condition, her limbs absolutely mangled. Miss Ivens had to amputate her left arm at once as it was only hanging on a thread, and her right leg seemed hopeless too. She is the bravest thing that ever lived, is Madeleine. As she was alone in this hut where it happened (at this work of hers each is alone), when she came to herself she dragged herself out along the ground until she was found! During the journey here and the painful dressings before and after amputation, never a murmur. She has a beautiful mind and keen intelligence, is full of appreciation and gratitude, in fact she personifies to my mind all that is best in the French woman's character. She is improving most marvellously, her legs are left to her and her right arm minus a finger and she is most grateful and says that she knows that there is work for her to do in the world yet. Her French is so beautiful and the way she expresses herself, and she is full of natural refinement.[36]

For all the patients at Royaumont – whether ally, civilian or foe – their stay there had been a significant experience in their lives. As Marjorie Miller wrote long afterwards:

We all remember with affection the souvenirs of 'yesteryear' –
the hundreds of very touching verses from our kindly and
very grateful poilus, verses that always evoke a smile, sometimes a laugh, pen drawings, water colour sketches, excellent
of their kind, sheets of paper on which dried lily-of-the-valley
(there was plenty of it at Royaumont) and other local wild
flowers, were gummed down in artistic form – all very
touching, but, alas, fleeting memories.[37]

❧

Among all the women at Royaumont who earned the affection and
respect of the *blessés*, there was also one man who was loved and
valued in equal measure by both patients and staff. This was
Monsieur l'Abbé Rousselle, curé of the nearby village of Asnières-
sur-Oise, and *aumônier* (chaplain) to the hospital. It is fitting to
conclude this chapter on the patients with a brief sketch of this
kind and brave man.

Perhaps his finest hour had come before the arrival of the
hospital, during the Battle of the Marne. In relating the story, Vera
Collum reminded her readers of the terrible fate that had befallen
the town of Senlis in the autumn of 1914. When the Germans
entered the town, the mayor counselled submission and, in good
faith, assured the Germans that the French troops had left. When
concealed French forces fired on them, the Germans believed the
civilians had deceived them. They took a terrible revenge. Using
civilians as a screen, they advanced to clear out the French troops.
Two of the civilians were killed. They then took the mayor and six
other civilians, chosen at random, marched them outside the town,
and shot them.[38]

All the neighbouring communes were in panic. At Asnières the
mayor and most of the male inhabitants fled the village. The curé
quietly assumed the office of mayor and each day, as the Germans
advanced and the sound of gunfire came nearer, he stood at the
crossroads on the boundary of his village, intending to plead with
the Germans if the need arose.

Collum told the story as she heard it from the old postmistress:

Dawn came, and M. le Curé and Mlle Baignières walked out to the crossroads, as all thought, for the last time. Would they save the village, or would the Germans treat them as M. Odent, the Mayor of Senlis was treated? It was dreadful to see them go, an old white-haired man, and a tall white-haired lady, walking with a cane – and yet – Oh it was fine! What a day that was – what suspense! No more refugees came through, no more troops, – only a straggler now and then. And in the evening the Mayor of Viarmes, M. Denain, came to tell M. le Curé that the Commandant had had marching orders which neither of them comprehended – for the troops were not to retire to Paris after all, but to swing across to Meaux. So the troops went, and we were left alone, and the sound of the guns crept further and further away. Gradually it dawned on us that a miracle had happened. For the Germans, after a week's occupation and a week's burning and pillaging, had evacuated Senlis, evacuated Creil, and their patrols had been withdrawn from the woods and from Chantilly. The menace to our own little village was removed – and we all felt very tired.[39]

The Miracle of the Marne had saved Asnières and the abbey.

Monsieur le Curé was 66 years of age when the war began. Through the long years of the conflict he never spared himself, showing unceasing devotion to the wounded throughout, and earning the admiration of all who knew him – not only for his charity, but also for his broadmindedness, and for his courage. Vera Collum wrote:

This simple and unselfish old man at once established his influence over the blessés by his practical Christianity. He never considered himself, and he made no difference in his attitude to wounded men who were theoretically anti-clericals, with the results that he disarmed them completely and they soon came to love the kindly old compatriot whom they all respected from the first. His attitude towards ourselves was equally catholic. He never thought of us as outside the church to which he belonged. He loved us because we were doing our best to heal and comfort.[40]

Others remembered him in after years. Dr Henry spoke of 'that dear old man who walked miles every day to Royaumont with his pockets full of cigarettes and candy, and his heart full of love and sympathy'.[41] And Anna Louisa Merrilees, who had been an auxiliary nurse, remembered how he 'went without a fire for two winters in order to have money to buy cigars for thè blessés'.[42] In 1915, when blood transfusion was still virtually unknown, he wrote to Miss Ivens volunteering himself as a donor: 'I offer you all the blood that runs through my body. Use it, I entreat you, to its fullest limit. You will make me happy, supremely happy, by accepting my offer.'[43]

The women were always aware how much they owed to their *aumônier*. In August 1918, when the hospital had been under great stress, Madge Ramsay-Smith, the administrator, reminded the committee:

> M. le Curé is a splendid old man who is devoted to the hospital and never spares himself on our behalf. He comes over most days to see the patients and writes letters for them ... as well as doing anything else he can for them. He never asks for a penny for his Church or for himself – and he is always so nice about the funerals – very different from the Maire [mayor]. Instead of paying him any fixed sum we have to ask him to accept a donation every few months to defray any expenses he may have incurred for the funerals ... Did the Committee only know M. le Curé as we do they would realize how much they owe him and what a good friend he is to the hospital.[44]

He shared in the rejoicings over the Armistice, and the orderlies showed their affection by chairing him enthusiastically all round the hospital. After the war he was awarded the medal of the Scottish Women's Hospital, and Miss Ivens used to visit him during her holidays in France. But by now his health had begun to decline, and he died on 11 September 1928. Quite by chance Miss Ivens came to Asnières on the very day of his funeral. She wrote 'how he had spent himself to the uttermost in bringing peace and comfort to the wounded soldiers of France. I left feeling that I and all of us, had lost a most faithful and sympathetic friend.'[45]

CHAPTER SIX

ᕿᕽ

1917: Strange Interlude

The 'rushes' experienced by the hospital during the great battles of the Somme were a direct result of the German strategy to 'bleed the French Army white' in the grim war of attrition around Verdun. The Allied offensive on the Somme had been intended to relieve pressure on the French in the Verdun sector.

The terrible conditions experienced by the French around Verdun through week after bloody week, month after bloody month, from 21 February to 18 December 1916, resulted in a collapse of morale. The French troops had experienced not only intense bombardment, but also attacks by the deadly gas diphosgene and by another hideous new weapon, the flamethrower, which resulted in terrible burns. Exposure to these horrors was unremitting, with soldiers enjoying few, if any, periods of relief behind the lines. For all their efforts and for all their suffering they could see little effect – and indeed there was very little.

French official statistics, notoriously unreliable, suggested total casualties at Verdun of 377,231, of whom 163,208 were killed or missing. For those who were wounded their care was totally inadequate. Alistair Horne writes:

> There were never enough surgeons, never enough ambulances, and often no chloroform with which to perform the endless amputations of smashed limbs. The dressing stations overflowed with badly wounded who had already been waiting for treatment for several days. . . . All the equipment was hopelessly inadequate – exacerbated by the poisonous environment virulently contaminated by thousands of puttrefying corpses.[1]

By the end of 1916, when winter put a temporary end to all but sporadic fighting, the infantry were beginning to question their role. They were depressed; they had lost faith in their leaders; they even began to resent their own artillery who, they felt, were not called upon to suffer anything approaching what they had to endure. Horne sums up: 'The great battles of 1916 were the seeds of mutiny, revolution and despair.'[2] The military deadlock was unbroken.

1917 dawned with no realistic prospect of any change. Neither the Somme offensives nor the operations around Verdun had produced results in any way proportionate to their costs. The troops were weary of being continually called upon to throw themselves against barbed wire and machine-gun fire. They knew better than their commanders how useless it all was. Stalemate, exhaustion and depression signalled the opening of 1917.

On 16 March 1917 the Germans took the militarily sensible decision to eliminate a big forward bulge in their front line and retreat to a shortened, straightened, well-prepared line. They destroyed everything in the vacated area: houses, trees, roads. They contaminated the wells and laid booby traps by the hundred. The ground for which the Allied forces had been fighting so desperately was now yielded up, but the Germans were stronger and the Allies weaker as a result. The disputed ground was so destroyed that any subsequent fighting there became almost impossible. It seemed the last straw to the demoralized French troops, but more was to come with the failure of an attack round Reims on 16 April.

In May mutinies broke out in 16 corps of the French army, and desertions rose to over 21,000 men. The men were absolutely disgusted with their commanders. 'We will defend the trenches, but we will not attack,' was a typical comment. 'We are not so stupid as to march against undamaged machine-guns,' was another.

It was a lesson for the leaders that they were forced to heed. Pétain was the man to save the situation. This was probably his greatest achievement in the war, for which he deserves great credit. Appointed chief of general staff, he spent a month visiting every division, listening to officers and men, and taking note of their grievances. He introduced reforms that attended to the welfare of the men, something that hitherto had been so badly neglected. He formulated the important principle that firepower should never be used indiscriminately, but only with the express object of conserving manpower. Any tactic that required the wholesale slaughter of men could never achieve a military objective – resources of manpower were not limitless and they needed to be conserved.

Gradually the French army regained some degree of confidence, but for many months to come its delicate state of health dictated that the main burden of the fighting on the Western Front was to be borne by the British. By August the French were beginning to recover their morale, boosted by regaining some ground that had been lost round Verdun. The recovery in October of the Chemin des Dames (a ridge that had always been of great strategic importance) was another big step on the road to increased confidence.

From May 1917 onwards Russia was weakening, and it was becoming clear that it would not be long before it was out of the war, and Germany would be strengthened by the transfer of troops from the Eastern to the Western Front. After the October Revolution, Russia sought peace terms with Germany. To offset this America had entered the war on 6 April 1917, though it would not be before 1918 that its contribution would have any significant effect on the course of the war. Nevertheless it was a great morale booster, and morale in the French army was higher at the end of 1917 than at the end of 1916. This, of course, was not the case with the British army, which had borne the brunt of the fighting throughout the year, culminating in the horrors of Passchendaele.

※

These events affected Royaumont to a very appreciable extent. The mutinies in the French army were a closely guarded secret; certainly at Royaumont they knew nothing of them. They could not understand why their hospital was now so quiet – why were they not receiving casualties? After the high excitement of the Somme 'rushes', life was beginning to feel rather flat. They knew that further north the British were having a terrible time. The

Third Battle of Ypres opened on 7 June – at first successfully, but success was short-lived, and it ended miserably in the 'bath of blood and mud' that was Passchendaele. At Royaumont many of the staff felt that they had outlived their usefulness where they were – and that they should close the hospital and move north to succour their own countrymen. There is an undated and unsigned letter, probably sent to the committee, that spells out their concern and dissatisfaction (remember they had no knowledge of the mutinies). They were seeking an explanation for their lack of activity. To quote the letter:

> I don't know if it has become common property or not at home, but there are strong reasons for supposing that all this District is now definitely out of the track of the evacuations of the wounded French.

Hospital trains were no longer coming to Creil, and all they were getting was an occasional trainload of evacuated patients, either slightly wounded or 'reported sick'. 'There are, of course, wounded, hundreds and thousands of them, somewhere. They don't come our way.' The writer had studied the railway map and speculated that their rail route was possibly being kept free for the transport of supplies, which always take precedence over the wounded. Another factor that she (or they?) thought might be responsible for the scarcity of cases was the new method of dealing with battle casualties. In 1916 they got their patients from Creil, usually within 48 hours of being wounded (90 per cent already infected with gas gangrene), and were able to save many lives and limbs. If Royaumont had not been where it was, and if the Royaumont surgeons had not been able to keep up with the flow by operating by day and by night, the casualties would have been faced with still greater delays, and certainly with greater mortality as a result.

The importance of avoiding delay in the initial treatment of casualties was, as a result of their experience, now recognized by both the French and the British medical services, and in 1917 a new system was devised and put into action. This was to erect very large wooden, barrack-style hospitals as close as possible to the front, where cases could be dealt with rapidly, though not necessarily definitively. For instance, wounds could be cleaned up, dead tissue cut out, drainage of wounds initiated and foreign bodies removed, provided they could be easily located. This undoubtedly decreased the development of full-blown gas-gangrene infection, and saved many lives that would certainly have been lost by the delays endemic in the old system, where the emphasis had been on transport to base hospitals before any but the most rudimentary treatment was given – in many cases just a field dressing. The medical authorities had had an erroneous impression that a 'rest' would be beneficial to the patient before transfer to hospital.

The writer of the letter reports that in December 1916 Miss Ivens had asked the Service de Santé that, if the distributing centre were to move, the hospital might be permitted to move with it so that it could continue to be useful. There does not seem to have been any response to this approach. The writer continued: 'Well, here we are, killing time, sitting idle almost, while the biggest offensive of the war is on, while England is sending out appeal after appeal for nurses, doctors and VADs.' The writer claimed that it was the general feeling among the staff that they should switch to 'our own people who are crying out for help'. Yet, she says,

> Miss Ivens persists in sticking to the French. Sometimes she is hopeful that if the head man at Creil were 'energetic' he would insist on wounded being sent round by his town in order to fill our District. Sometimes she thinks it is bad organizing... at other times she thinks it would be a pity to close Royaumont and that the Committee would like it kept open as a sort of convalescent home.[3]

Miss Ivens herself had a hunch that fighting would return to the Aisne region. She was of course quite correct. However, there was clearly some dissatisfaction among the staff, who did not want things to be too easy for them, and the idea of a convalescent home had absolutely no appeal.

Royaumont entered 1917 with the merriment that had characterized the party season in the previous two months. They celebrated New Year with a fancy-dress dance, and Orderly Dorothy Carey-Morgan (later a successul artist) displayed all her talent in organizing a show-stopper.

> This *pièce de résistance* was a performance of Three Blind Mice. Fat and with a round face, [Orderly] Berry was the farmer's wife armed with a large wooden knife covered with silver paper. The mice were clad in grey knitted helmets, long gray operation stockings, grey sateen costumes, tails of dressing gown cords, pink sateen ears, and – a gift from Michelet in the kitchen – whiskers from the straw casing of a champagne bottle. Holding each other's tails, and with Berry flourishing the knife, gleaming in sinister fashion in the lamplight, they burst into Canada Ward, squeaking with fright, leaping on and off beds, dodging behind tables and chairs, with Berry hacking at their tails. A moment's surprised silence, and then a roar of applause from the delighted patients.[4]

January set in with very hard frosts, and it remained bitterly cold for the whole of that month. Life wasn't all fun and games, as the staff settled down to steady, more routine, work: 'Useful, but a little monotonous,' as Vera Collum described it. 'We had won a high name for surgery,' she said, but now 'we received large convoys of sick and unfit men whose condition required surgical intervention of a more conventional order.'[5] With their spare capacity they were now treating many civilian patients.

Cicely Hamilton became the administrator in place of Miss Loudon, and was soon demonstrating her efficiency. She was concerned to be absolutely sure of her powers and sought guidance from the committee. She had run into difficulties with the kitchen staff and the chauffeurs. Miss Winstanley (now the matron) controlled the supply of orderlies, and also discharged some of the duties of housekeeper. It was agreed that Cicely Hamilton should have financial control, otherwise Miss Winstanley

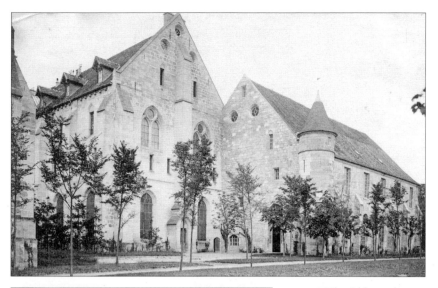

ABOVE. The Abbey of Royaumont, the location of a Scottish Women's Hospital throughout the First World War. Over 8000 wounded and sick soldiers were treated here. (Author's collection)

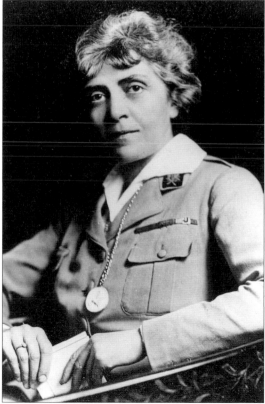

LEFT. Miss Francis Ivens, *médecin-chef* of Hôpital Auxiliaire 301 – as the Scottish Women's Hospital at Royaumont was known by the French military authorities. Round her neck hangs the Légion d'Honneur, one of the first ever to be awarded to a foreign woman. (By courtesy of the archivist of the Royal Free School of Medicine)

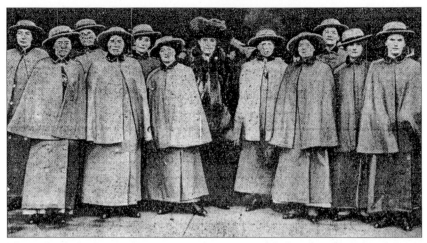

The Scottish contingent leaving Waverley Station, Edinburgh, on 2 December 1914. Miss Mair (centre, not in uniform), president of the Scottish Federation of the National Union of Women's Suffrage, sees them off. (Published in the *Edinburgh Evening News*, 12 December 1914. Author's collection.)

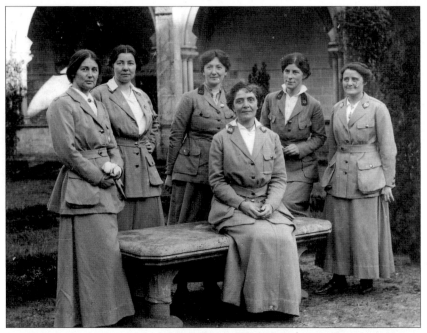

Les doctoresses in the abbey cloisters, 1915. Sitting, Miss Ivens. Standing, from left to right, Dr Savill, Dr Nicholson, Dr (Mrs) Berry, Dr Ross and Dr Hancock. (By permission of the Imperial War Museum)

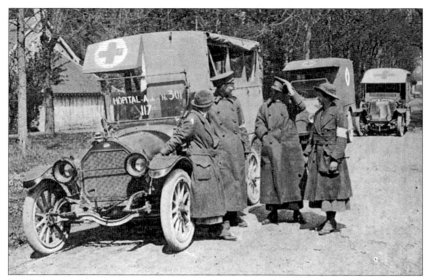

The hard-working ambulances were well cared for, but do not give the impression of great comfort. The one pictured here may have been converted from a private car. Later they were purpose-built. (Published in *The Sphere*, 12 June 1915. Author's collection.)

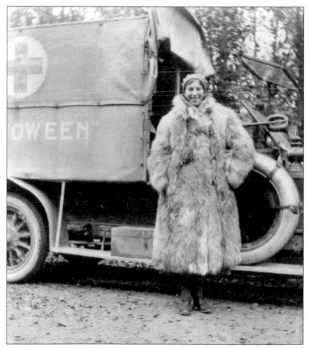

LEFT. Chauffeur Banks stands proudly in front of her ambulance. The drivers' khaki great-coats were replaced by goatskin coats in time for the terrible winter of 1917–18. (By courtesy of Dr I. Simmonds)

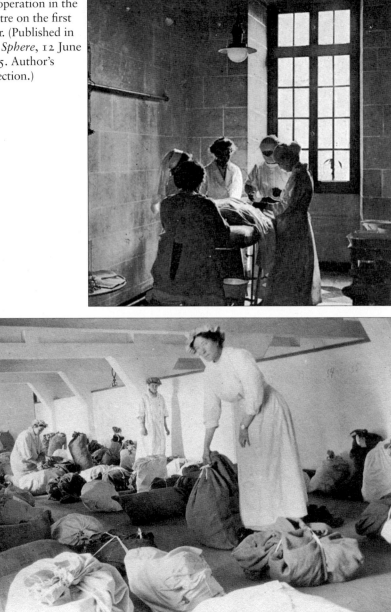

An operation in the theatre on the first floor. (Published in *The Sphere*, 12 June 1915. Author's collection.)

The job of the Vêtements Department at the top of the building was to sort through the filthy, tattered and bloodstained clothing of the injured. The work was made easier – if no less pleasant – after Orderly Gemmell devised a pulley to move the heavy sacks up and down the stairs. (By courtesy of Miss Helen Lowe)

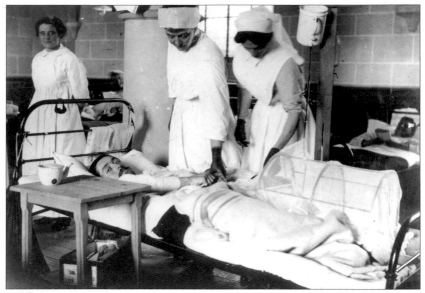

Miss Ivens on a ward round. Note the irrigation of the wound. (By permission of the Imperial War Museum)

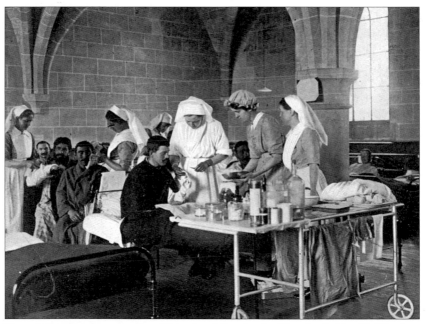

Nurses dressing the wounds of French soldiers in the Blanche de Castille Ward on the first floor. (Published in *The Sphere*, 12 June 1915. Author's collection.)

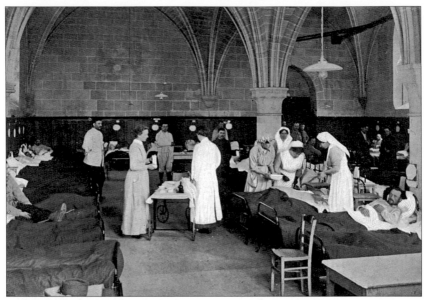

Another view of Blanche de Castille Ward. (Published in *The Sphere*, 12 June 1915. Author's collection.)

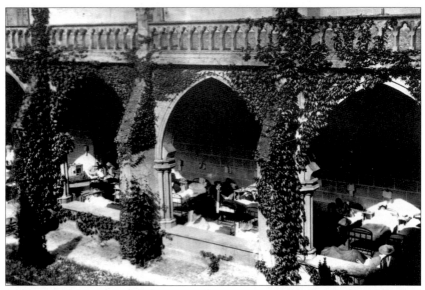

Patients were nursed in the cloisters in the summer months. Wounds were exposed to sunlight, protected by gauze soaked in saline solution. This treatment, combined with the peace and beauty of the cloisters, produced good results. (By courtesy of Mr David Proctor)

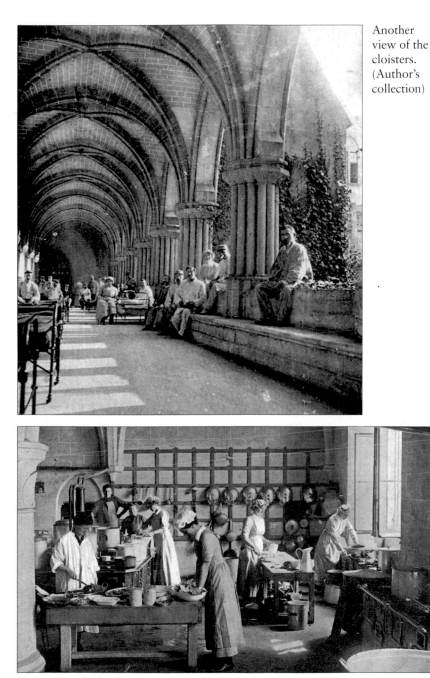

Another view of the cloisters. (Author's collection)

The kitchen. Note the heavy iron stoves that the cooks found so difficult to manage. (Published in *The Sphere*, 12 June 1915. Author's collection.)

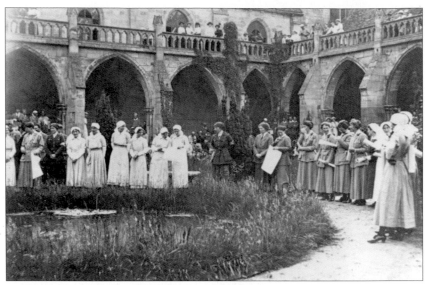

A decoration ceremony taking place in the cloisters. (By courtesy of Mrs Anne Murdoch)

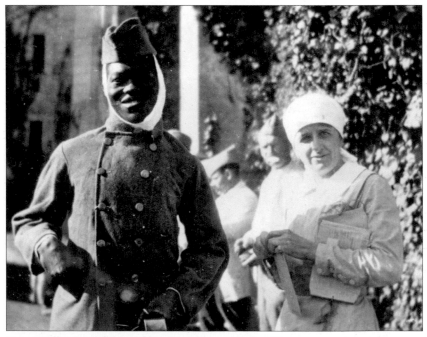

Sister Williams with one of her Senegalese patients. They were as devoted to her as she to them. (By courtesy of Mrs Crowther)

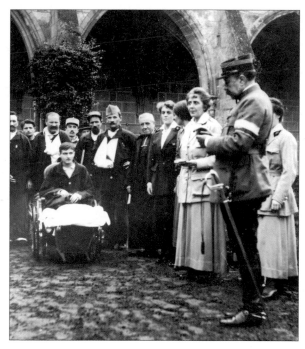

Miss Ivens looks on as a *poilu* receives a decoration. The Curé stands next to the soldier with his arm in a sling. (By permission of the Imperial War Museum)

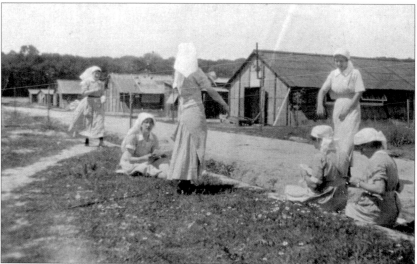

The arrival of the post at Villers-Cotterêts, the advance hospital set up in the summer of 1917, and dramatically evacuated during the German spring offensive of 1918. In this early photograph, the roofs are still under repair, and there is as yet no sign of either duckboards or rose bushes. (By courtesy of Mr David Proctor)

RIGHT. Orderly Proctor. Evelyn Proctor's letters home give a vivid picture of life both at Royaumont and at Villers-Cotterêts (pictured here). (By courtesy of Mr David Proctor)

BELOW LEFT. Miss Ivens, wearing her decorations, stands outside one of the wards at Villers-Cotterêts. (By courtesy of Miss Helen Lowe)

BELOW RIGHT. Miss Edith Stoney in her x-ray department in the Scottish Women's Hospital in Serbia, prior to her arrival at Royaumont. She is wearing a Serbian decoration. (By courtesy of the archivist of the Royal Free School of Medicine)

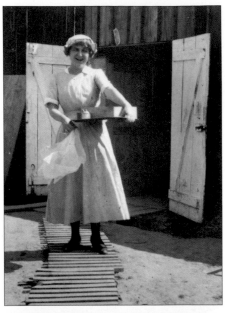

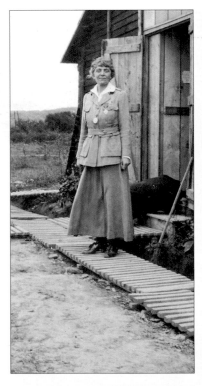

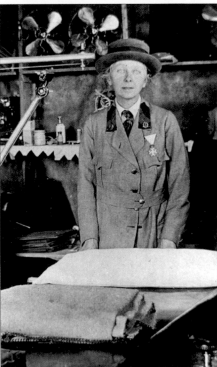

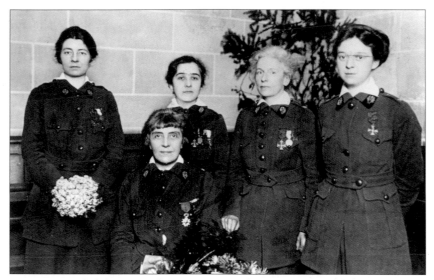

Doctors awarded the Croix de Guerre, December 1918. From left to right, standing: Miss Ruth Nicholson, surgeon, second-in-command; Dr Marie Manoel, Romanian bacteriologist; Dr Elizabeth Courtauld, physician and anaesthetist; Dr Leila Henry, assistant surgeon. Sitting: Miss Ivens, *médicin-chef*. Drs Berry and Martland were unable to be present at the ceremony. (By courtesy of Mrs Anne Murdoch)

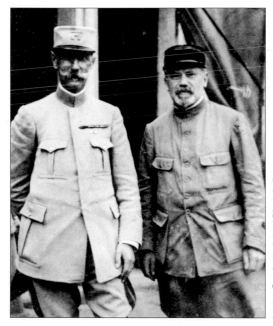

On the left, General Descoings – 'their own general' – and on the right, Professor Weinberg of the Pasteur Institute, whose research into gas gangrene was considerably aided by the clinical work carried out at Royaumont. (By courtesy of Mrs Crowther)

Dr Leila Henry, the youngest doctor, and Dr Elizabeth Courtauld, the oldest, on the terrace. (By courtesy of Mrs Anne Murdoch)

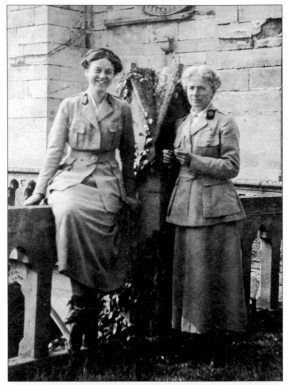

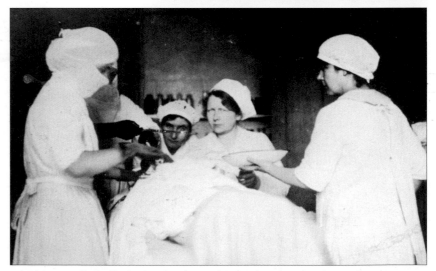

Dr Elsie Jean Dalyell, the bacteriologist, lends a hand in the theatre by giving an anaesthetic. (By courtesy of Mr William Dalyell)

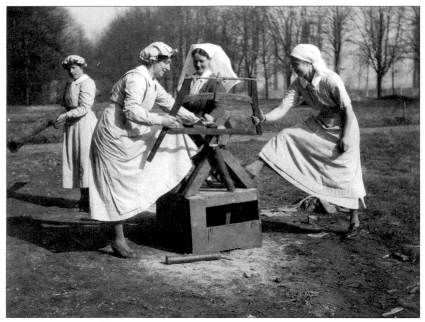

Sawing wood for fuel at Villers-Cotterêts, in the autumn of 1917 or the early spring of 1918. Orderly Violet Inglis is in action on the left, opposite a 'white-cap' auxiliary nurse. (By courtesy of Miss Helen Lowe)

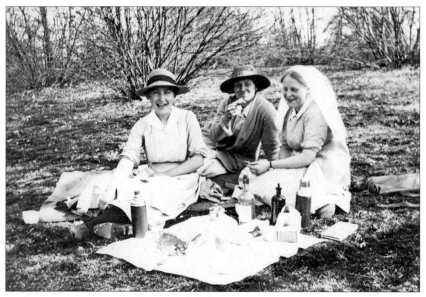

Staff enjoying a picnic in the grounds of Royaumont. (Author's collection)

Two *blessés* ('wounded') in drag, performing a skit. Entertainments put on by both patients and staff did much to maintain morale at Royaumont. (Author's collection)

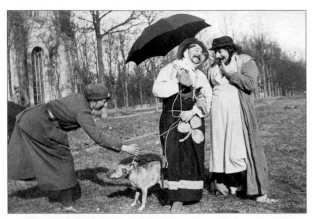

Staff with *blessés*. (Author's collection)

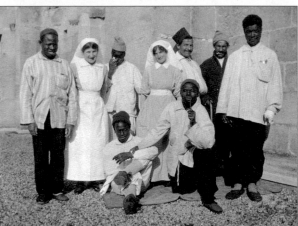

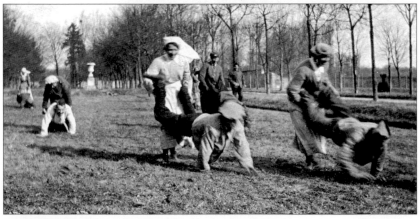

A wheelbarrow race at Royaumont. (Author's collection)

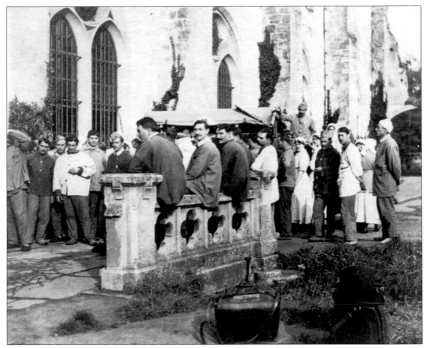

Soldiers about to leave Royaumont, 1917, having been judged fit enough to return to duty. For many, the hospital was 'paradise'. (Author's collection)

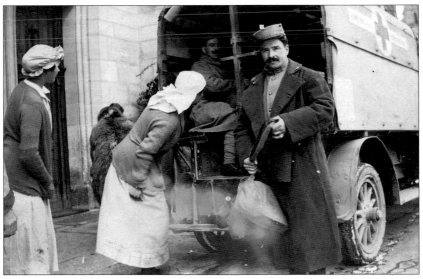

Departing from Royaumont. (Author's collection)

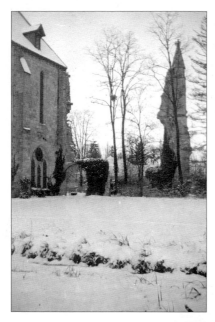

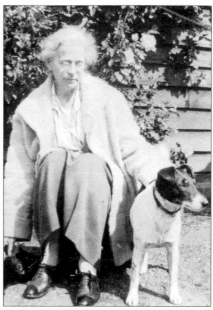

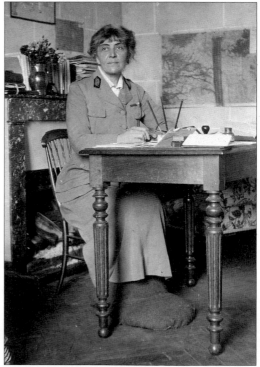

ABOVE LEFT. The abbey at Christmas 1917. (Author's collection)

ABOVE RIGHT.
Dr Courtauld as an old lady, with Spot, the mongrel fox terrier left at Villers-Côterets by British troops retreating before the German onslaught in the spring of 1918. (Author's collection)

RIGHT. Miss Ivens in her office. Note the economy – the fire is laid, but unlit, and her feet are in a muff. '*Quels yeux, quel esprit, quelle femme!*' as one of her French admirers put it – 'What eyes, what spirit, what a woman!' (By courtesy of Dr Christopher Silver) was to be in charge. All housekeeping departments were to report to the administrator on financial matters.

Cicely Hamilton had complained of the conduct of the chauffeurs. She spoke of their 'laziness and insolence' and told the committee that 'for the general comfort of the place it would be an advantage if the garage were a little more polite and obliging – good manners are not incompatible with good work and the ability to drive a car does not necessarily absolve its possessor from the ordinary rules of courtesy'.[6] There must have been a major row. Cicely Hamilton was known to have 'famous rages', but when the committee ordered that she should have authority over the chauffeurs on all matters affecting the administration of the hospital, she hoped for improved relations: 'The situation is difficult and the other day it seemed nearly hopeless, but I have been firm, and I believe tactful, obdurate but cheerful.'[7] We do not have the chauffeurs' version of these quarrels.

It was becoming difficult for some of the staff who had enrolled as volunteers to continue without any salary. They, like most of the population, had not expected the war to last so long. The chauffeurs in particular were now feeling the pinch. The nature of their work meant that they had many calls upon their purses that were unavoidable. They even had to supplement their uniforms. There was now plenty of paid work available for women chauffeurs, two of them at least (Young and McGregor) 'felt they simply could not continue to work voluntarily'.[8] Miss Ivens fought hard to retain them. In March she wrote to the committee requesting a salary: 'Their work here has made them expert and they are very important members of the Unit as they are very careful drivers and are known and trusted at Creil.'[9] In May she sent a telegram: 'PERSONALLY SUPPLEMENTING ALLOWANCE FOR YOUNG AND MCGREGOR CANNOT CARRY ON OTHERWISE'.[10] The committee were not moved. They would pay (at the rate of £12 per annum) for three months, but after that new volunteers must be sought. Miss Ivens was not pleased:

> I am extremely disappointed and worried by the refusal of the Committee to grant my personal request for the continued

services of our two reliable and skilful chauffeurs. New people are not the same as those who know everybody and who know every bump in the road. Miss H's personal dislike of the chauffeuses is very unfortunate but it is not likely that she can be very popular with them when they know she never speaks to them but in the most violent manner. It is an obsession. I believe they were inconsiderate but never swore, and their work is excellent. The manners of many members of the Unit leave something to be desired. But the important thing is that I do not want to be left stranded and should prefer the Committee to give me chauffeurs I know and trust rather than these helpless people who keep on coming out one after the other saying they can do things when they only spoil and ruin their cars and are a risk to the patients.

I have already stated the reasons which made me wish to have girls accustomed to the French rule of the road, Paris traffic and the transport of the wounded along bad roads. The length of our runs, and the fact that we have no mechanic also makes it essential that the chauffeuses should be capable of dealing with small adjustments that our old cars now require. I must reluctantly ask the Committee to be allowed to entirely disassociate myself from any censure from the French military authorities in the event of an accident, or responsibility should they in future decline to permit our chauffeuses to conduct the cars. It was with great difficulty that this permission was originally obtained in the Army Zone and I consider it most regrettable that the prestige of the hospital should be jeopardized for the sake of a few pounds a year, which I am quite willing to supply if there is such a shortage of funds. I am convinced the Committee does not realize the gravity of the situation![11]

She fought hard, but it was to no avail. Young and McGregor left in July to work with the Canadian army corps, though Young took the first opportunity open to her, in November 1918, to return to Royaumont, and saw the hospital through to its final closure.

Some odd jobs came their way. In early April they were requested to send a car to Amiens to help with refugees from the Somme fighting areas. Cicely Hamilton and McGregor took sacks of food and clothing and helped to distribute these in the town centre, where the Société de Secours aux Blessés was attempting to deal with over 2000 refugees who had lost their homes when the Germans shortened their front line and destroyed everything in the abandoned area. The sisters at Royaumont had organized a collection, and this money was spent on food for those refugees who had to face a further 24-hour train journey to unknown destinations.

The departure that spring of Cicely Hamilton, who had been with the unit from the beginning, must have been a blow to many. It is very likely that she was the author of the undated, unsigned memo already referred to, and she no doubt wrote it after discussion with other members of the unit. She now came to her personal decision. In April she was writing to the committee asking to be released. She 'was influenced in my decision by my doubts that Royaumont has outlived its usefulness'. 'The need is not pressing ... and it seems doubtful to me whether it will be pressing again.' She wanted more action and a change of work, but:

> I want you to believe that it is with a very full heart that I say my goodbyes to the Committee of the Scottish Women's Hospitals. I think that they have always understood that I was proud to be allowed to work with them; and I know that they will believe that I go from Royaumont only because it seemed to me to be right to go.[12]

She was to pass the remaining years of the war acting with the Lena Ashwell Players in northern France.

The departure of Cicely Hamilton prompted some fresh thinking about the post of administrator. Miss Ivens felt that the existence of such a post had only added to the difficulties of organization, and the idea had never been successful 'in spite of the personal qualities of the persons who had held that position'.

She felt a good secretary was all that was needed, and strongly recommended that:

> Miss Ramsay-Smith, who is 32, possessed of unusually good judgement, and who has been very well trained in the complicated office-work by Miss Hamilton should be given the post of Secretary at an increased salary (say £100). Her knowledge of French and book-keeping and her acquaintance with the intricate workings of the Croix Rouge Service de Santé and her knowledge of the authorities make her particularly useful here.[13]

Miss Ramsay-Smith was appointed, but the titles of secretary and administrator seemed to be used interchangeably in subsequent records. Whatever she was called, the appointment was highly successful.

As far as the rest of the staff were concerned, the departments were 'organized very completely under responsible heads who report to the Office'. The matron, Miss Winstanley, 'has the hospital staff in excellent working order and we have never been so comfortable as we are now from that point of view'.[14]

That May, during the lull, Royaumont received a visit from the poet Lawrence Binyon, best known for his poem 'For the Fallen', so frequently read at Armistice Day services ('They shall not grow old as we that are left grow old . . .'). Binyon was writing an account of the British voluntary hospitals for his book, *For Dauntless France*. He was struck by the beauty of the abbey and its grounds:

> There is a sense of old and large abundance in the surroundings, the heritage of peaceful centuries ... On this May morning, when the cherry was in clouds of white bloom, the impression was one of singular peace and beauty ... One receives an impression of airy cleanness and order.

The wounded were lying out in the cloisters, convalescents were strolling in the grounds, and a merry party was setting off in a boat on the lake. Others were fishing:

At Royaumont I was struck by the order and discipline that prevailed. The very fact that there are no men in authority over them appeals to the chivalry of the French nature ... One had a sense of happy cooperation between patients and staff.

He was impressed by their ingenuity, such as the pulley for the hauling up of the heavy sacks of clothing to the fifth-floor attics, and concluded:

The women of Scotland have cause to be proud of their representatives, who surely will leave a fragrant memory behind them in Royaumont ... If any male doubts the capacity of women to organize, administrate and create a cheerful order, let him go to Royaumont.[15]

Despite this tribute (and many others) to the efficient running of the place, there were nevertheless grumbles from some of the sisters – not about the hospital, but about the action of the committee at home. They strongly objected to the wording of an advertisement for nurses that the committee had published, which asked for 'some nursing experience'. To understand their concern one must realize that it was not until 1919 that there was any registration of nurses. Many of the sisters at Royaumont had been through a full three years' training at recognized schools of nursing, and were justifiably proud of their expertise. But nursing had not yet reached the status of a profession, and there was considerable disquiet that the hundreds of VADs who were nursing during the war would slip into civilian nursing after the war was over and dilute both standards and job opportunities for those who had come up the hard way. On 6 June the sisters wrote to the committee of their concerns:

We fully appreciate the difficulties the Committee may have in obtaining trained nurses for foreign service, and we have no wish to depreciate fever-trained nurses whom the Committee engage as such. We object to the 'not fully trained nurse with good general experience, and of robust health', who, very likely, has failed to get her three years' certificate, but who is apparently to be put into practice, and have the appointment of a sister. The point is we are anxious to raise and keep up a high standard in the nursing profession – and we hoped and expected the Women's Suffrage Movement to understand and help us to realize it. The advertisement in question is hardly likely to bring the best under the Suffrage banner – rather the contrary.[16]

On 31 July they wrote again:

The Trained Sisters at Royaumont have waited patiently for an answer to their last letter. As they have had no satisfactory answer to their protest anent the advertisement they now feel justified in sending the correspondence to the Suffrage and Nursing journals, drawing attention to their grievance.[17]

The committee evolved a scheme to settle ruffled feathers. Nurses, who had not had a full three years' training would be 'assistant sisters', and orderlies who were promoted to auxiliary nurse would be 'staff nurses'. New salary scales were introduced to take these distinctions into account:

Matron £120 Annual increment £10
Fully-trained nurses £75 Annual increment £5
Not fully-trained nurses £70 Annual increment £5

The fuss settled down. The sisters had made their point, and in 1918 they were so busy that there was never any time to return to the subject.

It seems strange that Miss Ivens, who was second to none in advocating the rights of women in the medical profession, was less than sympathetic to the anxieties of the nurses. She referred to this later as 'the agitation created by Sister McKnight', and she clearly found it rather tiresome.

Largely as a result of the mutinies, the French authorities were now becoming aware that something must be done to make life more tolerable for the *poilu*. This included the provision of canteens, until now seriously neglected. On returning from leave, the *poilu* was not entitled to any rations until he actually rejoined his regiment, and with badly coordinated troop movements this could mean considerable delay and long periods without food. Even if he had a bit of cash in his pocket (and we have seen how badly he was paid), the shops would often be shut and he would have to bed down where he could, tired and hungry. The lack of canteens was not only unjust, it was inefficient. General Pétain recognized this in the reforms that he was now introducing. The problem for the French was – who was to provide them? They turned to the London committee of the French Red Cross to ask the British to supply 40 new canteens. The SWH committee was approached, and they agreed to set up two canteens, one at Crépy and one at Creil. These did not involve Royaumont.

However, Miss Ivens was approached more directly. On a visit to Soissons she met the local commandant. He told her that in his opinion the most immediate and urgent need in Soissons was that of the *permissionaires* (soldiers on leave). He would take the opportunity there and then to beg the Scottish women to come to his aid. Vera Collum reported:

> Large numbers of soldiers returning to their sectors from leave passed through the town, and many of them had to spend a day and a night there. Being isolated from their regiments they were not entitled to draw rations. Soissons, he reminded them, was still within the range of the German heavy guns, and had only been completely restored to the French since April. There is not a house that has not been shelled; comparatively few civilians have gone back to their half-ruined homes since the German bombardment which followed the evacuation, hence there is absolutely no means of getting food. ... So, if the Scottish Women wished to help French soldiers here was the opportunity. Outside the Bureau at that very moment there were groups of men, haggard-

looking after a long journey and a sleepless night on an open railway station. Piled on the Commandant's papers were some loaves of bread which he himself kept handy for the more urgent cases, and more securely hidden there was a little heap of tinned sardines. He could do nothing as Commandant; as an individual he could, at least, distribute these to the more hungry. To make a long story short, Miss Ivens came back to Royaumont that night having committed herself and the hospital to come to the rescue, temporarily at least.[18]

She wired the committee to regularize her action: 'URGENT APPEAL FOR SMALL CANTEEN IN FRONT NECESSITY GRAVE WILL COMMITTEE UNDERTAKE STARTING PROVISIONALLY TOMORROW IS KITCHEN CAR AVAILABLE IMMEDIATELY WRITING'.[19] Her private comment was: 'Isn't it queer that the French women do nothing?'[20] The committee responded, authorized the canteen, and despatched the 'motor kitchen' as a back-up. This arrived in the first week of July.

It was good to feel, back at Royaumont, that there was an urgent task to be done, and the four women that Miss Ivens selected to go to Soissons were much envied. Florence Tollitt, the store-keeper, was to be in charge, assisted by three auxiliary nurses: Agnes Rolt, Marjorie Chapman and Etta Inglis (a niece of Dr Elsie). They loaded up the lorry with all the equipment they were likely to need and a small stock of provisions. This was just as well because, although they were authorized to order whatever they needed from military stores, the inevitable red tape meant a few days' delay before this could be put into effect.

They were given an abandoned schoolhouse, full of débris from the shelling, but – in contrast to the job of getting the abbey into order in December 1914 – a unit of soldiers was detailed to help them. Furniture was supplied by the mayor, and Tollitt was soon able to report back to Miss Ivens that they were getting 'comfortable'; they had planted salad stuffs in the garden, had been inspected, had served 797 meals (free of charge to the *poilus*) – and were greatly appreciated by the men. With so many shelled and empty houses they were able to raid the gardens for flowers and fruit. They did not confine themselves to the provision of food. A small bath and a piece of soap was placed in the yard by the pump, and newspapers, magazines and writing materials were also made available.

One visiting officer told the women they had no right to be there. The local commandant had exceeded his authority in inviting them to help in the emergency – only the Grand Quartier General* had that power! However, now they were there, he went on to point out that they equally had no right to leave Soissons.

Being close to where the action was, the four women experienced nightly air raids – they were never hit, but suffered several near misses, and had to sleep in the cellars. For them it was a new experience, and certainly exciting. After seven weeks of satisfying work, serving a total of 1681 meals, the women found the need for their services had largely passed: the military were now supplying lorries to take the men directly to their units after coming off the trains.[21]

୬୫

In June Dr Courtauld left Royaumont for Corsica, where she was temporarily to take over as chief medical officer of the Scottish Women's Hospital on the island, until a more permanent appointment could be made. The work at this hospital – for Serbian refugees – was very different from that to which she had become accustomed at Royaumont. It was mainly medical, with a large proportion of tuberculosis patients. Her experience was such that she was only too delighted to return to Royaumont, where she was reunited with her friends and the work that she loved so much.

Soon after Dr Courtauld's arrival in Corsica, Mrs Robertson (who was visiting the island on behalf of the committee) wrote enthusiastically:

The whole Unit is like a new world and Dr Courtauld's presence here alone for a few weeks, is just the last thing needed to complete the work. [The hospital had been through

* The GQG was the powerful body of military advisers who surrounded Joffre at the HQ in Chantilly. It came to be recognized that its influence on the war was not entirely beneficial.

a difficult period.] She is able to put into force the various internal improvements which no lay person can manage, and I think the Committee ought to write and thank her very gratefully for thus stepping into the breech and helping us.[22]

Later she wrote with a different view:

I had a long talk with her − about the possibility of her accepting the post of CMO here. She agrees with me about the inadvisability of it − i.e. she is not interested in this kind of work, does not recognize its value, has no sympathy with the Serbs, thinks Europe would be better if they were wiped out and is not a linguist. But quite apart from that she has no desire to leave Royaumont, or rather the Unit, and wishes to continue working there.[23]

Just before Dr Courtauld left Corsica in early August, Dr Erskine (also from the committee) wired back 'COURTAULD UNSUITABLE HERE'.[24] And so the interlude closed with satisfaction on both sides, and subsequent history vindicated the wisdom of this decision.

One newcomer at Royaumont, and a most welcome one, was Dr Leila Henry. She arrived on 27 July and remained to the end, a period which she later described as the happiest of her life. She had been the first woman to qualify in medicine in Sheffield in 1916, and had subsequently gained valuable experience in Sheffield Royal Infirmary dealing with accidents from the munitions factories − experience more appropriate to the work at Royaumont than could be offered by most women doctors at that time. Hers was a most successful appointment.

Throughout July and August the number of doctors fluctuated between seven and eight. Three more joined in the autumn: Dr Florence Inglis in September and Drs Walters and Manoel in October.

Dr Florence Inglis qualified in Edinburgh in 1914. She was a niece of Dr Elsie Inglis, the founder, and joined her two sisters, Etta and Violet, who were already working at Royaumont, respectively as auxiliary nurse and orderly.

Dr Enid Walters had qualified in London in 1908. Little is known about her early experience; possibly she had done some general practice work before serving with the RAMC in Malta in 1916. After a short period there she worked temporarily as an assistant medical officer in Hull.

Dr Manoel was a Romanian bacteriologist who had been working in the Pasteur Institute in Paris. Her specialized knowledge was of great value to the hospital, and she was subsequently awarded the Croix de Guerre. She seems to have fitted in remarkably well with the British staff.

With the temporary departure of Dr Savill in November, there were ten doctors working at the end of 1917, divided between Royaumont and its new outpost at Villers-Cotterêts.

❧

During the summer Miss Ivens was considering the unit's response to a request from the French medical authorities to organize and staff a new advance casualty-clearing station close to the front line. The purpose of such new-style hospitals was to provide early operative treatment and reduce the delays that so greatly increased the mortality from gas gangrene and other complications.

As early as April Miss Ivens was exploring possible sites. One of the chauffeurs – Marjorie Young – recorded how she drove Miss Ivens, Mrs Berry and Miss Nicholson to search for a suitable base.[25] On terrible roads they drove northward from Royaumont – first to a 16th-century chateau belonging to the family of a patient who had been in the hospital. Not surprisingly it turned out to be quite hopeless. Then they looked at a deserted hospital near Soissons, but it was too far from a railway. The *hôtel de ville* (town hall) in Soissons itself was in ruins after the recent shelling, as also was the Abbaye de Soissons. Another chateau and some 'indescribably filthy' old ironworks also proved impossible. Almost despairing, they came to the small town of Villers-Cotterêts, 50 miles northeast of Paris, and there they found a deserted woodenhutted evacuation centre right beside a railway station. This seemed to be the answer.

Vera Collum reported:

There our new hospital sprang up, mushroom-like. Nothing could have been more different than this ultra-modern baraque hospital from our own ancient Abbaye. Rows of wooden huts with oil-papered windows and composition roofs, on either side a new road sweeping through the camp to the railway line at the back, each with its smartly cut trench, its duck board and bridge. It made no mark to the eye at even a very little distance, the ploughland coming up to it in waves, the forest screening it.[26]

In July an advance party went up to Villers-Cotterêts, which was about 40 miles from Royaumont, to direct the necessary alterations and enlargements. They found two rows of huts, one behind the other. The wards in the front row were named after the Allies: Serbia, Belgium, Italy, Portugal, Romania and Britain. A covered way linked the wards to the railway station, so the wounded could be lifted directly into the hospital without exposure to the elements. In the second row of huts – also accessible by the covered way, there were three more wards – Russia, France and America – plus the operating theatre, x-ray installations, offices and staff accommodation.

On 2 July Miss Ivens was asking the committee for more staff. She wanted one doctor, three sisters, five orderlies and two more cooks. Later in the month she was able to report: 'They are working splendidly at Villers-Cotterêts, but of course it is hard rough work.'[27] She asked for another four-stretcher ambulance, as the authorities wanted them to be independent for transport.

On 8 August 211 beds were prepared, and there was still space for another 60. They had a staff of 33 and were expecting the first patients in the next few days. Another generator was needed urgently as the one they had was too small to cope with the x-rays. The hospital was now named 'Hôpital Bénévole 1 bis 6ième Région (SWH)'.

Madame Fox was proving 'a splendid quarter-master and tries to keep the German prisoners and infirmiers [French soldiers unfit for military duty] up to the mark. We are allowed 12 infirmiers and a caporal. They will do the rough work, but need a great deal of looking after.'[28]

Miss Winstanley was matron-in-charge, and on 12 August wrote proudly of the progress they had made:

> I have been four weeks getting the hospital ready and I do so wish the Committee could see it and hear a little of the praise we have received from several French generals concerning the transformation of the dirty barracks into a most beautiful hospital. The wards are really beautiful with their clean white-washed walls and red covers. We have had some difficulty with the sanitary arrangements but we are getting that well-attended to. The roofs have all been recovered and the theatre accommodation exceeds Royaumont by a great deal.[29]

Dr Savill had now returned and was supervising the preparation of the hospital as well as the x-ray equipment:

> Everything here promises well. Our great difficulty has been lack of men to do the work – General Descoings* came last week and commanded the various men here to leave all other work in the town in order to finish our hospital. The French authorities would have given us patients long ago had we been ready. That is the difficulty – to get ready when labour is so scarce. We have plenty of unskilled labour but so few skilled, so few who can do carpentering or plumbing. All the stoves and all the piping is being done by two men and all the working men are below par in health or would be in the Army. We have also ten German prisoners who work on the roofs. For the present most roofs are now – (at last) – water-tight with tarred paper covering but until all can be painted over with a layer of tar they cannot be guaranteed to stand much rain. General Descoings spoke most severely to the various men about, that it was a disgrace to the French that they had not finished the hospital long ago. He ordered an important

---

* General Descoings was their 'own' general – in charge of their area – and a great friend to the hospital.

Army man in the town to seek for us where we could have washing, milk, cheap meat and vegetables and every other necessity as rapidly as possible. We are to begin with water carried by the men daily in big tin reservoirs to each ward, and by Autumn a pipe *may* be laid from the big reservoir at end of camp to each ward – that is the only hope; but everyone is ready to work with the minimum of luxury. I have been a sort of Miss Ivens here. I go about all day between the huts and see how things are progressing, interview local authorities and military visitors – am referred to by plumbers, electricians, carpenters etc. Without Madame Fox, who knows every man's name, it would have been thirty times more difficult. She is a first rate aide. Dr Henry has now joined me to clear up the drainage system – most essential as we were eaten up by flies. The French have left some of the filthiest primitive cabinets we ever saw. No wonder we had flies. Our x-ray hut is huge, magnificent, all provided by the military genie. General Bon [responsible for distributing the *blessés* to the various hospitals] says we will be the show hospital of the neighbourhood. Though I have not had the rush of work I had expected I know I have been of some use in quite as important a way to Dr Ivens.[30]

In early September Dr Savill wrote privately to Mrs Russell of the committee:

I have installed a lovely x-ray room here and with the aid of a very smart mechanicien [*sic*] I have made such charming accessories at a few shillings cost. [Were these decorations to soften the clinical atmosphere, or technical improvements? Whatever they were, they do not seem to have impressed her successor in the x-ray department.] We shall get plenty of work here. It is going to be a very important centre. They mean to let us have grands blessés.[31]

Madge Ramsay-Smith, newly appointed as secretary, explains some of the feelings of the unit as they waited in October for action to commence:

At present there is a great lull – whether it is the quiet before the storm, or whether the French are not going to take the offensive after all [i.e. the expected attack on the Chemin des Dames] is a point none of us can quite make out. The only thing to do is to be ready for anything or nothing. If nothing comes our way it will be pretty sickening after all the preparations and the extra staff we have got out. On the other hand if there is a big attack I expect we shall need every ounce of personnel and material we can produce.[32]

She was right in this last respect – but their time of testing was not to come until March 1918.

Miss Ivens reported:

Hundreds! of inspectors have been and all seem to be pleased. We have a clearing station for patients arriving by car near the entrance to the hospital with a doctor (French, male) and 12 brancardiers [stretcher-bearers] to sort out the cases.[33]

The expected French attack on the Chemin des Dames did take place in October and was successful. Because of its success, casualties were rather fewer than had been feared, and Villers-Cotterêts, functioning as a reserve hospital, had only one busy week, when 100 *blessés* were received. Ramsay-Smith commented:

There have been a few cases sent to us since the attack but not the heavy work we expected, but then the French, fortunately for themselves, had very few killed or wounded altogether, and their preparation in the way of hospitals was on such a large scale that naturally each place only received a small number. Royaumont is really very much busier at the moment as we have quite a lot of malades [cases of illness] and also several very bad civilian cases which require a great deal of attention.[34]

One senses a little disappointment that they had not had a chance to show what their lovely new hospital could do.

Miss Ivens was balancing the needs of the two hospitals. For the time being Royaumont was short of actual beds as so many had had to be sent up to Villers-Cotterêts. 'There is no doubt,' she wrote, 'that the patients are extraordinarily happy and comfortable here' (i.e. at Royaumont). They had had a new *médecin-inspecteur* out from Paris who said it was 'a remarkable argument for feminism'. No wonder Miss Ivens declared him 'charming'.[35] He also said that he was considering asking her to move still further forward, which would mean that they would then be functioning as an 'ambulance of the front'. This, in the event, did not materialize, but indicated the confidence the authorities now had in the hospital and what women could do. An astonishing *volte-face* from their initial caution.

There were changes in the x-ray department. Dr Savill, who had seen to the installation at Villers-Cotterêts, had to return to her work in London. Vera Collum, who had worked so hard during the 1916 rushes, had returned home on the completion of her three-year contract. In November the x-ray department was joined by Miss Edith Stoney, who then served continuously until Royaumont closed in March 1919.

Edith Stoney was one of two remarkable sisters. They came from an enlightened family background. Their father and two brothers were all distinguished scientists and all three were fellows of the Royal Society. Their father had played a major role in giving women the opportunity to register to practise medicine by sitting for the licentiate of the King and Queen's College of Physicians of Ireland. This had opened the door to women, a door that had been firmly closed after Elizabeth Garrett Anderson had managed to obtain registration through the licentiate of the Society of Apothecaries. This was not to be tolerated by the opponents of women in medicine and for many years she and Elizabeth Blackwell were the only women on the Medical Register, and therefore legally entitled to practise. With such a father it was not surprising that Edith and her sister Florence received the best possible education (privately). Florence qualified in medicine and Edith went to Newnham College, Cambridge and graduated in physics. Both sisters were intensely interested in the recent discovery of x-rays and in their potential in medicine.

Edith Stoney had been a lecturer in physics at the London (RFH) School of Medicine for Women until 1915, when she joined the SWH unit going out to Guevgeli in Serbia, and later to Salonika, where she remained until the summer of 1917. Dr Isabel Hutton (née Emslie) knew her in Salonika. She described her as 'A learned scientist, no longer young, a mere wraith of a woman, but her physical endurance seemed to be infinite; she could carry heavy loads of equipment, repair electric wires sitting astride ridge tents in a howling gale, and work tirelessly on an almost starvation diet.'[36] Another commented: 'She gave the impression of a reed that might snap in two when the wind blew,' and 'She is a funny-looking frowsy old maid with untidy grey hair and large blue eyes – She is a most weird old person.'[37] Dr Henry left a little thumbnail sketch in a notebook:

> Grey uniform, grey hair, pale blue eyes, very slight, very intent on her job, – no special friend – no other interests, in and out of the x-ray rooms and developing room – like a moth.[38]

Edith Stoney arrived at Royaumont on 3 November and went up almost immediately to Villers-Cotterêts, where she was to be in charge of the x-ray department. She had come with a glowing testimonial from Dr Louise McIlroy, who was chief medical officer in Salonika: 'Her minute and thorough grasp of physics and electricity has made her infinitely more valuable than any graduate of medicine could have been.'[39] But she also came with a reputation of being a difficult person – although Dr Erskine (of the committee) met her soon after her arrival and reported: 'Miss Stoney is sweeter than honey. Long may it last!'[40]

When she arrived at Villers-Cotterêts, Miss Stoney was none too pleased:

> Very wet – drifting mist everywhere. I have not yet got the x-rays into working order – damp running down the walls and through the roof of the x-ray baraque – last night flooded the floor and put out the stove. I am very aghast at present at the makeshift way the apparatus has been put up. One is always frightened at a new job.[41]

Despite her initial misgivings, she was to work magnificently at Villers-Cotterêts and at Royaumont, as we shall see.

1917 had held its share of sorrow for the unit when they heard of the death on 1 August of Dr Wilson from acute appendicitis while she was on holiday in the Alpes Maritimes. She was only 36. It was, as Miss Ivens said, a great blow to them all:

> Her personal charm and extreme interest and solicitude for her patients gained her their affection in an unusual degree, and after their return to the front they not infrequently walked many miles and spent many hours of their short leave in paying her a visit. In spite of a frail physique, with an admirable spirit, Miss Wilson rose to the occasion during many periods of stress and fatigue – her loss has created an irreparable gap.[42]

After qualifying in Edinburgh in 1906 Dr Wilson had worked as a medical missionary in Jaffa and Hebron. She was a brilliant linguist, and was said to mop up languages as a sponge mops up water – French, German, Arabic, Latin and Greek. Had she lived she would have added Hebrew. She loved best physician's work, but her colleagues rated her surgical skills highly and these were much called into play during her time at Royaumont. She was said to be rather silent and reserved, with many friends but few intimates, but she had great personal charm. One friend wrote of her: 'She was so rare, she was so fine – and she had not the slightest idea of it.'[43] Another wrote that she had a special gift for 'helping men suffering from shock to regain their balance and control', and on hearing of her death, her patients subscribed 100 francs for a wreath. As for the man who presented it – 'Poor fellow, he could hardly speak.' Her name, together with that of Sister Grey, was later inscribed on the monument erected by the Royaumont Association after the war to commemorate those who had died in the hospital.

A happier event took place on 3 October when, with great excitement, the unit learned that their chief had been awarded the Légion d'Honneur – one of the very first to be awarded to a foreign woman. Miss Ivens maintained to her step-sister that 'she tried in vain to refuse it, but it was a great honour and earned by the whole staff'.[44] (Did she really protest? It seems a little implausible when it was such a mark of distinction for her beloved hospital!) She learned later that it was the *médecin-inspecteur général*, who was their chief in Paris during the Somme rush, who had proposed her for the award.

❧

In July a new orderly arrived at Royaumont. Evelyn Proctor was a prolific letter-writer, and her letters to her mother throughout her period of service (until March 1919) provide us with a fascinating view of Royaumont and Villers-Cotterêts from an orderly's point of view – although unfortunately (both for us and for her) a knee injury meant she had to be on sick leave during some of the most hectic times. Proctor was young and keen, and her enthusiasm spills over into her letters. Her change of attitude as she settled into the hard hospital life may well have been experienced by the many other young volunteers who had led a rather sheltered existence back at home.

Orderly Proctor's first comments to her mother after arrival at Royaumont bring us up to date with some of the domestic arrangements as they had evolved over the previous two and a half years:

I've completely lost track of days but I believe today is Friday, for which I am very glad as our washing comes back – By the way we have a clean sheet once a fortnight ditto towel, so we have to be careful! Did I tell you that the sole furniture consists of converted packing cases but we do get a bed and a mattress – I share a larger cubicle with a girl called Parkinson whom I met at the London office of the SWH before I left. She is quite nice – for which I am glad. I also have a window my side of the cubicle – my dressing table is quite smart as it consists of an old door that has been put on top of an old bagatelle table – and I have bought some stuff which I am going to hang round it. You will send me a bath as soon as possible, won't you? The country round here is perfectly lovely – I wish I had brought my bycycle [*sic*] with me, a lot of girls have them, it is the only method of propulsion to the nearest village, two miles, Viarmes – I wish we were not quite so cut off. I am in the ward called Blanche de Castille. It is a lovely ward with all latticed windows with creepers round and a vaulted roof. This is a *lovely* old place. Breakfast at 7.30 consists of bread and butter or jam and coffee. Then lunch [*sic*] at 10, the same, sometimes cheese instead. Lunch at 12.30, meat and generally fresh fruit or milk pudding. Tea – bread and jam – Dinner at 7.30, meat and fruit. It sounds more than it is and I am working as I have never worked in my life before and generally to be put to bed absolutely dead to the world – We never wear sleeves – which is nice in the summer only our arms and our hands are absolutely *disgraceful* to look at – We eat off enamel plates or the table (generally the table) and we drink out of enamel cups.

Everything is served on the side in the dishes they are cooked in and we grab what we can – food is served in a hut and we sit on forms – the sisters and doctors all feed together but the sisters have a separate table – we all smoke and it doesn't matter what one does – some of the people here have extraordinary manners, and are all between the ages of 24 and 30 ... The 'poilus' are the most charming people – so grateful and gentle – some of them have awful wounds – poor things – I am in the ward from 7.30 to 9 and get either from 2 to 5 off or from 5 onwards. The doctoresse of our ward [probably Dr Henry] is awfully nice, she is quite new – I do not care for some of them very much – there are ward orderlies (the same as VADs), kitchen orderlies and scullery orderlies – we are not always kept at the same work – Most of the orderlies are Scotch or Midland – some are quite nice, but the ones who have been here a long time are awful – But brothers and friends of people who are here – who come to visit – nearly all say, that we have to rough it here more than the officers in the trenches, specially in food and no tablecloths etc. [It

seems unlikely that these officers were in fact in the trenches
– more likely in comfortable quarters behind the line.] But it is
extraordinary what one will put up with when really hungry.
The Unit has started an advanced hospital at Villers-Cotterêts
near Soissons, and quite near the firing line, about 40 miles
from here – I believe we shall take our turn for a time up
there – it is near Crayonne, where the fighting is bad now – So
this hospital is only to have 250 beds instead of 600 as before
[it was actually 400 at that time] as there would not be enough
staff otherwise to go round. We hear the guns here and
especially at night and see the search-lights and yet *Paris* is only
40 miles away! Of course, I don't realize we are in the thick of
things at all, but I shall perhaps when I get home again.[45]

By early August she had had more time to look around her, and
on the 8th made these assessments of the medical staff:

Miss Ivens, the Chief, is a funny old bird … they say a marvellous surgeon, but rather an erratic temperament and she
changes her mind from one minute to another. Then there are
eight other doctoresses. Some are quite charming – and some
very odd appearances – typical suffragettes![46]

Proctor's letters also give us an orderly's-eye view of Villers-
Cotterêts in its early days. She was sent up on 9 August, only a
short time after her arrival:

It is considered by the French very near for women to go –
we are not far from Soissons, about 8 kms, which is under
fire. I am the most junior orderly here. There was an awful lot
to be done as the place was left in an awful mess and everyone
of us worked like the dickens with never a moment off to get
the place repaired. There is now a beautiful theatre and x-ray
department and the wards are awfully nice. Our first lot of
wounded came in three days ago – we opened three wards for
them – and I am the orderly for one of them. Each ward has
one sister and one orderly and one 'infirmiere' [*infirmier*, a

lightly wounded soldier who can do some work]. Really we are nurses and not orderlys [*sic*] and they call us nurse up here – So you see I am really doing the [same] work as people who have been out here for months as the other two orderlies on the ward are old hands – But I don't know how we are going to exist in Winter as we have to go out for everything as the huts do not communicate. I must have some warm clothes sent. I am hoping they will interchange us with people at Royaumont as camp life is much harder in lots of ways. This Hosp. is right on a little railway line and the wounded are brought straight from the clearing station here – Some of the wounds are awful, but they're wonderful patients. The British fought all over this country in 1914 – there are the most beautiful forests here that stretch for miles and miles.[47]

After a short spell in the wards she was moved temporarily to the scullery:

The girl at the head of affairs in the kitchen is an awfully nice girl called Jamieson [Anna Louise Jamieson] and we work together. But I shall be put back in the wards as soon as more orderlies from Royaumont come up, so Matron says. They are using us as a sort of clearance hospital as we are only allowed to keep the men for a month and get them straight. I don't like the present set of sisters up here very much but they soon change. The life is very hard but fascinating. The three Inglis sisters [Dr Florence, Etta and Violet, the latter being an orderly] are charming people, and all nice-looking and very well off.[48]

By 1 October the camp, she said, 'was beginning to look quite smart now as the gardens were growing up'. Mrs Berry (who was a farmer's wife when she was not being a doctor) had organized the planting of flowers and vegetables.[49]

The hard-pressed committee at home might have been surprised at the impression created on the young recruit that 'they were an enormously wealthy Society and they don't mind how much they spend'.[50] She could now compare life at the two hospitals:

The staff get really better done for up here as the life is supposed to be harder. I prefer it personally – as we did not get any comforts at Royaumont, but of course the place itself is so perfectly beautiful.[51]

By 11 October Proctor had clearly settled into the life at Villers-Cotterêts:

Am very happy here – play hockey when we can and dances and parties – wonderfully free – not a bit strict about uniform. Sisters keep more to themselves, but doctors and orderlies live together which is very nice as one realizes these women – extraordinarily brilliant women – are just the same as ourselves and are so simple and nice and kind – we call each other by our surnames – but we are otherwise entirely feminine! which might astonish some people who might imagine the Scottish women to be suffragettes of the most rabid type.[52]

(Compare this with the letter of 8 August.)

There seem to have been a few young men around – but the following is the only record of social life outside the hospital environment (apart from visits from brothers and other relatives) that has come to light:

There is a large Canadian camp near here [Villers-Cotterêts] and we often get the officers over, Canadian and Scottish, the Adjutant a Captain McNeill is an awfully nice man and sometimes takes us out in his car – a topping Sunbeam. There is also an American contingent at Longpont about 8 kms from here – they are a fine body of men but they are not too popular with the French, who seem to think they should have come into the war before and I am not sure that they are not right.[53]

Proctor wrote of the terrible noise of the big guns and the huts being shaken, and 'all day long yesterday drafts of wounded being brought in straight from the trenches, wounds not even dressed, half dead from fatigue alone'.[54] She found the cases nerve-racking, but she would soon get used to it: 'one does in an extraordinary way – specially when you get a ward full of bad first dressings and the men shrieking and groaning and taking about 6 people to do the dressing – and fearful blood and wounds and smells and rushing about with sterile instruments etc – that's when life ...' Here the letter becomes illegible, but she concludes: 'I quite see that they have to have young people for these jobs – one does not feel pain in the same way.'[55]

Later, in December, Proctor was working in a ward 'full of gassed men, 33 of them, all spitting and coughing themselves sick on the floor and running at the eyes all day – Some are pretty bad and are such an awful colour. There is very little to be done for them – and the worst part [for her, that is] is emptying their "crachoires" [spittoons]! poor things – such is life at the back of the front'.[56]

By now she was making plenty of friends: 'Inglis and I have been tobogganing up hill and down dale in the glorious woods with the deer all round and the sun shining furiously.'[57]

Dr MacRae, recalling her life at Villers-Cotterêts when she was Orderly Summerhayes, had vivid memories of the rats in the huts that provided their sleeping quarters:

> We slept on the floor as far as I can remember – I suppose we had a palliasse or something – something raised us a little bit from the rats. The things I remember about the huts were the rats. At night time the bombs used to drop [this was in 1918, but the rats were certainly in residence in 1917] – I didn't wake – awful noises they used to make – some not very far away – but if a rat came – just a scratch – I jumped up and threw my shoes all over the place trying to get these rats – I was much more afraid of the rats than the Germans.[58]

Some excitement was caused in December when a film crew appeared at Villers-Cotterêts. This had been 'ordered' by the British Ministry of Information as a propaganda exercise to show the French what the British people were doing for them. Times had changed since the War Office had done all it could to stop them going at all! Proctor told her mother:

> We had to fake all sorts of things, including an 'op' – it was too funny – I had to go out in the middle to produce a 'foreign body' which consisted of a piece of coal.[59]

(This film survives, but it is difficult to identify either Proctor or the piece of coal.) The unit's unanimous opinion when they saw the film after the war at one of their reunions was – 'atrocious'.[60] As for Miss Ivens, she said it 'made her blood run cold'.[61]

Proctor left a description of their 'top-hole' Christmas at Villers-Cotterêts:

> ... while we were having tea some beautiful carols were sung by 6 of the staff ... The lights were turned out suddenly and out of the darkness from double doors which lead from the refectory to the carpenter's shops lanterns came held by the carollers who were dressed in long military French blue waterproof capes with the hoods over their heads round which was [*sic*] put white cotton wool pieces so that it looked like snow and the storm lanterns were trimmed with holly and mistletoe of which there is an abundance here – They came singing and sang three carols and then walked out singing as they went through the hut with the snow and continued in each ward in turn. The men [Canadians] seemed quite touched. We forget they are so far from home and things like that must bring it very near to them.

This was followed by a concert with pierrots, Père Noel and presents for all. There was more next day:

> On Boxing Day there was a staff dinner party with a fancy dress dance afterwards – Mrs Berry ... was dressed as Cardinal Wolsey awfully good get up ... Everything of that kind involving any kind of entertainment is of a high standard out here and always original – there are so many really clever

people altogether – I don't say all but the standard of intelligence is so much higher than in an ordinary crowd of women anywhere ...[62]

Back at Royaumont Dr Henry recalled many memories of Canada Ward in the old Refectory:

But none more beautiful than in Christmas Eve 1917, as I stood in the music gallery at the North end ... All 100 beds were occupied, the only lights came from two flickering candles on an improvised altar at the base of the pulpit where the old Curé from Asnières-sur-Oise was celebrating Mass. The silence was broken by the choir of orderlies beside me.[63]

And so a relatively quiet year drew to a close. The war was far from over, however, and once again they must have wondered what the new year would have in store for them. But with their two hospitals in good working order they were set to meet the challenge.

※

CHAPTER SEVEN

1918: Their Finest Hour

As 1918 opened, the balance of power on the Western Front was changing.

The Germans were reaping the advantage of the ending of the war with Russia: peace talks had been started in December 1917, and the Treaty of Brest-Litovsk signed in March 1918. Between those two dates, large numbers of German troops were transferred from the Eastern to the Western Front, where it was estimated that the strength of the German army increased by 30 per cent. To set against that, the capacity of Germany's industrial base to maintain military supplies was deteriorating, and shortages of all kinds were becoming a serious problem. The entry of the United States into the war would, from now on, provide more troops and more resources of all kinds for the Allied forces, and in spite of all the tragedies of 1917, a year which had been a very grim one for the British in particular, there was a certain renewal of hope and a lifting of morale among the fighting troops. The US troops arriving in Europe, raw and untrained though they were, were getting ready for action, and more and more fresh troops were arriving every month.

It was clear to the Germans that if ever they were to make a decisive attack and bring the war to a victorious conclusion, they must launch a major offensive in 1918, and as soon as possible. Never again would they have as much manpower or military material. For them time was running out. It was now or never.

With his clear numerical superiority, General Ludendorff, the German commander-in-chief, planned an offensive in three different sectors: the attacks in the Lys and the Ypres areas would be primarily against the British; the third in the Champagne would be primarily against the French. It was this great 'spring offensive' that would result in dramatic events at both Villers-Cotterêts and Royaumont.

The first of the attacks was launched on 21 March, and by 27 March the Germans had reached Montdidier, where the railway line to Paris was cut. By 30 March they were on the outskirts of Amiens. The battle came to an end a few days later, a heavy defeat for the British. Further attacks followed on 9 April on the Lys Front, and continued until 29 April.

The big German breakthrough came at the end of May. Up till then, all seemed quiet on the Aisne between Reims and Soissons. US commanders had predicted an attack on the the strategic ridge of the Chemin des Dames, but the French did not believe it would come, stating as late as 25 May that 'In our opinion there are no indications that the enemy has made preparations which would enable him to attack tomorrow.' Even after a warning given by two prisoners on 26 May that the Germans were about to attack, it came as a complete surprise to the French when, at 1.30 a.m. on the morning of 27 May, a bombardment of unparalleled ferocity burst on the Franco-British front between Reims and Soissons along the Chemin des Dames – just as the US commanders had predicted. The bombardment lasted for three and a half hours, and by midday the Germans were pouring over the Aisne bridges, which the French had failed to blow up. In one day the Germans had advanced an astonishing 12 miles. Liddell Hart wrote of 'the helpless endurance of the Franco-British troops amid the ever-swelling litter of shattered dead and untended wounded made more trying by crouching semi-suffocated in gas-masks'.[1]

On 29 May the Germans made another big advance, captured Soissons, and on the 30th reached the Marne. On 31 May they turned westwards towards Paris, and penetrated right up to the Forest of Villers-Cotterêts. This proved to be the limit of their advance, and was the climax of this Second Battle of the Marne.

On 1 June Pétain ordered up reserves. The advance was checked, and the Americans, now operational, attacked fiercely and successfully at Château-Thierry – 'an indestructible moral tonic to the Allies'. By now the morale of the German troops was beginning to slip, as what had seemed to be an inexorable advance ground to a halt.

Villers-Cotterêts was destroyed, but Royaumont survived.

The French regrouped, and more than 20 divisions (mostly French, but including two American) were now hidden in the forests round Villers-Cotterêts, along with 350 tanks. On 15 June the French counterattacked at Noyon. The result was indecisive. On 15 July the Germans attacked again; the French counterattacked once more. All these attacks and counterattacks resulted in enormous numbers of killed and wounded – French, British, American, Canadian, Australian, German. The flow of wounded into Royaumont was continuous.

Ludendorff called 8 August the 'black day' for the German army, for it was then that it became clear that it had been decisively beaten. Although the battle went on until 21 August, Ludendorff told the Kaiser that the war must end. In September the alliance of the Central Powers began to crumble; the final assaults of the Allies at the end of that month broke through the defences of the Hindenburg Line; the Germans were in retreat. On 28 October a naval mutiny broke out at Kiel, and socialist governments were installed in Munich and Berlin. The people were sick of war. On 10 November the Kaiser retired to Holland, and on 11 November the Armistice was signed in the railway carriage at Compiègne.

❧

One may be sure that the new year did not come in unmarked by the staff at Royaumont or at Villers-Cotterêts, though no record of any celebration has come down to us. What did not go unrecorded was the terrible cold of that winter – said to be the coldest since 1870. On 1 January Orderly Proctor was writing home from Villers-Cotterêts:

We have had 22 degrees of frost in our cubicle [the cubicles were partitioned off within the wooden huts, and were just big enough to contain a bed and a shelf for a jug and basin].

Sponge, toothbrushes, soap, all frozen hard. Water absolutely hard, even hot water bottles – I believe my hair froze the other night! – But weather is lovely, bright sun on the snow – which is quite deep. I believe people at home would call it hardships [*sic*] and I suppose they are but no one ever thinks of grumbling – Frozen tea is a funny sight but frozen café au lait is rather nice! Have you ever had a frozen face? ... It's such an odd sensation.[2]

Auxiliary Nurse Etta Inglis described how:

Our breath froze to the sheets, our hair to the pillows, our rubber boots to the floor, our sponges would have seriously hurt anyone if by chance we had used them as bombs, and hot water spilled on the floor would in five minutes be frozen solid. The camp was under snow for three months and huge icicles hung from the roofs of the huts.[3]

Although the staff could take it pretty lightly, it was a serious matter for the troops in the trenches as they shivered on opposite sides of No Man's Land. In a strange repetition of the Christmas truce at Mons in 1914 the two sides agreed they would not fire on men bringing up rations provided they were unarmed.

'Guten tag, Fritz.'
'Bonjour, monsieur.'
'Kalt.'
'Ya, pas chaud.'
'Et tes officiers?'
'Quand il fait froid, officiers sont pas la; ils boivent du champagne.'
'Böse Krieg.'
'Et pas finie!'[4]

Such was the solidarity and mutual understanding existing between those at the bottom of the military hierarchy. From their level of hardship they would have envied the night orderlies at the hospital who carried food around the wards 'in icy gales, with snow whirling round them, the night as black as pitch, – impossible to keep clear of the deep ditch'.[5] At least they could slip into the wards at intervals to warm themselves at the hot stoves. In spite of the cold they were exceptionally healthy at that windswept barrack hospital, more so in fact than at the low-lying hospital at Royaumont.

Mrs Robertson braved the cold and paid a visit to Villers-Cotterêts on behalf of the committee:

> I am very much delighted with this as a whole. I should think the standard of efficiency was a high one. The patients seem most comfortable and well-cared for and the cooking is excellent. Jamieson [Anna Louise Jamieson, head cook] is splendid. Jamieson has pigs and chickens. One of the pigs was killed and we are at present eating Louisa, who is very good – the hens are laying and Jamieson is setting eggs for her chickens. The men put up both bee-hives and pig sties. It's all quite after my own heart and very well-managed. Sister Lindsay makes a capital Matron, and things seem very happy.[6]

The hospital produced as much of their own food as possible. As soon as they had arrived the previous summer they had planted vegetables and flowers, with much rivalry between the wards. Reporting on Royaumont at the same time, Mrs Robertson said:

> Royaumont may cost us a lot but there is no doubt that it is the best fed [since Michelet was in the kitchen] and the best-managed hospital in France.[7]

On 7 February Miss Ivens was reporting:

> We now have nearly 300 beds at Royaumont but always keep at least 50 empty – and if a big convoy comes in evacuate in a day or two – Our numbers have never been so high as during the last weeks when the French ambulances in the St Quentin section were evacuated for the British.[8]

The committee were rather alarmed to hear of 300 beds – they had not given permission for so many and felt they could not be responsible. Little could they imagine the streams of casualties that would shortly be pouring into Royaumont. However, Miss Ivens was now disposing her forces before the big German offensive that many were expecting to begin at any moment.

Foreseeing the heavy demands ahead, Miss Ivens must have been very thankful when Dr Helen Lillie arrived on 28 February, thus increasing the complement of doctors serving the two hospitals to eleven. Dr Lillie had qualified in 1914 from Aberdeen University and had distinguished herself as an exceptionally able young resident in Sheffield Royal Infirmary. Probably because of wartime conditions in civilian hospitals she gained extensive surgical experience. When she left Sheffield she went to the Scottish Women's Hospital in Ostrovo in Serbia. There she collected material for a thesis on malaria, which she submitted successfully for an MD degree after the war. Dr Bennet, under whom she served in Serbia, described her as 'the right sort', and said she 'had never seen a woman do an operation so deftly and so quickly'.[9]

On 5 March Miss Ivens recalled all doctors who were on leave, and asked the committee to send out another doctor. On 15 March, still conscious of a shortage of medical staff, she recalled Dr Martland, in spite of the fact that Miss Aldrich-Blake, the eminent surgeon, had declared she was unfit to return. She also sent for Vera Collum, now an expert radiographer, who had returned to Britain after serving a full three years at Royaumont. Miss Ivens explained to the committee:

An Army order now makes it imperative that all cases must be operated on 24 hours after admission. That is why we must have our own x-ray installations fully equipped and a good personnel and enough doctors to operate within 24 hours.[10]

On 20 March bombs began to fall on Paris; some also fell close to the abbey, breaking some windows. The German offensive that started the following day in the Montdidier and Noyon sectors resulted in a rush of work. On 27 March the number of patients was drastically reduced to make room for the expected run of casualties: they were down to 25 occupied beds at Royaumont and 29 at Villers-Cotterêts. Miss Ivens asked for, and obtained, formal permission to move forward if necessary. On 10 April the Service de Santé asked for 100 more beds at Royaumont (which they would supply). Royaumont was now officially recognized as a casualty clearing station (CCS) for French and British patients. (The British were now sharing a section of the front with the French.) Wounded were arriving steadily, bringing the total of beds occupied by 17 April to 190 at Royaumont and 77 at Villers-Cotterêts.

Vera Collum returned to France in early April and was distressed to see the enormous numbers of civilian refugees as she made her way, by a circuitous route, back to Royaumont. On 11 April she wrote:

> The fierce fighting on the Western Front has had a very marked effect on the work at Royaumont. They are now a First Line Evacuating Hospital and streams of wounded are constantly passing through. The staff is working night and day and fresh workers are being sent out to cope with the rush. ... French and British alike are coming to Royaumont. It is a deep satisfaction to the staff and to the Committee to know that for the second time the Scottish Women's Hospitals are serving British officers and soldiers.[11]

Apart from the treatment of the casualties there was a heavy workload for the chauffeurs:

> The car work had changed from the time when we got in about a dozen patients every day – now they come 40 to 70 at a time, and we often have to send out 30 to 40 convalescents over the whole day. We also have to help Creil to evacuate other hospitals so that it can be done more quickly.[12]

One of the two new chauffeurs (probably Katherine Fulton) described how, having had no previous experience of active service, she had 'dropped right into such an intimacy with war as I had never dreamed of':

> Troops and guns streamed along the roads, newly cut trenches disfigured the fields. Bomb holes gaped with awful reality within a few hundred yards of the Abbaye itself, and wounded poured in continuously. We were at work night and day: it was like a never-ending nightmare to a newcomer, and what sleep we did get disturbed by constant alarms and air raids. For ten days I lived on my ambulance, and worked like one in a dream. Nothing seemed real, there was nothing familiar for my mind to grip, and as at night I tore along without headlights through the soft blackness with a heavily laden ambulance, or helped to load and unload countless stretchers with their groaning burdens, I used to bite my lips till the blood came to convince myself of the reality of it all.[13]

On 25 April Miss Ivens sent details to the committee of the work actually carried out. In the month 23 March to 23 April 437 patients had been admitted, of whom 8 died; 369 operations had been performed; 851 bacteriological examinations, 404 x-ray photographs, and 371 x-ray screenings carried out. (It was not surprising that the radiographer Marian Butler was suffering from x-ray burns.) The peak period for admissions was 7 and 8 April when 165 were admitted and 80 operations performed, with a further 34 operations on 9 April. The cases were all *grands blessés* who could not travel any further.[14] The beds now numbered 400. It was clear that a much bigger staff was needed, especially doctors and orderlies. Miss Ivens reported:

> The work here is very heavy and at any minute Villers-Cotterêts may be deluged. We have got through so far very well as everyone has worked at full pressure and extremely well, but several are showing signs of collapse.[15]

On 10 April she was asking for ten more doctors. These clearly could not be supplied. Dr Logan was the only one who arrived in

April. She had qualified in 1912 and gained her London MD in 1916. She had experience in obstetrics and gynaecology – the usual specialty for women at that period. Unfortunately, as will be related later, her time at Royaumont was not a particularly happy one.

Things quietened down to some extent in mid-May. Miss Ivens reported to the committee that 'the patients (the very bad ones) are just beginning to look a little bit more like Royaumont patients'. Staff, she said, were getting a little rested now, but the cars were still very busy. 'It is rather a comfort at HAA 30 [Villers-Cotterêts] that we can do nothing but be in bed as there is nowhere else to go.'[16] It was not to last.

Some of the over-worked doctors at Royaumont went up for a 'rest' to Villers-Cotterêts, the advance hospital, which had been relatively peaceful during the rush, and some of the fresher doctors came down to Royaumont to share the burden there.

Dr Elizabeth Courtauld, who had been administering anaesthetics for days and nights during the rush, as well as looking after a ward of seriously wounded men, was rejoicing in a half-holiday in the surrounding woods with a piece of bread and cheese when she wrote to her sister on 25 April:

I am sending you a blossom of pulsatilla [pasqueflower], I picked it this afternoon ... they grow on a warm bank skirting the forest, and are quite abundant ... we are no longer having hectic days, but fairly steady work. In fact my ward is now quite reasonable, so I can begin to enjoy life and the patients again. I like it much better than the rushes, though the younger ones seem to like the excitement of a rush. [Dr Courtauld, at 50, was the oldest of the doctors, and probably the oldest of the whole staff.] We are having dreadfully bad cases just now and have had 8 deaths in the past month's work. We get men sent to us with bits of shell and bullets in most difficult and dangerous parts, but so infected that an attempt must be made to remove them ... In spite of the cool weather they had to put 60 beds in the cloisters, and for three weeks the staff had had their meals outside in the cloisters, sometimes snowed upon and often disagreeably cold ... If it is at all mild I like having meals out. Many of our cases are so smelly that to breathe fresh air at intervals is refreshing.[17]

Three other doctors arrived in May: Doctors Dobbin and Richardson on the 4th and Dr Adams on the 23rd. This brought the complement of doctors up to 14, certainly fewer than Miss Ivens would have wished – but she was nevertheless delighted with them: 'We like the new doctors very much, especially Miss Richardson and Miss Dobbin who is a charming little thing.'[18] Dr Adams and Dr Dobbin had both qualified in Belfast in 1917 – presumably they had decided to volunteer together. Dr Richardson was older, having qualified in Edinburgh in 1907, and had worked as a medical missionary in India.

※

Although the work at Villers-Cotterêts had been lighter than at Royaumont through much of the spring, it had certainly not been uneventful. Severely wounded men were coming in, though not in the large numbers that were flowing into Royaumont.

The hospital, formerly known as 'Hôpital Bénévole', was now to be entirely under French army orders and to be known as 'Hôpital Auxiliaire d'Armée No 30 (HAA 30)'. In the event of the 'deluge' that Miss Ivens was anticipating (correctly as it turned out), a selected number of staff were warned to hold themselves in readiness to move at two hours' notice with a pack of essential belongings.

There are few records available to supply details. Orderly Grace Summerhayes, working in the theatre, remembers one particular night – probably the night of 6/7 April. She describes it as 'that bloody night'.[19] Dr Henry left among her papers a little fragment of a diary she kept at Villers-Cotterêts – just a page torn out of a notebook:

17 May. Air raid. 4 admissions. 1 officer aviator and his pilot both went up with Boche before and behind. Engine stopped, avion came down. Officer fractured spine. v. ill. Pilot fractured ankle.

18 May. 2 other admissions, men bombed at the factory. – [illegible] officer operation laminectomy [an operation to remove the lamina of a vertebra], died later. Valette died. Resection of head of femur.

19 May. Miss M[artland?]'s birthday ... [words missing] ... Air raid. 2 admissions.

20 May. Funeral après-midi Madame V[alette?] heart br ... Officer's funeral ... picnic ... Enjoyed being alone ... V C tonight – wish I were back at R. feeling the heat very much. Whit Monday.[20]

The staff had been distressed when tired British troops, retreating from the German advance, rested for a while at Villers-Cotterêts, amazed to find British women stationed so close to the front line:

They left behind them a memento – a little old fox terrier dog with an unashamedly vulgar tail that curled over his back. The battery passed on; the little dog was missing and could not be found. Hours later he was discovered, draggled, caked with mud, curled up on the bed of the young 'Vague-Mestre' [the orderly in charge of the post, Miss Kitty Salway] who promptly adopted him as the hospital mascot.[21]

The fox terrier retained the important post of hospital mascot until the end of the war, and eventually returned to civilian life in Britain accompanied by Dr Courtauld.

❦

When the beginning of the great German offensive was signalled by the massive bombardment in the early hours of 27 May, Miss Ivens, at Royaumont, 'happened to hear quite unofficially of the attack'. She made immediate preparations to take all available staff up to Villers-Cotterêts during the afternoon. 'When we arrived at Villers-Cotterêts it was very strange – they had heard nothing although so much nearer [40 miles nearer the front line].'[22]

Why, one might speculate, did Miss Ivens only hear 'unofficially'? And why had no warning been sent to Villers-Cotterêts – which was now, after all, 'directly under the Army'? If Miss Ivens had not arrived with reinforcements, the staff would have been in great difficulty. This lack of readiness on the part of the French command seems even more inexplicable given that the army had decided some considerable time earlier that the location of Villers-Cotterêts was so advantageous for a casualty clearing station that they were building another large hospital alongside. At the crucial time, however, this was not ready. Villers-Cotterêts stood alone.

Miss Ivens' accounts of the work of the hospitals were always straightforward, factual, usually brief, and certainly not given to hyperbole. She wrote to the committee on 30 June apologizing for being 'very neglectful', but 'I know you will realize that we have been working at the highest pressure and that it has taken us all our time to get through'. It is worth quoting her report in full:

At 5 p.m. May 27th some badly bombed cases arrived [at Villers-Cotterêts], and at 4.30 a.m. on Tuesday morning May 28th, the stream of wounded began to come in by car. Refugees poured in by every kind of vehicle and on foot, and during the night all the medical staff of a hospital nearer which had been forced to evacuate. We worked practically continuously, and yet the receiving ward was always full. During the few days, more than 3,000 wounded passed through the centre, and we had 127 of the worst, as the big hospital was not yet equipped for work. At mid-day the Médecin-Principal came to me and said he had very bad news, and that we must be preparing to evacuate. We were dreadfully disappointed but as it was perfectly clear that the wounded could not be kept there, I simply said we should do as we were told, but wished to remain until the last possible moment that we could render service. He said it was inevitable and that we must pack up, and be ready to go and form a hospital on the other side of Paris from Royaumont. I gave orders accordingly, but in the evening he came to me and said that as no other hospital was in a position to work, and as no confirmation of his order had been received, would we stay, as a great many cases were expected during the night. Of course I said we should all be delighted, and the theatre unpacked and the x-rays were put together again in about an hour's time, and work was resumed and went on during the night until the middle of the next morning [Wednesday 29 May]. It was an appalling night. We had to work almost in total darkness for from early in the evening, air fights had been going on and we were a target. Tremendous explosions came from a train of ammunition which had been hit by a bomb, and the whole sky was illuminated. The patients were thick both on the beds and the stretchers in the receiving ward 'France' and we kept on tackling the worst cases. No one showed the slightest trace of nervousness in spite of the horror of the night. I lay down for half an hour but was soon called up by the arrival of more and we began again on Thursday morning [30 May]. I was in the middle of operating when the Médecin-Principal walked into the theatre and said we must be getting ready to go and must not attempt to do any more operations. A train was expected to evacuate the patients, but did not arrive. When it did only half ours could be put on. The telephone was cut the day before. However, during the morning I had sent down to Royaumont for every available car to come up, sending down at the same time a batch of the younger orderlies, and all the important archives. At lunchtime I told the staff to pack up their valuables to take with them, and the rest of their possessions in their trunks, and to dress to be ready to start at any minute. We then devoted ourselves to getting the patients dressed so that they could be sent off as soon as the opportunity occurred. A train came in, and I was allotted 70 places for the 120, which left me with 50 to dispose of. I accordingly sent off all our three cars with wounded to a little town about 15 miles behind, with instructions to return for more as soon as possible. Then three cars from the American section were placed at my disposal, and I filled them up with wounded. At last our cars from Royaumont began to arrive, very late, owing to the condition of the roads, and we were thankful to pack up the rest of the wounded in them. They were to be taken to S[enlis] – each car took a sister. A little before I had started off a considerable number of the orderlies and doctors [began] to walk as it was quite clear that it would be night before the cars could get back for them, and they would be picked up as opportunity offered. During the afternoon the shells began to whistle overhead, and the American car drivers told me that it was quite time for us to go as the Boche were only 5 kms away and were coming on very fast. At last all the staff and wounded were off. – We kept the little lorry, and Moore [Miss Evelyn Moore, chauffeur] loaded it with petrol which at that moment was our greatest need, and we started for C[répy]. On the way I met several of our returning cars and sent two or three of them on with orders to help with the evacuation of the big hospital, and if not, to bring any valuables they could. I decided to call at C. where we had sent some wounded, to see if they had left in a train, or what arrangements had been made. It was a station more bombed than any other behind the lines, and a great hole in the station yard greeted us – We looked about and found several of them [the staff] still there, including Mrs Berry and, I think, [Orderly Florence] Tollit. We continued our journey to S. The country was illuminated. It was just like gigantic fireworks, for air raids were going on in every direction. As we got into S. there was a block – all lights were out. However as we had to pull up, an army doctor came out, – We then made for the hotel where I expected to find most of the nurses. Twenty one were there, and I was very cross on finding them in their beds instead of in the cellars, as the raid was on. We decided to make for R[oyaumont] by a quieter road as we could see the bombs dropping over the one we generally took. It was not a happy selection from that point of view for we met a continuous stream of Foch's reinforcements and understood that was what the bombs were trying for. It was a most reassuring and impressive sight – silent dark shapes moving slowly along towards us in the night with quantities of guns and cavalry. Not a sound and hardly a light (I saw, I think, two cigarettes). After a detour we reached R. at one o'clock, and a very short time after Murray [Elizabeth Murray, chauffeur] arrived with four patients from Villers-Cotterêts – The following morning May 31st I returned to S. to see for myself the Médecin-Principal. I arrived during a conference of all the medical authorities involved. S. was to function as a clearing station. We were to fetch and receive our patients from there and HAA 30 [the Villers-Cotterêts unit] was to work at Royaumont. It was all fixed in about 5 minutes. We got a load of wounded and took them back with us. Two extra theatres were arranged. Matron Lindsay took charge of one, and our theatre sister [Sister Everingham], from Villers-Cotterêts, was to do the night work.[23]

Other members of the unit also recorded their experiences, giving us a very complete impression of the days leading up to the evacuation, and the evacuation itself.

Dr Courtauld had been working at Villers-Cotterêts for about three weeks when the German onslaught began. Since the patients had started coming in, 'one has lost count of time more or less, for the staff has been working pretty well night and day. Noise, dust, bombing going on night and day almost so if one did get to bed for an hour or two unless one was dog-tired sleep was out of the question, and one never felt it desirable to undress.' She continues:

When the first order to evacuate was cancelled and the new order came on to stay we were glad. It seemed horrid to be told to go and leave things working behind us. All night long we were hard at it, and working under difficulties. Terrible cases came in. Between 10.30 and 3.30 or 4 a.m. we had to amputate six thighs and one leg, mostly by the light of bits of candle held by the orderlies, and as for me giving the anaesthetic, I did it more or less in the dark at my end of the patient. For air raids were over us nearly all the night and sometimes we had to blow out the candle for a few minutes and stop when one heard the Boche right overhead and bombs falling and shaking us. However our camp remained intact. Next morning about 11 a.m. we were told the whole place must be evacuated and all as fast as may be. Patients had come in all through the night, some practically dying, all wanting urgently operating upon. But we had to stop operating, dress the patients' wounds and splint them up as best we could and all day ambulances came up and we got the patients away. A hospital train was also made and a lot went by that. But heaps of really badly wounded had to start to walk. We also got away a good many of our orderlies and younger doctors and nurses. We sent off a party of lusty young ones walking, just carrying what they could in their hands. We had all been provided with what we called a 'retreating ration' the day before, for emergencies, two hard boiled eggs, one orange, a bit of cheese and a bit of bread. [Another account mentions brandy in the ration pack.] By the evening Miss Ivens, myself, the Matron and only a few orderlies and sisters were left, and only 9 extremely bad patients. At supper came the order that the whole place was to get away as fast as it could. Our Royaumont lorries and ambulances had been sent for ... so directly our patients were got on to stretchers and met the ambulances we rushed to our barrack, picked up our handbags and knapsacks and came straight down in the lorry to Royaumont. I got here about 11.30 p.m. It was an exciting journey part of the way. For reasons which seem pretty clear now, but we did not know last night, the road was likely to be bombed, and at a certain place the car got into the midst of it. The moon had not risen. Our camion [lorry] is a great heavy thing and can't go very fast, and though it seemed dark to the driver (for we had no lights on) yet the road showed as a white line among the dark forest surroundings, and evidently was a good mark for the Boche. Anyway we had a few sharp minutes and I didn't think we should get through unscathed, but we did, but the brutes seemed to follow along from above. And even when we got here bombs and barrage were booming away all round the district. Royaumont has been almost emptied of patients during the last few days, but I think now we are going to get a lot of these poor things who were evacuated by necessity from the hospitals nearer the line – For five days we have lived through a lot and had hardly any sleep. It is simply horrible leaving so much behind. Things packed up and lying just outside one barrack by the side of the railway ready to come but unless we can get them soon they will be looted. I was there only three weeks and took only a few clothes and have not left much behind, my rubber bath being my most important loss.

She had one other regret:

I wanted to dig and burn up all the masses of vegetables the staff have grown, but hadn't a moment. Had picked a bed of radishes for supper, but had to retreat before we could eat them.[24]

Dr Henry remembered those four days 'when time did not exist'. The wounded men coming in were the most severe cases. 'Their wounds were terrible, and in most cases they arrived at the hospital minus even a field dressing.' As for the staff:

For four nights and three days they worked without ceasing except for meals. We began to lose all sense of time, and worked like machines. On the last morning when we stopped for breakfast Theatre Sister went fast asleep sitting bolt upright upon a bench, and she had to be shaken before she could be awakened – That last week at Villers-Cotterêts will ever be remembered by the staff as a terrible nightmare ... The saddest sight of that last week – was the seriously wounded men streaming along the roads dead tired, and in many cases, almost unable to drag themselves along.[25]

Dr Henry was one of the more youthful doctors who set off with a party of the 'lusty young ones' to walk back the 40 miles to Royaumont with orders not to spend the night in any of the villages en route:

We joined the refugees. We were on the run. Presently an empty train car rolled along the railway line, we crossed the field and signalled. Do you remember the French wagon labelled 'Trente hommes ou Huit Chevaux [30 men or 8 horses]'? That was ours. It was very dirty but we climbed in and sat on a tightly packed row on the floor, our heads nodding in our tiredness. So we arrived at Senlis where our wounded had been dumped on the station platform.[26]

As an old lady, her daughter tells us, Dr Henry still had nightmares about that evacuation journey.[27]

An orderly, acting as second sister in the theatre, described those days to Vera Collum:

A hell and a shambles. Nine thigh amputations running; men literally shot to pieces: the crashing of bombs and the thunder of ever-approaching guns; the explosion of a train of munitions on the line; next, the destruction of a level-crossing keeper's cottage within a stone's throw of their own siding; the operating hut with its plank floor and the tables and the instruments on them literally dancing to the explosions; the flickering candles, the anxiety lest the operated cases might haemorrhage and die in the dark; the knowledge that the next bomb might get them; the still more awful fear that the French had miscalculated – that the door might be thrown open and a German officer walk in on them.[28]

Maud Smieton remembered how she and her fellow orderly Etta Inglis were seconded to the theatre, where Inglis held a candle at one side of the operating table while she stood at the other 'trying to keep our hands steady while loud explosions went on outside':

The whole place was a shambles with men lying on the floor everywhere. It was so dark – that it was difficult to know if a man was dead or alive. On our last morning, when we were feeling at our last gasp, Miss Ivens said to me: 'Smieton, go and find another blessé. I shall do one more operation'. There were so many wounded still lying on the floor, mostly badly wounded, it was difficult to know whom to choose. However, I saw a man with a tourniquet on his arm so I had him moved into the theatre.[29]

Miss Ivens remained unflappable throughout, Orderly Georgina Cowan describing her as 'Just as cool as could be'[30], while Sister Goodwin remembered her as 'a Rock of Gibraltar'.[31]

Radiographer Florence Anderson was summoned up to Villers-Cotterêts on 28 May. After taking a devious route via Paris, and very tired after many nights of bombardment at Royaumont, she arrived in the thick of the packing and unpacking, and the hectic work that followed. In her account:

Wounded came in all night. The ward next the x-ray department was a nightmare. Black blankets on the beds. On each men were dying, screaming, unconscious and delirious, the Sisters doing their work the best way they could with lanterns – Miss Ivens operating, operating, operating by candle light. Six amputations of the leg, and all the time the horrible bang bang of the bombs and the munition train, and shrapnel falling sometimes on the roof. Then the weariness! – With a train full of wounded, we got, six of us, to Chantilly, from whence we got a trap. But that road from Villers-Cotterêts to Crépy! Soldiers, transports, refugees, crowds of wounded all on foot, poor fellows, all hanging on to any vehicle they could. In the train we were in a horse box with wounded and refugees.[32]

Another (unnamed) member of staff at Villers-Cotterêts wrote:

To appreciate what the work meant it must be realized that at the same time as the wounded were pouring into the hospital, men so badly wounded that every one of them needed immediate skilled attention, the camp was also a thoroughfare past which streams of civilian refugees were pouring, pushing their possessions in front of them on little barrows, or driving in carts of every kind, and was a refuge for the staff of more than one hospital which had to evacuate in the minimum of time. One company of people in this plight had not even time to get all their clothes, but had to leave in a condition of semi-undress. A party of evacuated nurses were given shelter in our hospital, while the staff of another hospital were given rough lodging in tents by the adjacent French HOE [Hôpital d'Evacuation].[33]

One member of the unit, looking back from 1968, remembered the descent of these fugitive ladies upon Villers-Cotterêts:

> They floated around in high heels, complete with voluminous veils and Red Crosses and heavy make-up and had no intention of soiling their hands with hard work. They fell foul of [cook Eva] Ashton in the kitchen who afterwards used to refer to them briefly as 'the dam' rouges'.[34]

While the nursing staff attended to the patients, Ashton and the other cooks not only fed the refugee guests, but also provided an emergency canteen for some of the streams of soldiers passing through.[35]

One of the other cooks, Helen McLeod, looked back on those days three decades later:

> Could one ever forget the one candle in a bottle for light to cook by, the rats slipping out from under one's feet, the windows and doors that opened and shut when no one was there? Miss Ivens appearing from the blackout at 4 a.m. and sitting at the orderlies' table discussing the events of Villers with Jerries hovering overhead. Could one ever forget?[36]

On the evening of the 29th, when the hospital was ready to begin work again after the order to evacuate had been rescinded, the unidentified member of staff continued her story:

> As far as the difficulty of the work was concerned that was the worst night we had to cope with. The blessés began coming in

between 8 and 9 at night, and almost immediately began a violent air raid. The men were among some of the most terribly wounded we had yet received and in the middle of taking them all in the 'All Lights Out' order was given, and we had to carry on by the light of a few heavily shaded lamps, with the whirr of enemy machines overhead, and the heavy b-o-o-o-mp, b-o-o-o-mp of bombs dropping nearby. The raiders were so persistent that it was found to be impossible to delay the operations till they had passed over, and at the same time the raiders were so near that it would probably have meant disaster if a light had been allowed to be shown anywhere. The solution to the problem was that work in the operating theatre was resumed by candlelight.

About 10.30 the order came to prepare the patients for evacuation. In the air raid of the night before the station of Villers-Cotterêts had been bombed, and was still filled with debris so that no trains could pass through it till the debris had been cleared away. Consequently the 'trains sanitaires' which should have taken away the wounded were not available, and the problem of how to get the men removed had to be met. The less seriously wounded men who had been spending the night at the French HOE [evacuation hospital] were started out to go on foot till they could find some better means of transport, but not one of the men in the Scottish Women's Hospital could possibly go anywhere on foot, so Miss Ivens sent for the cars to come up from Royaumont and take the blessés from Villers-Cotterêts to the first available hospital further back. The result of this arrangement was that everyone without exception in the Scottish Women's Hospital was evacuated safely, and in addition the Royaumont cars were able to help to transport some of the men for the HOE. The British staff, who, according to first military orders, were to have been taken by train with the hospital equipment, were now deprived of that means of transport. Like the blessés and the civilians there was nothing for it but to start on foot, and hope to get some better means of transport further on. So a large party of doctors, nurses and orderlies were sent off about midday to find their way as best they could to Royaumont, leaving behind everything except what they could carry.

Those who did not go with the first company remained to help to look after the blessés till they left, and to attend to the final packing of the hospital. By six o'clock in the evening there only remained 8 blessés in the hospital, and nearly all the staff had left. The end of the evacuation was very sudden. Two American cars drove into the camp with the news that the German advance was becoming more rapid, and about the same time we heard the screech of shells for the first time. The result was an instant order for the blessés to be put into the American cars, and for the staff to get into the Royaumont lorry which had just then appeared. When Miss Ivens drove out of the camp about 8 p.m. the evacuation of the blessés and the staff, both English and French, was completed.[37]

Miss Stoney had won everyone's admiration for her work during the rush, and it was characteristic of her and her devotion to her beloved x-ray apparatus that she made superhuman efforts to save as much of it as she possibly could. She had packed up the apparatus carefully and methodically on the first order to evacuate, but she had to work fast to get the equipment operational once more:

The blessés were already pouring in again. Thanks to the ready and skilled help of my helpers, [Orderly Patricia] Raymond, [Orderly Marian] Butler and [Orderly Florence] Anderson – thanks to the help too of [Hilda] S[meal], the chauffeuse who had sometimes helped me before, and of the infirmiere [*infirmier*, i.e. French male orderly] Defarge we got all the electrical wiring replaced and the Gaiffe apparatus fully functioning by 11 p.m. Villers-Cotterêts [i.e. the town] was blazing – a woman and children were killed at the corner of our hospital. We dared show no light. But Miss Ivens, Miss Martland, Mrs Berry and the other doctors operated all night by the light mostly of a 50 candle-power electric lamp I had stuck in a cocoa tin to shade it – or candles. The engine had to be run for the x-rays – and the electrician had fled to the fields – we had also to see to the engine. I was sent to bed at 4 a.m. and Berry and Butler were working on when I came on duty again three hours later. We worked on till 4 p.m. Thursday seeing x-ray cases. Then the order came to pack up finally. At 1.30 p.m. Miss Ivens sent off the younger doctors and orderlies walking, and hoping for odd lifts – this included my three assistants, Anderson, Butler and Raymond. Then my last helper, the x-ray infirmière [*sic*] was needed to carry the blessés – and help with the wounded – the doctors and nurses remaining were desperately busy with patients. The whole of the x-ray equipment was however repacked by 6 p.m. and we went to supper. During supper the shelling began, and the splendid American ambulance men came along for the last of our blessés whom we had not yet been able to evacuate in our own cars. And this left our returning cars free for the last of us to luxuriously drive to Royaumont. We were heavily bombed on the way.[38]

'We were on the road all night', wrote Hilda Smeal, one of the 'shovers':

It would have been very thrilling if it had not been so unspeakably tragic. The roads were quite a sight to behold, simply black with troops, convoys and big guns going in one direction and in the other, refugees and the poor blessés who were forced to go on foot as all the cars were needed for the stretcher cases. Some of the poor souls had trudged along for miles and miles, and they did look so dusty and weary – a truly pathetic sight.[39]

One further tale must be told of the evacuation of Villers-Cotterêts. Despite the efforts of 'La Colonelle' to ban all pets from the unit, a brace of canaries (one called Jimmy) had been surreptitiously hatched at Villers-Cotterêts, actually within the operating theatre – presumably the warmest spot in the hospital during that bitterly cold winter. When the final signal to abandon the hospital was given, the Germans being within 4 miles, the canaries had to be left behind:

> When all the Villers-Cotterêts people had returned to Royaumont, the malade [patient] who had been identified to act as theatre brancardier [stretcher-bearer], failed to appear. There were those who in their thoughts accused Dominique of base desertion. But one day, when Inglis was in the hall, she saw a dusty weary figure stumbling up the path – it was Dominique, with a birdcage in his hand, which he flourished triumphantly, calling for 'Sistaire'. He had walked the whole way from Villers-Cotterêts, carrying the birdcage with Jimmy and his brother.[40]

In due course the canaries returned to England with Sister Everingham – whose theatre had served as their incubator.

The safe return of all the patients and staff to Royaumont was not the end of the Villers-Cotterêts story. Early the next morning (Friday), Miss Stoney, along with Madge Ramsay-Smith (the administrator) and Orderly Tollitt, returned to salvage what material they could – every item would be desperately needed at Royaumont. Shelling began almost as soon as they reached the hospital. They loaded the car with all it could carry while they themselves walked. With the help of occasional lifts they were almost back when they met two Royaumont cars and returned once more to Villers-Cotterêts. Miss Stoney did her best to make up a complete x-ray apparatus to take back with her. Renewed bombing on the road on the way forced the second car into the fields till morning, but they got through. Miss Stoney went back yet again and it was only on strict orders that she ceased in her efforts. In spite of that she had her x-ray equipment at Royaumont set up and working within 24 hours.

Although she had striven heroically to salvage what she could, Miss Stoney was still troubled by what she had been unable to achieve: 'I trust the Committee will realize the difficulties before blaming me too much for the heavy loss of apparatus entrusted to my care.'[41] She wrote to her sister Florence what a privilege it was to help in such work, and later she told Mrs Laurie, the treasurer of the committee:

> It was nice in that cold bracing forest air! I loved Villers-Cotterêts ... one is so eaten up these days with dread of not getting useful enough work that it has been of the deepest pleasure to me to be on the Western Front these days – and where such very excellent help was given when so desperately needed ...[42]

This was in spite of the fact that she felt she had been very overworked all the winter:

> The engine was old and out of work constantly – and there always seemed to be burst pipes to be soldered – kitchen drains to be seen to – broken windows in the men's barraques to be mended etc – and it was cold – colder even in a way than December 1915 in Serbia ... I was without an orderly, we were so short of staff – and the stove had to be lit – the floor washed etc – my hands gave out – and it is not easy to write with one's hands bandaged up.[43]

We will leave Dr Courtauld to speak for many of those who participated in the Villers-Cotterêts adventure:

> None of us would have missed the last week's work for a good deal. What we are rather proud of is that when the great need began to come, we Scottish Women were apparently the only hospital in full working order and I think we really have done some good work there.[44]

Those who had been left behind at Royaumont had been very anxious during this tense time. They had had no news for two days after Miss Ivens and her reinforcements had left for Villers-Cotterêts on 27 May – the day the great German attack had begun. Then they heard – with relief – that the hospital was to be evacuated to Meaux.

This, of course, did not occur, but Miss Ivens sent them an order to empty as many beds as possible. Vera Collum, who was one of those still at Royaumont, takes up the story:

> Then silence. On the 30th the news in the communiqué was so bad that we felt justified in fearing that Villers-Cotterêts was already in German hands. We had spent the night of the 29th and the early morning of the 30th in evacuating the wounded from our hospital; I think we had reduced our number to 16! Then came a message from our Médecin-Chef, laconic, unembroidered: 'Send up all cars you possibly can immediately to evacuate hospital.' So they were still there! And the enemy, for all we knew, on the point of entering the town. How our remaining chauffeurs worked! For the two who had taken up staff had not come back.
>
> Afterwards we learnt that they had been commandeered by the authorities to help evacuate Soissons. We beat up every car that could crawl. Our chauffeur, with mumps, got up and took the lorry. The mechanic took the big American car known as the 'elephant' – we have dropped the adjective 'white' – which holds 12 stretchers. Orderlies who could drive took out other cars. Our Secretary went up in one car to see what could be saved of the equipment. An orderly went in an old car that won't go unless someone sits and pumps petrol all the time, so the hall porter went along as a pumper. – I do not know how much they all exceeded the speed limit that evening on the stretches of road that were clear. There were miles when they had to creep in and out of more slowly moving convoys. As they neared Villers-Cotterêts they met unceasing traffic – the mixed sad traffic of a forced retreat. The Germans were already shelling Longpont, 7 kilometres distant by forest path from the hospital camp.[45]

She continued:

> At about 10 p.m. the first of the refugees got back [to Royaumont]. They reported that some had reached Senlis

and some Chantilly, some were on the road, and Miss Ivens and her little band were still at Villers-Cotterêts. I thought they might not be able to leave until late, and might have to walk, so I got a man to take me in a big brake [a four-wheel horse-drawn carriage] along the road to Senlis. We hadn't gone a mile when Fritz paid us his almost nightly bombing visit, but as he was giving it hot to a certain town through which we had to pass, I confess I felt rather queer. The mare felt queerer, and tried to bolt. So we had to turn back. Just as I was about to go back to the Abbaye, I heard a car pelt up to the garage with lights out. It was the lorry from Villers-Cotterêts. Our people on the lorry had run right through a certain town in the thick of the raid – running into it before they were aware – being shouted at to douse their lights – and then going hell for leather, the bombs dropping along after them, but always running. Fritz was following the white ribands of the roads, which show plainly through the dark forest, and bombing at low elevation, anything he could see, in the hope of a convoy of troops.[46]

One of the new chauffeurs recorded her impressions of the evacuation, compared to which the previous 'rush' she had experienced 'paled into insignificance':

Everything on wheels was commandeered for that evacuation. Some of the cars, hastily patched for the occasion, held together as by a miracle, and our journey from Royaumont to Villers was a hairbreadth escape from beginning to end. For miles we had to creep in and out of slowly moving convoys, on the clear stretches of road we defied all speed limits, and as we neared Villers the road became choked – The town had been bombarded by night and by day, but the hospital had escaped miraculously. The shelling was continuous when we arrived and the town partly in flames before we left, to be heavily bombed from the air all the way back on our return journey.[47]

It was not only the staff concerned with the transport, reception and treatment of the wounded who were working at high pressure. On the night of 29 May, Vera Collum recorded:

> The office staff [at Royaumont] had sat up till 4 a.m. getting the papers done of the men in our hospitals whom we had orders to evacuate. We got away all but 7 immovable cases on the 30th. Then no one much got to bed that night, what with our staff from Villers-Cotterêts arriving and the awful raid.[48]

Royaumont was having its share of nightly bombings. Collum continues:

> When a big bomb fell in the field just behind us [the crater is still there], and a big machine just skimmed the ruined tower above our heads we plunged into the old monkish cellars beneath the Abbaye and waited tensely ... Instead of a bomb we heard the welcome hum of our own lorry's engine, which came creeping in, all lights out, into the garage yard. All our cars were in by 5 a.m., and all had had adventures.[49]

To integrate two hospitals at any time is something of a challenge. To have to do so at the shortest of notices during a headlong retreat, in the fog of war, under aerial attack, was an extraordinary achievement. To quote Vera Collum again:

> On the 31st of May began for us at the Abbaye the period of the greatest stress and strain our staff had ever known. During the First Battle of the Somme we had the consciousness of meeting the crisis fresh, with something in hand. There was never any danger of our organization being strained to snapping point. This time we were tried up to and beyond our strength. And we started tired. The Villers-Cotterêts Hospital was officially evacuated on to us, and carried on in amalgamation with us. Somehow or other we managed to provide 480 beds – they even stood in serried rank[s] all round the four sides of the Abbaye cloisters.[50]

Orderly Georgina Cowan wrote 'Where everybody is going I don't know – I am in a barn for six.'[51] Day and night staff were sharing the same beds, and many of the extra staff had to sleep on chairs.

There was no rest for Miss Ivens, and the very next morning (31 May) she drove up to Senlis to discuss the changing situation with the medical authorities there. In five minutes everything was arranged: HAA 30 (the Villers-Cotterêts hospital) was to work in tandem with Royaumont; wounded were to be collected directly from Senlis, which was now the clearing station instead of the more vulnerable Creil (though slightly further from Royaumont). She then and there took back what wounded they could carry and arranged two extra theatres, to be under Matron Lindsay and Sister Winifred Everingham (theatre sister from Villers-Cotterêts).

For the next two weeks the chauffeurs had to face daily bombing on their trips to Senlis to collect the wounded, and many of them also made tip-and-run raids to Villers-Cotterêts to salvage what equipment they could until they were forbidden to take such risks. Fortunately by this time they had been issued with tin hats. In spite of their efforts a vast amount of equipment had to be abandoned.

It was not only hospital equipment that was lost. The staff at Villers-Cotterêts had packed their trunks and stored them in an empty hut, but, as Orderly Simms reported:

> After we left the French Army got in and looted everything. One of the wounded arrived here [i.e. at Royaumont] the other day in a lady's chemise so it looks rather fishy. The chauffeurs brought back the remains of our luggage, but there wasn't anything much worth having. I got my trunk, a pair of socks that I was knitting and a vest, and another girl found nothing but her bathing dress!![52]

Grace Summerhayes lost her precious patent-leather shoes, which had been hanging above her bed out of reach of the rats. She firmly believed that it was the local townspeople who were the guilty ones.[53]

In response to the requests of local commanders, Miss Ivens

agreed to increase their beds to 600. Huts, beds and bedding were all to be provided by the French army, and the whole hospital was to be entirely under army control. Neither Monsieur Goüin, the owner of the abbey, nor the French Red Cross were happy at this expansion of beds, but Monsieur de Piessac, a good friend of the unit at the War Ministry, 'represented to them that it was the fortune of war and politely hinted not to be officially disagreeable and unpatriotic'.[54]

In the light of the fluidity of the military situation, Miss Ivens suggested to the committee that they should consider providing a mobile hospital, fully equipped, in tents, 'otherwise when the Army moves we shall be left high and dry – in the present we shall just go on working here'.[55]

Vera Collum continues the story after the return of the Villers-Cotterêts unit to Royaumont:

In three days we were full to overflowing. In 15 days we had brought in, x-rayed and operated on, 1000 wounded men. On several days our six drivers brought in 100 cases from Senlis and evacuated another hundred to our new HOE [evacuation hospital] for the northern front, 8 kilometres in the opposite direction. I do not know how many men were brought in during that first 24 hours of 31st May – but I know that I personally, made 85 x-ray examinations, and that neither my assistant or the developer in the dark room got to bed until dawn. I went on until the assistant from the Villers-Cotterêts hospital relieved me at 9 a.m., and did not go on duty again until noon. We worked at this pressure in the x-ray department until the 4th June when the Villers-Cotterêts radiographer rigged up the salved outfit and started in to help us. The heaviest week for the Villers-Cotterêts équipe [team] was the one that followed, from 9th June until the 15th, in which period they made 164 examinations, – Our own Abbaye équipe, from the 31st May until 13th July [the period of the Aisne fighting] made 1100 x-ray examinations, against 9000 of its entire 3½ year career, the total figures bringing that total up to 1680 examinations for 6 weeks.

The x-ray and theatre staffs, after the first two or three days, when they fared equally badly in the matter of sleep, roughly organized themselves into shifts working eight hours and resting six. Thus we were able to cope with it but at the cost of much physical and mental strain on those who were already tired with two or three years' work at the hospital, that some of them were worked out by August who might otherwise have carried on till the end of the war. However, they coped with it, and that was the main thing ... Two extra emergency theatres were opened. With three theatres working all day and two of them all night it can be imagined how the surgeons were pressed, and how near the anaesthetists came to being anaesthetised themselves. I do not think the Médecin-Chef or the Second in Command Miss Nicholson ever got more than three hours rest in the 24 during that first strenuous fortnight.[56]

On 4 June Madge Ramsay-Smith, the administrator, wrote:

The work here is unending and the cases are so bad that it is heart-rending to see them. The staff is working at full pressure night and day in order to treat as many cases as possible and get them sent on to other hospitals. We have received over 400 in three days and we evacuate as quickly as we can and there is hardly ever an empty bed – using sphagnum pads whenever possible – dressings very heavy – many men have several wounds and as they discharge need very large dressings.[57]

(The committee had been getting worried about the quantity of dressings required. They urged using more sphagnum moss, which cost nothing.)

During the month of 31 May to 30 June there were 1240 admissions and 891 operations, but only 44 deaths. This does seem to be a remarkably low mortality rate considering the severity of the wounds and the pressure under which the staff was working.

Writing on 30 June, Miss Stoney tells us what Vera Collum herself does not:

Collum has been so badly burned with the old Butt Table's want of adequate protection that she could do no x-ray work. I am very thankful – very thankful indeed – that those working the Butt coil have now a better protected table in this new Gaiffe table.[58]

Collum was not the only one to have trouble from exposure to x-rays; Marian Butler was similarly affected. When the pressure of work was very great, some of the diagnostic work had to be done by screening rather than by photographs, which meant a greater danger for the operator. It emerged later that Collum had suffered more than x-ray burns; her blood had also been affected by the heavy x-ray exposure. Professor Salouraud in Paris, whom she consulted in August, forebade her to go back to x-ray work for at least ten years.

Two decades later Collum wrote a moving tribute to Frederick Butt, who died at the age of 60 after years of acute suffering resulting from over-exposure to x-rays. He 'paid with his life for the too scant attention given in those earlier years to protection for the operator'. She reminded her readers that:

> ... more than one of the 'Salle Radio' staff suffered from lack of protection in the little Army pattern 'mule-back' Butt installation with which our hospitals started work and carried on, not only through the 1916 Somme push, but in the heavy work of 1918, when a second and French apparatus was in use. Butt, as a designer and builder of apparatus for war conditions, concentrated on portability and reliable foolproof functioning. Thousands of wounded men have cause to be grateful for the reliability of his apparatus, which never let the radiologist down mechanically, and showed none of the 'temperamental' qualities of, for example, our own more beloved Gaiffe installation.[59]

Looking back on the month of June, Miss Stoney felt:

> It has been huge luck to me to be where help was so needed and so ably given by the surgeons, but that we have had over

1200 x-ray examinations in a month is some excuse if the x-ray staff are tired.[60]

She pays tribute to Orderly Patricia Raymond and the cook, Eva Ashton, 'who gallantly and most ably helped us in the worst of the rush when we had night work with the lights not able to be shown because of raids overhead. She has gone back to the kitchen. Anderson (the masseuse) [not certainly identified; could be Mary Anderson, 'dispenser', or Alison Anderson, orderly] has mostly taken charge of the Butt apparatus – [Orderly Katherine] Grandage has developed photographs from 8 a.m. to 10 p.m. day after day.'[61]

Edith Stoney's sister Florence, who was in charge of all the radiological work in the Fulham Road Military Hospital in London, wrote proudly:

It is a marvellous performance. When she wrote [i.e. to Florence from Royaumont], she was waiting to examine another case – she had started on duty at 8 a.m. and had been continuously on duty for 30 hours and was soon going off. She feels very old and tired, but she says she seems to stand it as well as some of the younger ones. The wounded keep pouring in all the time, night and day. She says the surgeons must have saved many lives from gas gangrene by their work. Their hospital was the last to be kept working at Villers-Cotterêts. And she says what a privilege it is to be able to help in such work. We may indeed be proud of them all but I fear there will be a heavy aftermath to pay for the great overwork they are undergoing. Here, in London, we think we are busy, but it is a backwater compared with Royaumont.[62]

There was a welcome increase in the medical staff in June, bringing the total number of doctors up to 16, its peak level. Recently qualified (from Glasgow in 1917) and recently married, Dr Jessie Grant arrived on 6 June in that first hectic week after the evacuation. Dr Gladys Miall-Smith joined the unit on 26 June. After attaining a first-class BSc degree, she had qualified from the London (Royal Free Hospital)

School of Medicine for Women in 1916. Dr Edna Guest, with some years of surgical experience behind her, came on 16 June. She had qualified from the London (Royal Free Hospital) School of Medicine for Women in 1908, and gained her London MD in 1914. From 1912 to 1915 she was on the surgical staff of the Christian Medical College at Ludhiana in the Punjab, founded in 1894 by Dr (later Dame) Edith Brown, one of the pioneer women doctors. From Ludhiana she went to Malta, and then to Egypt, 'attached' to the Royal Army Medical Corps. Most women who served in this way keenly resented the low status and discriminatory treatment meted out to them by the army authorities.[63] After the war – indeed for long after – this was one of the many unfair practices medical women had to fight. After leaving this 'attachment', Dr Guest worked as chief medical officer in the Scottish Women's Hospital in Corsica from October 1917 to 9 June 1918.

It seems that Dr Guest joined the unit almost by chance. She had come over to see Miss Ivens at Royaumont on 16 June, and found the unit so extraordinarily stretched that when Miss Ivens asked her to stay on she 'had no doubt which path she was to take'. A few days later she wrote to Mrs Russell:

> The doctors and staff all looked very tired out and still the wounded poured in night and day and everyone worked with no time to rest. Until two days ago I just helped wherever I was needed – did dressings, gave anaesthetics or helped to operate. Now Miss Ivens has given me charge of the evacuation ward which before no one had time to organize, and it seemed really to fill a gap when I took it on. The 'admission' and 'evacuation' wards are lively spots in a hospital as near as this [i.e. to the front line]. One has to judge whether cases are fit for the journey and [one] is responsible that they do not die en route or haemorrhage or get anything serious – and still must keep them moving in order to have a 'bed and a welcome' for all who are sent down from the ward preparatory to going. We have only got cases that needed operations at once – or were too seriously injured to go any further – since the advance.[64]

With a wide experience of war service behind her she was able to say with some authority:

> The Scottish Women have every reason to be proud of their work here. A Military Hospital who, 'on active service' has much waiting to do would be justified in waiting four years for the work of the past four weeks alone ... I have the greatest respect for Miss Ivens – and in the same breath for Miss Nicholson, the whole medical staff is good, but *several* are exceptional ... I have always felt proud, *really* proud to belong to the SWH. They have such a dignified capable reputation everywhere I have been, in England or abroad, here or in America.[65]

Although she was only able to stay until 5 August, her help at a very critical time was crucial.

One doctor, during that hectic month of June, chose to send in her resignation to the committee. This was Dorothy Logan, who stated that 'she was not satisfied with the kind of work Dr Ivens had given her'.[66] Dr Logan also criticized the conditions of work that prevailed among orderlies and nurses. She left on 27 June. Miss Ivens responded vigorously. Her version was that she had dismissed Dr Logan because, she said, she had refused to give an anaesthetic when asked to do so. If this was so, it could be considered a serious offence in the conditions then prevailing. With two to three theatres at a time in operation, and the usual anaesthetics being open ether or chloroform, regular anaesthetists were working very long hours, with heavy exposure to the fumes. 'I am very glad to have her out of the hospital,' she wrote. 'At any rate she did not overwork.' She also referred to 'poisonous remarks like Miss Logan's about "sweating"'.[67] (Of course they were all 'sweating' then.) Despite the cloud hanging over her departure, Dr Logan was present at the celebratory dinner in London in 1919, and remained a member of the Royaumont Association until 1954.

Miss Ivens had some other personnel problems during this stressful period that she could well have done without. One of the most unpleasant incidents that afflicted the hospital, fortunately unique, occurred at this time. The story is worth recounting as part of the history of the hospital for two reasons. Firstly, it throws some light on the sanitary and domestic arrangements; and secondly it demonstrates the spirit and the ethos of the hospital.

Perhaps the committee at home had been hard pushed to find staff of the necessary calibre, and had not been as careful as they might have been in checking the attitudes of candidates. In any case, one of their new appointments, Doris Stevenson, arrived as an orderly on 19 May. Ten days later she wrote to the committee, 'horrified at the quite unnecessary bad conditions which prevail'. She went on:

> This hospital, I understood, was near Paris and had been stationary for three years. I presumed, therefore, that I was coming to a more or less hygienic and well-organized institution – I likewise understood Royaumont was administered by gentlewomen and worked almost entirely by them.[68]

She painted a grim picture of the salle des bains – 'absolutely disgusting', she fumed, just four WCs for the use of three wards of over 100 beds, two baths scarcely curtained off, etc. Then there was the lack of a kitchen in Millicent Ward, only a small table upon which 'dirty instruments and mattery tubes are washed, milk, sugar, eggs and drinking water laid down', while milk and water for the wards was kept in stuffy cupboards, and so on.[69] She complained of lack of method, illogical moving of patients up and down stairs, a lack of consideration for the health of the orderlies, and unsuitable baths for the staff (this at least was freely admitted). What was more, the supply of drinking water was inadequate, the hospital noisy, and 'appears to be a school for women doctors at the expense of us orderlies of good will and intention'. She admitted the food was excellent but doubted whether – even in France – a sanitary inspector would pass the drainage and unhygienic conditions. On 8 June, with the staff reeling under the continuous inflow of casualties, she wrote to Miss Ivens:

> I *cannot* be associated with an institution representative to the French of British enterprise, so instantly and so lacking in

organization and discipline as the domestic side. It is also most unfitting that white women should attend to natives in the ways we orderlies have to, as it will tend to lower the prestige of the white woman in the East, as anyone who has lived in India well knows.[70]

There was no regret at her departure. Matron reported that she was 'absolutely useless as an orderly'.[71] Miss Stevenson, however, was not finished. After leaving the hospital, she wrote again to the committee:

The whole spirit of Royaumont is ludicrous to the few of its members who have seen something of the world, the spirit is positively Prussian in its puffed-upness. The lack of humane-ness, civilized spirit or even common politeness is very astonishing to a newcomer, who is supposed to be educated and sometimes well-bred.[72]

Her racist views were expressed more forcibly:

Anyone who has lived in the East knows well that it is not fitting for white women to wait on natives. In practice they are even less ready than the rest for Christianity, and it will only retard matters by lowering the prestige of the white woman in the East. May I quote an instance, in the ward 'Elsie' an Arab got up and simply made use of the floor, after which an orderly had to clear up. In the East this is the work of the lowest and outcast woman. The French *lady, (and infirmière)* will not wait on her countrymen in the particular ways the Royaumont orderlies do, and with good grace, in spite of the lack of means towards modesty – I ask you is this quite fair to the French lady or ourselves?[73]

This can be contrasted with the attitude of another orderly, Grace Summerhayes, to a similar incident. In a personal communication with the author, she described how she went into a bathroom one night and found a North African defecating on the floor. 'So what happened then?' 'We got a shovel and shovelled it up and put it into the little loos and whoops it came back and was just on the floor again [hoots of laughter] – it wasn't a very good system!'

Miss Stevenson also criticized the reception of the wounded: 'never have I seen such lack of organization. The wounded lay in the halls and passages for hours – many of the men were in the hospital twelve hours without food of any kind'. She had not been involved in the Villers-Cotterêts evacuation but that did not prevent her from carping about the way it had been handled, and among other things she charged that some of the wounded had been left behind in spite of one car leaving empty.

It is not surprising that Miss Ivens reacted angrily 'respecting the malicious charges made by orderly Stevenson':

> With regard to the one that wounded were left at Villers-Cotterêts I consider it sufficiently damaging for me to place in the hands of the Medical Defence Union [a body providing legal support to doctors whose competence has been questioned]. It is absolutely untrue. – It is quite true that Royaumont has no modern conveniences, but the sanitation, if a little old-fashioned, has given excellent results. Single cases of infectious diseases have repeatedly occurred and have, so far, never given rise to any epidemic – when the hospital is full I myself order the clearance of the cesspools at very short intervals.[74]

Later she gave the committee further details:

> With regard to the latrines! They are just ordinary water closets, and can be kept in perfect order if the orderlies burn rubbish instead of putting it down them. The infirmiers [unfit soldiers] clean them and the renowned Salle des Bains, which is simply the basement room open to the top to the skylights where a marmite and two baths boarded in are installed. The infirmiers have cleaned the Salle des Bains and water closets since the arrival of the HAA 30 [i.e. the Villers-Cotterêts] infirmiers at the beginning of the rush and the 6 infirmiers we

have borrowed from Creil – were fully occupied (to breaking point) carrying coal and burning rubbish as well as stretchers innumerable. Since then they have done their work under the supervision of the Matron who is after them all the time. I have been in the Salle des Bains at all times and hours and have never found the dreadful conditions described by Stevenson. [Grace Summerhayes provided some confirmation that the Salle des Bains was not all that salubrious. She recalled to the author that when she cleaned it the grease got under her nails.] I have placed her case in the hands of the L and C Medical Protection Society. One infirmier is now attached to each ward. – Nearly every statement is inaccurate – The orderlies are supervised and their health is considered in every possible way, but in the pressure of work there is great difficulty in giving individual attention to the delicate ones, – I cannot see in any way where the doctors benefit at the expense of the sisters and orderlies. I consider such a statement as merely malicious and devoid of fact. The doctors have worked fully as hard if not harder than others both night and day.[75]

When the contents of Stevenson's complaints were heard by the rest of the unit, they were as indignant as Miss Ivens herself. Agnes Anderson wrote on behalf of the orderlies: 'They felt,' she said, that Stevenson's letter 'is in no way representative of the feeling of the orderlies as a whole.' Regarding the Salle des Bains, she pointed out that a curtain was provided for the baths, but it is not always used:

Some of the new orderlies find it difficult at first to realize that the French attitude towards these matters is entirely different from the British [Anderson had been an orderly since April 1915 so had plenty of experience of French attitudes towards personal modesty], but as the patients are, for the most part, uneducated Frenchmen, it is easier for us to adapt ourselves to their attitudes than for them to understand, for them, a prudish British one.[76]

This seems a commonsense and eminently practical point of view. She responded equally practically to the various other criticisms, and also explained that the health of the orderlies was very well looked after, although 'Royaumont is not a place for delicate people or those who tire easily – we do not expect to be mothered here, there is no time.'[77]

The orderlies waxed particularly indignant when they read of Stevenson's remark on the 'Spirit of Royaumont': 'In three weeks she can scarcely be expected to gauge that.' Anderson's comments on the treatment of the North Africans are worth quoting:

> Once a soldier comes into hospital he is merely a patient and is treated as such regardless of nationality and colour. It has always been the pride of Royaumont that the orderlies have been able to do for the Frenchmen and others what their own countrywomen would not or could not do for them. The French themselves realize this and are respectfully grateful – The Director of the Service de Santé had asked other Médecins-Chefs at a recent meeting to 'model their hospitals on Royaumont'. The care given to the Arabs can in no way endanger the prestige of white women, French or English.[78]

Sister Jean Thom had more understanding of the North African who had so offended Stevenson for 'using the floor':

> He was a head case, operated on the previous night and not responsible. We have a number of Arabs in the ward, all of whom behave very well indeed and give sisters and orderlies no trouble in any way. The Arab Miss Stevenson speaks of is now one of the most helpful and obedient in the ward. In my experience here I find the Arabs in every way as modest as the French.[79]

Miss Lindsay, who had been matron at Villers-Cotterêts, was indignant at the charge that patients had been left behind:

> By the evening every patient had been evacuated. As Miss Stevenson was never on the Villers-Cotterêts staff I fail to see how she dared to make any statement about our hospital there.[80]

The committee did, however, respond to the complaints about the baths – complaints that had been endorsed by the staff. They ordered 12 canvas baths which would be much easier to fill and empty, bearing in mind that all water had to be carried. They also suggested that the feasibility of erecting a bath house might be looked into, thus picking up an idea from the difficult Miss Stevenson. There is no record that this ever materialized.

❧

The shortage of doctors, and indeed of all staff, was becoming acute after the amalgamation of the two hospitals. Miss Ivens sent repeated telegrams for more staff: on 6 June 'WORK COLOSSAL'; on 13 June 'ENORMOUS PRESSURE STAFF INADEQUATE THOUSAND PATIENTS IN A FORTNIGHT 630 OPERATIONS'; and on 25 June 'STAFF COLLAPSING SEND REINFORCEMENTS'.[81]

She could be forgiven for feeling a little aggrieved when she sent a further telegram: 'STAFF OVERWORKED LONDON OFFERING NEW HOSPITAL IN FRANCE CAN THEY NOT SUPPLY STAFF FOR ROYAUMONT INSTEAD'.[82]

The explanation is a curious one. 'London' refers to the London sub-committee of the Scottish Women's Hospitals committee, which was based in Edinburgh. The sub-committee had a good deal of autonomy and were very good at fund-raising. They were responsible for the 'London' units, which operated in Romania and Russia, and later for the 'Elsie Inglis' unit in Macedonia.

The offer of a new hospital in France had apparently been made by this sub-committee to Monsieur de Piessac in the French War Ministry, and it was on the basis of this offer that M. de Piessac invited Miss Ivens to take over the hospital in Troyes. He assumed, naturally, that Miss Ivens – whom he knew well, and for whom he had the greatest respect – knew all about it and would be prepared to take over another hospital. When Miss Ivens explained to him her serious staffing problems at Royaumont, he was 'very puzzled', as she was herself. She was also resentful that in London they had so little appreciation of the tremendous strain under which the staff at Royaumont were working. The 'unit' proposed by London must have been a myth, she finally decided, and she wrote along those lines to Mrs Russell.[83]

There was now a pressing need for more ambulances to deal with the unrelenting flow of patients into and out of the hospital, and to meet the demands of the army authorities to help out in other areas. The x-ray car was no longer required as a mobile unit, as now all the hospitals in the neighbourhood were equipped with their own machines. So this car was adapted as an ambulance to carry four stretchers. Similarly the kitchen car, which had been so useful in the Soissons canteen, was now transformed into a lorry. The 'elephant' – which before the evacuation had been regarded as of the 'white' variety – was now coming into its own, as it could carry 20 patients at once. Always ready to use all the talent that was available, Miss Ivens applied for the permanent attachment of a patient who had great mechanical skills. This *méchanicien* was very skilled at keeping their somewhat aged fleet of cars on the road.

With so many very bad fracture cases in the hospital, a portable x-ray apparatus for use in the wards was becoming necessary. Miss Ivens and Dr Courtauld went ahead with the purchase, making use of money donated directly to the hospital. Miss Ivens felt she could not ask the committee, 'having lost so much'.[84]

With so many mouths to feed, it was not surprising that stresses and strains arose in the kitchen. These came to a head when Peternia Simpson, one of the chief cooks, asked, and was permitted, to leave before completion of her contract, having repeatedly quarrelled with Michelet. Miss Ivens, recognizing that the great chef was not easy to deal with, had asked Simpson to make allowances for his 'temperament and nationality' – not easy when one is tired and overworked. Simpson accused him of frequent drunkenness, though she later moderated the charge, saying instead that he was 'excitable'. (For her part, Miss Ivens maintained that Michelet had never been incapable.) Among her complaints about Michelet, Simpson told the following story. During the rush the matron had asked the locally employed kitchen women to wash their own floor, thus relieving the orderlies who were required for the unending tasks in the wards. When Simpson made these arrangements, Michelet responded by spraying the floor with grease (so Simpson claimed), declaring that he would tell Miss Ivens if she enquired that matron had refused to have the floor washed, and 'he did not care if it should lie so for two months'.[85] (Perhaps he was 'excitable' at the time!) Miss Ivens thought Michelet's health and temper would benefit from a long convalescence, and sent him off, but was annoyed that Simpson then refused to take charge even with Michelet out of the way. Moreover she would not allow Simpson to work in other parts of the hospital as she wished to do until her contract was completed. Instead she dismissed her. Simpson told the committee that 'she loved her work and felt that her dismissal was unjust and quite uncalled for'.[86] She may have had a point.

When the committee asked Miss Ivens if Michelet was really worth all this trouble (Simpson was not the first cook he had quarrelled with), Miss Ivens stood up for him:

> If you had been here from the beginning you would know that the cooks had always quarrelled [some of these she detailed]. The usual cooks sent out are not capable of running efficiently alone such a big establishment, and chefs are at a premium. Michelet has his faults but cooks meat splendidly, and is devoted to the patients.[87]

She did not give in to the committee, but nevertheless made alternative arrangements that she hoped would solve the problem: the kitchen hut would be used for the staff and the night cooking, and, when Michelet returned from leave, he could have sole charge of the men's catering in the main kitchen.

On 30 June the steady, almost overwhelming, inflow of patients suddenly ceased. Miss Ivens went up to Senlis to find out why. She learned from the consulting surgeon of the army that they wanted beds reserved – possibly 300 – for fresh cases from the front line. This was the period of attack and counterattack. It was agreed that they would do so – the beds officially numbered 600 – with the proviso that the whole hospital would now be completely under army control. Reporting all this to the committee, Miss Ivens added: 'For the present we shall just go on working here ... but we should be ready to partially close down here and move when necessity arises.'[88]

During that first month – and longer – they had to work under conditions imposed by the nightly air raids. As Vera Collum remarked, 'They interfered considerably with our work.' She continued:

> It was impossible adequately to darken vast, ecclesiastical windows, hence we had to put out all lights in the corridors, halls and stairways. Imagine an inky dark corridor full of stretchers of newly-wounded – more stretchers being carried up pitch-dark stairways from unloading ambulances: more stretchers being carried out of theatres with unconscious men on them – the groping in the dark, with the noise of the guns all round, and then the shattering crash and dull quaking of a bomb! And in one of the huge wards [Canada Ward, formerly the monks' refectory] – a vast building in which one could place a parish church, with as many lofty windows – and in the half-open cloisters, nurses groping about in the dark, and men beginning to haemorrhage.[89]

As an orderly Grace Summerhayes remembers how they were desperately short of linen to cope with the unending stream of casualties. 'You put someone into bed with bloody sheets from the last man – without time or sheets to change – that kind of thing.' She concluded – and would have agreed with the difficult Miss Stevenson – that hygiene left much to be desired, but unlike Miss Stevenson she took it in her stride: 'Well, what did she expect?'[90]

Writing to her sister on 27 June, Dr Courtauld gives us some insight from a doctor's point of view. She had been called from her bed at 5.45 that morning to see one of her patients and was using the short space of time available before the daily rounds began again:

> Many of my patients are so bad that calls from one's bed to urgent cases are not infrequent – We had a tremendous noisy raid in these parts last night ... the noise was tremendous with

guns far and near and now and again the rattle of the mitrailleuse [machine-gun], and in the lull – we hear the horrible little 'hum-hum' of the Gothas [German bombers] hovering round. And my room got full of powder, reminding me of the taking of wasps' nests.[91]

A major French counterattack had been launched on 15 June, part of it from the forests around Villers-Cotterêts. Royaumont was still getting wounded, a score or so a day, but the wounds were rather less serious and they arrived with only a few hours' delay. They were also getting some German prisoners; Dr Courtauld had two very badly wounded in her ward ('quite decent youths') and a German officer ('perfect terror'). She was much moved by a young American aviator who died in her ward with his young wife of only two months beside him.[92]

When Dr Courtauld wrote again on 16 July the hospital had begun to empty – they had evacuated almost half the patients, in response to the request to hold beds ready for the next attacks. 'We are ready for anything next,' she wrote, but in the meanwhile she was 'enjoying the lull immensely'. Her remaining patients were really bad fractures with 'awful wounds'. This work was very time-consuming.[93]

Miss Ivens, recognizing the need to relieve the stress, was trying to arrange for the staff to get short periods of leave while the respite lasted. This would also relieve some of the overcrowding experienced by the staff: the younger doctors and the new arrivals were sharing rooms, and a house in Asnières was rented for the night staff to let them rest away from the daytime bustle and noise of the hospital. The lull also allowed for a welcome (albeit shortlived) resumption of a Royaumont tradition, when on 14 July, Bastille Day, a ward concert took place in the cloisters.

Understaffing in the x-ray department – two radiographers were *hors de combat* with x-ray burns – was giving Miss Ivens cause for anxiety. She asked Dr Savill – who had been ill, and who was looking 'absolutely cadaverous' – to return to help out. Just after her arrival in July Dr Savill was able to write:

I am glad to say that I have arrived at a quieter time when all are tired. Poor Miss Stoney went off duty with a bad varicose leg. She had worked like a Trojan, and what an amount of abstruse knowledge she possesses. We are a very harmonious and congenial x-ray department now. [This last comment was perhaps a sting in the tail as Miss Stoney was known to be difficult to get on with.] My Mrs Large [Ruby Large, her radiographic assistant in her London practice] is a great success – liked by everyone and good at her work too. As no blessés are well enough to help now we have Smieton and Salway to run all the messages, fetching cases and cleaning generally. Anderson is first rate and delightful too. We had the two rooms going today. The tales I hear from all of Miss Ivens' courage, steadiness and superhuman physique in carrying on day and night without rest are really of a super-human creature, and she looks well, handsome and obviously cheerful and happy.[94]

However, on 30 July, Orderly Simms was writing: 'Poor Miss Ivens, she has more than she can do now, she is looking dreadfully worn and haggard.'[95]

The long months of strain on top of four years of hard work had finally broken Mrs Berry, who had to be sent home on 7 July with a complete nervous collapse. Dr Martland was the next to break down, and had to go home on 9 August. She had responded to Miss Ivens's appeal in the spring and returned to duty in spite of doubts that she was well enough. Apart from the physical strain, the emotional demands on all those in direct contact with the wounded must have been great. The doctors, sometimes regarded as 'hard', were not exempt. Orderly Simms reported that after the particularly sad death of 'a dear, very badly wounded but so brave and grateful' young American, that *'even the doctors wept over it'*.[96]

In mid-August Miss Ivens, with four doctors ill, was becoming desperate and asked the committee to try again to recruit more doctors, even if the appointments could only be temporary.[97] The committee wired to three doctors, but the only response was from Dr Lena Potter. This, however, was very welcome as Dr Potter had considerable experience of battle casualties in very bad conditions with the Scottish Women's Hospitals in Romania with Dr Elsie Inglis – who had described the work there as a nightmare. Dr Potter arrived at Royaumont on 16 August.

On 29 August Miss Ivens wired for five more doctors to come immediately – those already there were on the point of breakdown. Dr Grant had given notice, and Dr Walters was also feeling the strain and had to go home on 2 September. A replacement came for her the next day in the person of Dr Grace Hendrick, an American who had been working in the Medical College for Women at Vellore in southern India and who had been one of a group of American women who had visited Royaumont the previous May. The medical staff was now down to 14 in August and 13 in September. Miss Ivens felt that the minimum number should be 17. They never reached that total.

⁂

A welcome return (from the chronicler's point of view at least) was that of Orderly Evelyn Proctor, who had recovered from her knee injury and now resumed her work at Royaumont – and her letters to her mother. She recounted the evacuation from Villers-Cotterêts and how Miss Ivens was 'operating to the very last absolutely at her own personal risk – they say it was the most marvellous thing'. She had changed her mind from her original impression of the 'funny old bird' and had fallen under her spell, flattered that Miss Ivens wanted her back. She compared Royaumont as it was now with her happy memories of Villers-Cotterêts – 'although I like this place it is not half as nice as up at Villers-Cotterêts – we were just one big happy family up there – here it is different – military huts in the grounds to accommodate 250 blessés'. 'Several of the nicest doctors have absolutely broken down and have had to go home.'[98] (She was particularly attached to Dr Martland and Mrs Berry.) She went on:

> We have been fearfully busy here – having had convoys of blessés in every day for the last week – the poor theatre staff

195

have been working day and night without ceasing – two poor things died before they could be relieved or undressed – one of our 'babies' died yesterday, poor fellow, it was very sad as he was the only child and such a splendid person – he had shrapnel in his legs, and they at last took him down to the theatre to operate as a last recourse, but he died under the anaesthetic. We are very busy and now we only keep them till they are well enough to be moved – the men come in direct from the line and have their ops done here and are then sent out.[99]

Proctor was now working in the cloisters, 50 beds with a staff of five – one sister, a senior orderly and herself, plus two other orderlies, quite new, who had never even been in a hospital before. They had one male orderly, but he had only one arm:

We have nothing but heavy surgical cases and the shrieks and groans that go on sometimes are too awful – it's awful to see a strong man yelling with pain at the top of his voice like a demented thing. – Miss Ivens is looking very well, much better than when I came home [in January]. She is a most indomitable worker and has done and is doing marvels – so are all the staff.[100]

There were, however, some compensations which must have made her mother green with envy in war-starved Britain: 'Being "militaire" we get all the food we want – little white grapes, peaches, nuts, melons and pears. Butter and sugar are rationed in the hospital but we can buy in the villages.'[101]

Dr Courtauld takes up the tale on 28 August:

I haven't written much lately. One is busy all day, and sometimes most of the night, and hitherto when one does get a moment one is far too witless to write a letter. The French are not making any special attack on our part, so for that reason, and also because we have hardly an empty bed, we have had no new patients for the last two or three days. [After 8 August, the 'Black Day' for the Germans, the front line was moving quite rapidly away from them.] But the wards are full and heavy, and one keeps on from morning to late evening, before one can get a moment to oneself as a rule. We are planning a big evacuation soon, 150 patients or so. Then Miss Ivens can ask for a train, one which has a doctor on board, so we can evacuate quite bad cases. So in a few days' time my own patients may diminish from 60 to 30 or 40.

... An American boy in my ward who was terribly wounded died the other morning, and I had two days later to conduct the funeral, the second American I have had to bury. It is so difficult to get a Protestant clergyman here, so one of us has to read the service or part of it at the graveside, and just see the coffin lowered. Generally when I have done it one or two of our French soldiers are being buried. We try to fix the time that my car with the Protestant coffin should come to the cemetery just as our other car with the French soldiers' coffins has emptied itself from the church, and their service finished. But we meet sometimes, and yesterday I joined up with the French party, and after that was over, conducted my Protestant funeral, and in this case had quite an audience, as all the villagers, who had turned out as they always do in a kindly way for our French soldiers, stayed for our American soldier. Of course I read in English so I don't suppose much was understood. A new addition to the village cemetery has had to be made these last two years, and is for soldiers only now; French, a few English and American, a few Arabs and niggers are there and two Germans. The Arabs lie by themselves with their graves dug in the proper way, the head, I think, facing Mecca, and they have Arabic words and a crescent on their stones. The niggers have nothing, only a mound. All the French have stones.[102]

The names of 93 soldiers who died at Royaumont are now commemorated on a memorial in the cemetery at Asnières. This represents about half the deaths that occurred at the hospital.

In October, with Drs Berry, Martland and Walters all having broken down and returned home, the remaining 12 doctors were soldiering on, but the strain was telling. Dr Savill – already very unwell when she had returned to help out in July – struggled on till the end of September. Miss Stoney was back from sick leave but found her staff were almost completely new and in need of much training. She had to check personally all localizations (of shrapnel etc. in the wounds) for the surgeons, and for over five weeks could not get even half an hour out. It was too much, and she became ill – possibly with influenza. She had also had an argument with Miss Ivens (unspecified, but, she maintained, justified), and she could not get on with the senior sister in the x-ray department. Miss Stoney was always very sensitive about her lack of a medical degree, and this seems to have been at the root of the problem:

> The sister did not like to work under me as I was not qualified
> medically – it is a funny world – that I have four university
> degrees would count nothing to her even if she knew it.[103]

With her asthma, she could not face the thought of the 'wet of Royaumont in winter', and went to Cannes for a well-earned holiday. However, loving the work at Royaumont as she did, and in spite of the personality problems that beset her, she could not refuse Miss Ivens's invitation to return. She saw the hospital through to the end.

Miss Stoney was not alone in suffering from *la grippe* – influenza. A form of flu had hit the armed forces in July, but this had been relatively mild. However, in October the desperately serious 'Spanish influenza' swept through France, Germany, Britain, the United States and most of the world – a true pandemic. It continued unabated, well into 1919. The death rate was enormous: there was no effective treatment, and infection spread like wildfire. It was reported that 70,000 American troops were hospitalized with the disease, of whom one third died. Many of the staff at Royaumont became ill, but, as Dr Courtauld reported, they got off comparatively lightly:

I am convalescing from an attack of 'grippe', which I had the bad luck to succumb to about a week ago, after two days' work here only. [She had been on leave.] I took over ten sick staff among whom there were a dozen or more [*sic*] grippe cases, but of course it is everywhere about here as elsewhere. I have had a slight attack and came back out of isolation to a room with a fire yesterday to my own quarters. It is nice to get independent again – the staff is shorthanded as you can guess with so many ill and some really bad so there was a lot of staff isolated and nursing the sick staff. Doctors are rather short – and the hospital crammed just now. 200 patients poured in all the night before last, none, or very few of them really bad ... but taking notes, examining wounds, dressings, x-rays, operations (if needed) even on light cases take up hours and hours when patients flood in like that. – Our idea here is that directly a flu person is well enough she rises from her bed and crawls along in the sun in the garden and retires back to bed if need be, for there is no sitting accommodation provided when one is isolated.[104]

At least the outbreak did not hit them when the worst of the rush was on. Their policy of isolation seems to have been relatively effective, and perhaps they had the advantage over most of the population, at least in Western Europe, of being well-fed.

The number of patients was declining, but all through October and into November remained round the 400 mark. It was typical of Miss Ivens that as the war was drawing to a close she expressed a wish to 'honour at the Festival of All Saints the memory of the soldiers of the Allied Armies who had died in the hospital at Royaumont' in order that 'the tribute of our admiration and the expression of our sorrow should be brought to those who had fallen in this the most noble cause'. The ceremony took place in the local cemetery, and also provided an 'opportunity for the families concerned – and of the entire country – to express their gratitude to the Ladies of Royaumont – whose self-abnegation and boundless devotion call forth our admiration'.[105]

Finally the day they had all been waiting for for so long was approaching, the day of the Armistice. Dr Courtauld:

Well, what can we say more about these gorgeous times than has already been said? I have never lived through such a fortnight. The suspense of last week as the climax was gradually reached. The three days of thrilling suspense during which the fate of the Armistice was in the balance. The gorgeous news which we got here, thanks to our General [Descoings] who came over himself about 8 a.m. on Monday morning to tell us. 'La guerre est finie [the war is over],' he said. The Germans had agreed to sign an Armistice and at any moment a message might come through that it had been signed. Doctors, sisters, orderlies went from ward to ward to spread the news. In less than an hour the telephone rang. We heard the Armistice had been signed at 5 a.m.

Then the hospital let itself go! From ward to ward went processions of orderlies waving flags, singing, cheering, and beating anything that made a noise. And cheering men greeted them everywhere. 'Vive la France!' 'Vive l'Angle-terre!' 'Vive les Alliés!' Impromptu concerts began in odd corners and never ceased till all were in bed by midnight. The rope of the bell on the roof comes down by a patient's bed, and I don't think that bell ceased for five minutes except when food was going. How the cook managed it I don't know, but by 5 p.m. we had an extra spread in our great Canada ward, when nearly every patient in [the] hospital, nearly 300, came in on beds or sat at table, scores of staff and odd maids also, so we must have had 5–600 there. Such a sight of flags and colour and merriment. General Descoings appeared also. Two of his daughters had been placed with us as orderlies. The fun went on fast and furiously. Miss Ivens and two others who have been here from the beginning [Miss Nicholson and 'Disorderly' Gray] were chaired round the place, then M. le Curé, then the cook [Michelet], then the General, all this done with our enthusiastic orderlies. The men had champagne to drink to victory and the General sprang on a chair and made an excellent little patriotic speech. Then the Marseillaise and 'God Save'. I have heard them often here shouted out by hundreds, but last Monday night it was grand. The General stood at the salute at the time we were singing 'God Save'.[106]

There followed an impromptu ceremony that may seem somewhat tasteless to modern sensibilities:

Then the staff and all the patients who could streamed out into the rose garden. There in a large open space had been erected a huge pile of faggots and straw and on top a huge effigy of the Kaiser. Miss Ivens set a match to it and soon the pile was blazing. It was a sight; the straw and wood flamed up high into the air. Then the Kaiser caught. His helmet flamed. A huge ring of a hundred or more went round and round the pile. It was a lurid scene. At last the Kaiser fell backwards and a perfect howl of hate rose from the patients. Some jumped as soon as the fire was at all low on to the burning remains of the Kaiser and tramped him out with curses and execrations. I fancy the French are a more revengeful race than the English. In fact we have often been laughed at for feeling so little personal spite, but then the English have not had the cause the French have.[107]

The evening finished with a concert in Canada Ward.

Dr Courtauld was not the only one to spare a thought for the prisoners-of-war who were patients in the hospital. She and Miss Ivens went in quietly to give the news to one of them, an Austrian. They felt sorry for the man, with his eyes full of tears and looking very depressed. He rallied well enough, however, and in a few days was almost smiling and asserting that the crown prince must be killed and the sooner the better. Another prisoner put on fancy dress and enjoyed himself mightily with the French patients.

Amidst all the rejoicing, Dr Courtauld was conscious of the fact that she had come through all the years of the war well fed and without a scratch, and having had congenial work to do:

... no sacrifice at all on my part – all on theirs. Two little mutilated boys in my ward who must die and till then a

201

paralysed life as they have dragged out since last June are examples of the end of the war between them and me. One wept, when we were all rejoicing, poor little chap!

I tell Sister MacGregor, the one in my ward, Queen Mary, that when the last patient has gone, I and the staff of my ward shall salute the 50 empty beds, salute the flags which have hung there the last four years and then walk out solemnly.[108]

※

CHAPTER EIGHT

Aftermath: From Armistice to Closure

The Armistice was signed. It was time to start looking to the future, although there were still many patients to be cared for. It was also the time to recognize the valuable work that had been done. The French were generous with decorations, and on 20 November the newly promoted Marshal Pétain signed the order for the award of the Croix de Guerre to 23 members of the staff at HAA 30 (the Villers-Cotterêts unit). The ceremony took place on 12 December:

> Today Royaumont was en fête ... it was a singularly pictur-esque ceremony, the beauty of the ancient Abbaye lending a touch of enchantment to the scene, indeed, for where in the annals of history before these last four revolutionary years is to be found any instance of a Women's Unit receiving military decorations at the hands of a foreign government for direct participation in war?
>
> At two o'clock in the afternoon all the staff were gathered in the great hall now known as Salle Canada. The beds had been cleared away from the centre of the ward, but there still remained a row of them down either side. The staff stood at the far end, with those who were to receive the Croix de Guerre in a line in front. On the right hand side was the band of the 12e Bataillon de Chasseurs Alpins. On the left the infirmiers attached to the hospital were drawn up. General Nourisson, Général Commandant Direction des Etaples de l'Ouest du Groupe d'Armée Maistre, was to give the decora-tions.[1]

Perhaps they were a little disappointed that it was not their own General Descoings, but he had been posted to Alsace, the province newly returned to France. Dr Courtauld painted the scene:

> All the staff who could possibly leave [their duties] ... stood en bloc ... the blue and white of the gowns looking lovely ... the Chasseurs' band has a most taking way of giving a swing round and round high in the air to the trumpets which have gay tassels, before beginning ... Full uniform being the order of the day we were as alike as two peas.
>
> General Nourisson and his staff arrived at 2.30, heralded by a fanfare by the Chasseurs with the double flourish of their trumpets above their heads. Then followed the Marseillaise with all the military party standing at the salute. Next, another fanfare and the citation for Miss Ivens was read out. The General stepped up to Miss Ivens, pinned the Croix de Guerre avec palme on her coat, and kissed her on each cheek.[2]

Then came the turn of the doctors, who also received the kisses on each cheek and the Croix de Guerre avec étoile pinned on. The recipients were Miss Nicholson, Mrs Berry, Dr Courtauld, Dr Henry and Dr Martland (neither Mrs Berry, who was then seriously ill, nor Dr Martland, who had had to go home before the end of the war, were able to receive their decorations in person). Dr Manoel (head of laboratory services) and Miss Stoney (head of radiological services) were also honoured, as were Matrons Lindsay and O'Rorke, Sisters Goodwin and Anderson, and Orderlies Smieton, Salway, Armstrong and Daunt. The work at the Soissons canteen was not forgotten, and awards went to Auxiliary Nurses Inglis, Chapman and Rolt. Orderly Tollitt should have been included here, but she had been recalled home to look after ailing parents. Vera Collum, the assistant radiologist, also received a medal, as did Madge Ramsay-Smith (the administrator), and finally the gallant chauffeurs, Elizabeth Murray, Katherine Fulton and Hilda Smeal.[3]

After the decorations, citations, kisses and handshakes, the Marseillaise again, the general's speech, God Save the King and a salute, the staff and the many guests filed up to the empty Blanche de Castille Ward, to a tea of scones and shortbread and wonderful plum cake. 'The French always love our Scotch teas,' said Dr Courtauld, 'and try to pronounce "scone".'[4] The band played on down in Canada Ward, photographs were taken, and conversation made (tiring for Dr Courtauld, whose French was never all that good).

After the Armistice there were still 141 wounded patients to be cared for and also, with their surplus capacity, they were once more admitting civilians from the neighbourhood. These were now 'flocking in', as Dr Courtauld wrote, 'to take advantage of treatment before we close'.[5]

The remaining doctors carried on their routine medical duties, but also had to tackle stacks of paperwork to satisfy the military authorities. These were the dreaded *'feuilles d'observation'*, which had to be drawn up for each patient who had passed through the hospital. They had to follow a rigorously defined format. There were 'thousands' to do, Dr Courtauld reckoned:[6] 10,861 patients had passed through the hospital by the time it closed, and although clinical notes and army records had always been kept carefully, it is likely that a large number of these still required their *'feuilles'*.

Two of the chauffeurs (Monica Yeats was one) responded to an appeal from a French corporal attached to the hospital to rescue his wife and a friend who had been imprisoned by the Germans. They were now free but isolated in the little village of Fourmies, eight miles from the Belgian frontier. On 9 December the two chauffeurs set off with a car and some provisions. Their route took them through Villers-Cotterêts, Soissons, the Chemin des Dames (the scene of so much bitter fighting, and from where they had received so many wounded men), and Laon:

Villers-Cotterêts was much damaged and Soissons was in ruins. We passed through the Chemin des Dames and had lunch by the roadside and inspected some of the trenches and dugouts. This part of the front was by far the worst which we saw during the whole run – shellholes quite 30 feet deep and the whole countryside torn up and stripped of its trees, which are only blackened remains. Between Soissons and Laon the desolation was appalling, and all the villages which we passed being just heaps of stone and debris.

Refugees with hand baggage were tramping along, worn out, begging for a lift in the cars which passed. One cannot imagine what these poor people would do when they reached their destination for not a single house was habitable. Also, if they do discover the remains of their village, they will most likely find it a heap of stones and rubble with no place to give them shelter and no possibility of buying food. From Laon to Fourmies, the country and villages are intact but these places were entirely cut off from railway communication and transport, this part being the invaded country.[7]

Arriving at Fourmies that night, the corporal and his wife were reunited after their four-year separation. The chauffeurs found they were the first British to enter Fourmies after the Armistice; they shared their food with the villagers who, in turn, found them a few blankets for the night. Next day, returning by another route, they found the road so bad they had to stop off in a village for the night where they had the choice of a cave, a ruined house or a stable. There was no water – they had to use the water in the car radiator to make their tea – 'and it was good tea too'. Another long drive took them through St Quentin, 'completely destroyed, the railways all blown up and the road for miles around had been ruined every 300 yards and blown up'. German prisoners were mending the roads, filling in mine holes with stones and planks of wood, but they had to make many detours:

> The desolation of all the places we passed through is past description; churches, cathedrals, raised [*sic*] to the ground, and all damaged beyond repair. At intervals along the roadsides, we came across lonely little graves of soldiers who had been buried where they had fallen.

They were distressed that there seemed to be no organization to help people 'returning to what had once been their homes, without transport or supplies of any kind or means of building or remaking'.[8]

Their report seems to have had an influence on some of the unit, as a number elected, after their work at Royaumont ended, to work in the devastated areas. The committee were also moved and voted £100 for Miss Ivens to use for individual refugee relief. They were all curious to see the scenes of so much fighting, and now some of them were able to satisfy this curiosity – and who can blame them now that the country was at last cleared of the invader?

Dr Courtauld, with Dr Henry and Madge Ramsay-Smith, the administrator, took a short holiday. With rucksacks on their backs, bread tickets and *permission* papers they set off by train from Creil to Compiègne, and then on to Villers-Cotterêts. There was no trace of the former casualty clearing station, only a few shell holes – 'not a patch of our garden to be seen – just waste land',[9] though Orderly Proctor reported there was one mud hut with poppies growing on top, where they used to keep butter and vegetables:

> The beautiful forest of Villers-Cotterêts as we knew it in 1917 was ruined, leaving an occasional shell-torn tree, and scattered graves of Scottish Highlanders and English Guardsmen.[10]

(The forest had sheltered large contingents of Allied troops in the Summer of 1918 when the Germans had retreated from the immediate area, and before the June counterattacks were launched.)

They moved on to Longpont, but it was not the Longpont they had known in early May 1918. Then it had been a

> ... lovely little village with a beautiful ruined Abbaye, a chateau adjoining, a lovely rural scene of buttercups and water meadows, wooded hillsides and funny little cottages – Now it is dreadful. I think there are three families returned, each to a room in a ruined cottage, the rest all shelled and a tumbled mass of ruins.

An unexploded shell still stuck in the wall of the old Abbaye, and there were stray graves of German and French soldiers. Above the village the real battlefield was

> ... strewn with every sort of munition exploded and un-exploded, and graves, German, French, and possibly English scattered about, lots with crosses and names, lots without, and often a post with a helmet stuck on top.

They explored the ruined farms:

> Dumps of bayonets, helmets, rucksacks, guns, shells, bullets, clothing, German grey, French blue, English khaki, all mixed together. In one mouldy unwholesome, shell-worn dug-out we found a copy of 'John Bull' of last June and tins of Rowntree's cocoa and Crosse and Blackwells' potted meat, and could easily trace English there.

They reached Soissons and recalled how the first intimation they had had the previous May that the Germans were really in Soissons was from a patient who had a huge iron bolt sticking out of his smashed hand – the bolt had come from the Pont des Anglaises in Soissons, where he had been engaged in hand-to-hand fighting with the 'Boche'. Further on, they came to a big village, now a

> ... great desolate heap, not even a car. I don't think I have ever seen such desolation of walls standing in dead silence, and just tree stumps and broken wood on every side. – A steep bank full of dugouts of the weirdest aspect looking across a steep valley to a ruined village – and graves by the roadside and graves even in the dugouts. Germans mostly just here. It is funny somehow to see side by side 'mort pour la patrie' ['dead for one's country'] or 'Gefallen vor den Fater-land' [*sic*; the correct German would haved been *Gefallen für das Vaterland*, meaning the same as the French phrase] written up roughly on bits of poles, or shell cases made into crosses. One often sees 'les soldats inconnus ['the unknown soldiers']'.

By this time they were on the edge of the Chemin des Dames. There were miles of desolate, treeless country all around, 'just going on and on' – trenches, graves, barbed wire, great dumps of German, French and English munitions. Beyond the front-line trenches there was nothing but broken-down wire and shell holes, some small, some vast craters, and every sort of debris half-buried in the mud. This was No Man's Land.

They came to the crossroads at Laffaux, where so many of their patients had fought:

> An awful scene of desolation – all one great upheaval of earth, – shells and shells and shells – bullets, gas masks and water bottles and boots and clothing and wire and bits of gun carriages and armoured cars trodden into the mud ... and here and there a bit of a cross or a hole showing a grave.[11]

Such were the memories they brought back with them, and never forgot.

As it turned out, they were lucky that they managed to return at all. Dr Henry, the young one of the trio, had collected sundry pieces of military hardware in her haversack. Later, as they relaxed beside the fire in a nearby inn, she showed her trophies to an officer, and was taken aback when he grabbed them, rushed outside, and threw them into the nearest pond. They were live hand grenades.[12]

Even after the Armistice, Miss Ivens was still asking for more orderlies – she had enough doctors and nurses for the reduced demands of the hospital, but orderlies were, in many respects, the backbone of the hospital. They could put their hands to a multitude of different tasks – and with impending closure there were still many tasks to be done.

The planned closure was to take place, officially, on 31 December. On 30 November Mrs Laurie wrote to Miss Ivens on behalf of the committee:

> Is there no possibility of M. Goüin in any way disposing of it [i.e. Royaumont] to Government or French Red Cross for

convalescent purposes, such as a home for limbless French soldiers or TB cases or anything of that sort? It is so beautiful and permanently fitted up with its operating theatres, steri-lizers, kitchens, with the system of electric light we have put in, along with the sanitary improvements and all the stoves in the different wards, not to speak of the operating tables and instruments, drugs, x-ray rooms and labs. To scrap all these seems such a waste ... to hand them over intact as a gift to be retained in the Abbaye de Royaumont would be a tangible and surely desired gift to the French Nation in acknowledgement of their kindness and graciousness to us during these four years of war.[13]

On 13 December Miss Ivens wrote back:

I have had an interview with M. Goüin and he has no intention of establishing any kind of home in the Abbey after we leave. He wishes us to remove everything we have put in (electric installations, stoves, laboratories, fittings etc).[14]

They therefore had to consider the disposal of all their equipment. Mrs Laurie again:

It should be donated in a handsome way as a lasting memorial of what the Scottish Women have done in the Great War, – it would perpetuate a memorial of Royaumont in a fitting manner.[15]

After enquiries had been made, and with the advice of the French Red Cross, it was decided that all the hospital equipment should go to the main hospital in Lille. Lille had been occupied throughout the war by the Germans, and when they evacuated the hospital they had taken almost everything with them. Not only had they removed all the brass, copper and glass utensils, along with the bedding and other equipment, but they had also broken up the bedsteads and smashed the floors of the wards. The purloined equipment could have been of use to their deprived hospitals back in Germany, but the smashing of bedsteads and floors looked like sheer vandalism. In February 1919 the 'Commission Administrative de Lille' wrote to Miss Ivens thanking her for the gift of 20 railway wagons of equipment for the Hôpital Sauveur.[16] The gift included 400 beds and quantities of medical, surgical, x-ray and bacteriological equipment, together with other stores. One microscope and a special air pump went to the Pasteur Institute in Lille and another microscope to the Pasteur Institute in Paris. All the non-medical equipment – bedsteads, tables, cupboards, etc. – was sent to Villeneuves, one of the devastated villages, after the final closure of the hospital at Royaumont in March.

Royaumont being Royaumont, it was thought only fitting that the festivities to celebrate the first Christmas in peace-time for five years should be of an exceptional magnificence. On Christmas Eve, with all the patients in bed, all the lights were extinguished, and then three heavy knocks heralded the entry of the carol-singers, each carrying a lantern. They were followed by Father Christmas on a sledge, who brought a present for every man, then at midnight some of the orderlies sang Mass in one of the empty wards.

On Christmas Day itself the doors of the abbey were thrown open to welcome the locals to the great Christmas pantomime – one that was to eclipse all previous pantomimes. Preparations had been intensive. The show was *Cinderella*, and it had been written by one of the orderlies – all in French. There was a host of talent available. Two of the orderlies had been trained by the opera singer Marchesi, and another, Irma Minchin, was a principal in the Margaret Morris School of Dancing. 'There is nothing,' Evelyn Proctor told her mother, 'she does not know about stage management and make-up and scenic effects, and her own dancing simply brought down the house and the men simply screamed for more.'[17] There had been a sudden panic when the horse's head could not be found. Etta Inglis and Marjorie Chapman had *always* played the horse. The whole of Paris was ransacked for a replacement head – with ultimate success. Tradition could now be maintained.

As in all good pantomimes, there was plenty of variety. A succession of songs and ballets: Widow Twankey (Irene Howard-

Smith) riding astride the Inglis-Chapman horse – 'honestly a second Dan Leno' – and when the horse collapsed in a helpless heap with Widow Twankey underneath – 'simply killing'. There was a splendid pirate scene in which the prince dashes in killing the pirates and the wicked baron; a court scene with an orderly dressed as a wandering minstrel who played the violin 'absolutely divinely'; there were minuets and Scottish reels; and, as a grand finale, a tableau 'victory' – 'A very good-looking sister, all draped in white, with green palms in her hair and holding a shining sword which scintillated and looked dramatic.' Beneath the jollification, more poignant emotions were never far from the surface. Proctor recorded that 'Many people wept.'[18] Nearly a thousand people saw the pantomime; it was a grand ending to long years of effort.

The official closure came on the last day of the year, when 200 men were moved on; only one ward, with seven patients too ill to be moved, remained open. For these men and their carers, the following six weeks witnessed – to use Proctor's picturesque phrase – a *'lutte contre mort* [struggle against death]':

> It is rather wonderful that these last dreadfully ill patients are being entirely nursed and looked after by us orderlies – all the trained sisters with the exception of the Matron who was at Villers-Cotterêts were sent home, even the theatre sister, and we have had five operations – three of them amputations since. Of course there are none but the very ablest orderlies left who are auxiliary nurses and most of them have been out for three years and are covered with Croix de Guerres and other decorations – but still it is rather wonderful – isn't it! I am the most junior orderly again! There are only twenty of us left! [She was writing some time in January] – And up to a little time ago I was among the seniors![19]

Meanwhile, Miss Stoney was having problems in the final clearing of the x-ray department. Somewhat characteristically, she managed to make things more difficult for herself than perhaps they need have been. She had handed in her resignation and left Royaumont on 24 October, feeling very unwell after flu and bronchitis. She 'dreaded the wet of Royaumont in winter'. But she had another reason:

> I could not have worked with the Senior Sister – she used language I could not have passed over when I tried to show her the Gaiffe apparatus and other French things we have – new to her – which she therefore naturally could not work without getting it out of order. As I was likely to have to go in any case on account of my own health I thought it easier to go than complain and so force her to go. I don't want you to think that I left everything at sixes and sevens – I went over everything very fully with the x-ray orderly, Low [Catherine Lowe], who will be the person to keep the apparatus in order. She is excellent.[20]

However, after a holiday in the south of France Miss Stoney felt able to respond to Miss Ivens' invitation to return if she felt well enough. She came back, but it was a period of great frustration for her, as she told Mrs Laurie after she left:

> It was a great rush at the end in the x-ray department – hampered by frozen water etc and my assistants had to go on to other work long before we had got through the x-ray prints of all the four years – no regular record had been made before and one was necessary in case of questions re pensions etc. The War Museum of the College of Surgeons is wanting copies of all the stereo plates I was able to save – but it was a great disaster at the close – Miss Ivens put the x-ray plates out of my charge and into those of Sister McAlister – she had not the necessary education to see their great value or to keep the card indices etc and Miss Courtauld has a story of seeing boxes full of plates thrown out and broken. This was while there was still a great deal of x-ray work going on and I had all I could do – but after the Armistice then seeing how things were going on of course I took over the plates again, but nearly all the stereos had been spoilt – The sister seems to have thought they were duplicates and destroyed one of each pair. You must have thought me very slow and careless in

closing up – but I got bronchitis after influenza and that made what depended on me slower – I had no trained assistant then – Knowing Royaumont you will understand the delays caused by the cold in January – The water wheel froze – the sluice gate was allowed to freeze on a very cold night. This meant no water or electricity for the printing as for the other things. An emergency operation had to be done on one of the five patients who could not be moved when the hospital officially closed on December 31st. The want of water made it unsafe to heat the theatre by its own fires under an empty boiler – so the chief x-ray room with a good fire had to be cleared and cleaned out in a desperate hurry – It is, of course, all in the day's work in a front hospital. But I am only trying to show you why I was so slow.[21]

It must have been a shattering blow to a conscientious scientist, as Miss Stoney certainly was, to lose all this valuable material – which would also have provided clear evidence of the quality of the work that was achieved by the unit during the war. One might, however, speculate, that Miss Stoney – with her difficulty in getting on with people and her own sensitivity – could have averted disaster if she had explained what stereo x-rays were all about. But Miss Stoney was also capable of seeing the bigger picture, and in her letter to Mrs Laurie paid fulsome tribute to the unit:

Your surgeons are wonderful – and I think the way Ramsay-Smith and the matrons and cooks managed with that great increase of work and staff was grand.[22]

After Miss Stoney's final departure in February her sister Florence wrote to Mrs Laurie:

She is not at all well – it is the price she has to pay for the help she has given during the war. Few people realize what the constant strain of x-ray work in the dark and stuffy atmosphere and with the x-rays about – mean to the worker – If she had been in the Army she would have had a pension, but that is one of the things where it is hard to be a woman.[23]

Edith Stoney was certainly a complex character, and had many problems with her colleagues – often of her own making. Dr Henry records that she and Mrs Berry never got on together:

I remember Mrs Berry taking me aside one day and begging me to take Stoney for a walk in the forest. 'If you do, I shall get you an egg for breakfast, and if you take her for a walk and lose her, I'll give you two.' And that was when eggs were scarce.[24]

Nevertheless, Miss Stoney served Royaumont devotedly, and even the exasperated Mrs Berry, a generous and kind woman, kept in touch with her after the war and, as minor irritations faded with the passage of time, described her as 'a saint'.[25]

❧

At long last, in February, Miss Ivens was able to take a proper holiday, her first real break since her arrival in 1914. She went to the south of France with Miss Nicholson and two other doctors – an indication of the strength of the friendships that had built up in spite of being cooped up together for so long and sharing so many stressful events.

For her part, Dr Courtauld was formulating her plans. Her first decision was to take charge of Spot, the mongrel fox-terrier with the comic tail who had been left behind at Villers-Cotterêts by a British battery whose mascot he had been. Kitty Salway, the devoted orderly who had looked after him, could not take him home with her. Dr Courtauld negotiated his quarantine, and they settled down together for many years at her home in Essex. Her other decision was to 'work for a month or two amongst the devastated villages':

I have had a fine three years' work with the Unit, and from one point of view it is a grievous business finishing it up and severing connections with one's fellow workers. But the experience will always be something worth remembering. My new work is to be under the American Fund for French Wounded which now really means work among the refugees. I am to be taken to

Cambrai next week with a bed and a few household utensils and a dispensary outfit, and, I think, a nurse and an 'aide' are to accompany me. We are to set ourselves up in a ruined village called Caudry, somewhere near Cambrai, and make that our HQ and work other villages from there – giving material as well as medical aid. There are already some workers in Cambrai, so I hope to find out from them how to proceed. It will be rather an 'adventure' and I hope I shall be able to carry on alright. At present the people are coming back to their district, and there is practically nothing for them to set up house with, even if they have sufficient shelter. But in some districts already things are looking up a bit I am told – French doctors coming back and transport getting better, so help from the Allies will not be needed much longer.[26]

After all the adventure, excitement and freedom of their lives at Royaumont some of the orderlies were reluctant to return to a more mundane life at home. Some, like Dr Courtauld, worked for a time in the devastated areas. Others went to join the Cologne Leave Club, where Lena Ashwell's Players were entertaining the occupying troops. Cicely Hamilton was there, and her reputation was still high at Royaumont.

Three orderlies – Lucy Cranage, Netta Stein and Grace Summerhayes – entered the London (Royal Free Hospital) School of Medicine for Women and subsequently qualified. Others continued to work for the SWH, some in the London office, some in the SWH hospital for tuberculosis patients at Sallanches, France, and some in SWH hospitals still functioning in Serbia. A number of orderlies obtained jobs in Paris, postponing their return to a possibly less exciting life at home. As Evelyn Proctor said, 'The Scottish women are very much sought after as we have a very good name and a good tone.' For her closure was

> ... desperately sad to think of and we all feel it most frightfully. Life here has been a wonderful experience and one never to be forgotten and funnily enough Royaumont has closed at the height of its fame, which is a good thing in its way.

She, for one, was now absolutely convinced of the quality of women doctors:

> I could not bear the idea of them at first but that was only from ignorance and prejudice – I expect the idea of women doctors seems awfully odd to you [her mother], specially such young ones, but they are a splendid lot of women out here and work frightfully hard all the time.

Like many of the orderlies, she had matured – 'Women must do more now.'[27]

Marie Descoings, the daughter of their 'own' general, who had been permitted to work as an orderly (foreigners were not normally employed), wrote with Gallic fervour of the 'deep regret' she felt at having to leave Royaumont:

> You cannot believe how grateful I am to all and what deep remembrance I keep in my heart. I have passed the happiest years of my life at Royaumont. The union was perfect, all the English were like sisters to me. France will never forget ...[28]

It was the treasurer, Mrs Laurie, who summed up the contribution of Royaumont to the war effort when she wrote:

> It seems curious that Royaumont is of the past. Despite the hard work and many discomforts it has had a wonderful and glorious record of war work, along with Villers-Cotterêts. I do not think even the Committee or public realize what extraordinary heroism and valour were displayed and hardships endured by the staff during the terrible retreat and ensuing weeks of work.[29]

And one patient, desperately ill, must surely have spoken for many when he said: '*Il y a des choses qui ne s'oublient pas*' – 'There are things that are never forgotten.'[30]

ॐ

The Hospital: An Assessment

The hospital at Royaumont was unique in many respects. Above all else, it was entirely staffed by women – apart from the two male chauffeurs employed at the beginning, the chef Michelet, the occasionial *mécanicien* (mechanic), and the *infirmiers* (unfit soldiers) who in the last two years helped to carry stretchers, deal with the rubbish, clean the 'cabinets' and do other unsavoury jobs – though female orderlies still had to do their share of the unpleasant tasks. A further unique aspect was that unlike other British voluntary hospitals, Royaumont was under the French Red Cross, and latterly under the French army; it had no connection with the British medical services. Again unlike other voluntary hospitals, during slacker times the unit at Royaumont treated civilian patients.

Royaumont was in continuous action throughout the war, from January 1915 to March 1919. At its peak it was the largest of the British voluntary hospitals in France, with 600 beds. Only the St John's Hospital at Etaples approached it in size with 520 beds, and, apart from St John's, it seems to have been the closest to the front line.

Royaumont and its advance hospital at Villers-Cotterêts were in due course classified as casualty clearing stations (CCSs). According to the official history,[1] these were 'the pivot on which the whole system of collecting and evacuating sick and wounded turned'. In the early years this was their primary function. Later, as the importance of early operative treatment came to be recognized, their function changed and by later 1917 they could hold casualties for up to a month before transferring them further back to the base. This new policy is thought to have saved many lives.

If one compares the work of British CCSs from later 1917 with the work done at Royaumont in the critical periods of 1918, one can see what an exceptionally formidable team Miss Ivens had gathered around her.

By 1918 the British CCSs were getting larger – up to 1200 beds (compare Royaumont at its peak – 600). During a battle, operations went on continuously day and night – as they did at Royaumont. The major difference was that the medical staff in the Royal Army Medical Corps (RAMC) could be supplemented if need be from base hospitals. This was not possible at Royaumont. Similarly, base hospitals could send forward more orderlies for stretcher-bearing and other duties. At Royaumont orderlies and chauffeurs had to carry on regardless. In the British CCSs they worked a shift system: for the first 24 hours of a battle they worked in the theatre continuously for 16 hours; this was followed by eight hours off; subsequently they worked 12 hours on, 12 hours off. This was a far cry from the hours worked by the Royaumont women. For instance in the Somme rush (Chapter Four) several had no more than 16 hours' sleep in eight days – and three hours' consecutive sleep was an almost unbelievable luxury.

In the RAMC the record number of operations carried out in 24 hours was held by No. 3 CCS in August 1917. This was 103 – and the maximum was seldom over 80. Operations were carried out by a team of 12 to 16 surgeons. Compare this with the number of operations and staff available to carry them out at Royaumont in 1918. For example:

7–8 April (24 hours): 80 operations performed.
Between 23 March and 23 April: 437 patients admitted; 369 operations performed.
Between 31 May and 30 June: 1240 admitted; 891 operations performed.

In April there were 12 doctors in all, shared between the two hospitals. In May there were 14, and in June, when the two hospitals were combined in the abbey, there were 16. Of these, 11 were surgeons.

In the British army a scheme was evolved whereby any one CCS was required to admit a total of 150 cases when a battle commenced. When that total was reached, all further casualties were switched to another CCS in the area, so the staff of the first could concentrate on follow-up treatment. A further improvement was then made, whereby two adjoining CCSs shared the first 200 cases, so that both were fully occupied from the beginning of the battle, and not sitting idle while the other filled up. There was no relief of this sort at Royaumont. The flow of casualties remained continuously high for at least a month after the withdrawal from Villers-Cotterêts. As they evacuated patients, they filled up again immediately. The casualties received at Royaumont and at Villers-Cotterêts were as serious as any that reached a CCS.

There seems to be no record of how many of the medical staff in the British forces broke down under the strain. Given the intensity of work at Royaumont in 1918, it would have been surprising if there had been no breakdowns, especially as there were no relief arrangements – unlike in the RAMC. That there were only three who broke down is a tribute to the remarkable stamina demonstrated by the majority. Some of the women probably did not realize themselves how much stamina they had. Certainly they made it difficult for sceptics to maintain that women were too weak for the heaviest demands in wartime conditions. Miss Ivens herself was a perfect example of stamina in the face of great challenges, but there were also others, particularly Miss Nicholson – on whom fell, with Miss Ivens, the greatest burden of the major surgery.

The total number of patients treated between Royaumont and Villers-Cotterêts was 10,861. Of these, 8752 were soldiers, among whom there were 159 deaths: a death rate of 1.82 per cent. In all, 572 civilians were admitted, and a further 1537 were treated as outpatients. Of those admitted, 25 (4.5 per cent) died. They were probably older, less fit and less well-fed than the soldiers.

Although the great majority of soldier patients were battle casualties, there was also a range of other conditions requiring surgical treatment. At intervals there were some admitted sick. Among the civilian patients, women and children predominated, and some small rooms were set aside for them if admission was required. There was also the occasional civilian casualty from the munitions factories (Madeleine in 1916 was one of these).

Compared to today, during World War One medical science could do relatively little for the battlefield casualty. The type of injury had changed from previous wars: more wounds from shrapnel and machine-gun fire, and fewer from single bullets or hard steel. New techniques had to be learned. Moreover the conditions in which wounds were received had not been met in previous wars, or indeed in any of the other theatres of war in 1914–1919. The well-manured and heavily contaminated soil of northern France – all too often a sea of mud – harboured the bacteria responsible for gas gangrene, tetanus and streptococcal infection, to mention only the most deadly. How to deal with these and other infections was one of the most urgent tasks facing the medical services in that pre-antibiotic era.

The use of antiseptics against bacterial infection was soon abandoned as it proved positively harmful. Various fluids, delivered through tubes, were used for the continuous irrigation of wounds. At Royaumont they experimented with a number of different fluids, all of which were being used in the British army, and after extensive trials settled on their own preference of 5 per cent saline with 2.5 per cent carbolic acid. The surgeons at Royaumont soon learned the importance of various techniques, especially the excision of damaged tissue and the free drainage of wounds, all to be carried out as early as possible.

Anaesthetics were usually open ether, or sometimes chloroform, though later on nitrous oxide and oxygen were used. The relief of pain was generally inadequate: aspirin, morphia or a general anaesthetic were all the surgeons at Royaumont (and elsewhere) had to offer. They followed a routine of frequently replacing dressings, which must have been very painful – nowadays such a frequency might be considered excessive and possibly unnecessary. Their surgical techniques would appear to have been of a high standard, and they earned the respect of medical visitors and inspectors.

The surgeons at Royaumont realized the importance of following new developments – Miss Ivens recalled later how they all studied Sir Robert Jones's classical paper on the treatment of fractures, and how it was referred to again and again. They all became adept in the use of the Thomas's splint, which did so much not only to promote healing of lower-limb fractures, but also to reduce pain and mortality. Miss Ivens recalled their distress when a consignment of badly needed Thomas's splints finally arrived – only to find they were all children's sizes.[2] In training the staff, Miss Ivens was careful to emphasize the importance of avoiding pressure so as to prevent the worst consequences of gas gangrene. The doctors were encouraged to follow their patients to the x-ray department whenever possible to learn, among other things, the way to detect gas in the tissues. When a new technique of 'primary suture' of wounds was introduced by the French Professor Tuffier in 1918, Miss Ivens adopted it in very carefully selected cases. This technique depended not only on very meticulous bacteriology but also on close observation and very sound judgement.

'Masseuses' (the old term for physiotherapists) were employed from the autumn of 1915 until January 1919, and they came under the supervision of Dr Savill (who was also responsible for the x-ray department). Their techniques were less evolved than those employed today. Certain forms of electrotherapy were used for the stimulation of damaged muscles and nerves; and movement, both active and passive, was encouraged. Mrs Berry was recognized as being particularly skilful and patient in the manipulation of damaged fingers and restoring movement. Where apparatus could not be provided, they improvised – for example, by utilizing an old treadle sewing machine and a dwarf harmonium to create an apparatus for actively exercising the leg muscles.

It is difficult to judge the quality overall of the nursing care. In the beginning a number of the nurses could not adapt themselves to the very different work – and working conditions – of a hospital in the unforeseen conditions of wartime. However, the quality of nurses showed a steady improvement as time went on, although recruitment of new nurses became increasingly difficult in the last year of the war, when nurses were in very short supply everywhere. Miss Ivens met some of these difficulties by appointing the best and most intelligent of her orderlies to be auxiliary nurses, and this was highly successful. Throughout there were always some senior nurses who were of very high quality; they worked particularly well in the rushes of 1916 and the prolonged stress of 1918. Many of these went on after the war to rise high in the nursing profession. We know that the medical documentation of the wounded was carried out meticulously, as Dr Henry included many nursing charts in the MD thesis she wrote after the war on gas gangrene,[3] and Miss Ivens was careful to ensure that vital medical records were sent back to Royaumont when it became clear that evacuation from Villers-Cotterêts was imminent.

One aspect of nursing care must have been a real problem for the nurses in 1918. Dr MacRae (née Summerhayes), looking back in her 99th year to her time as an orderly in 1918, felt that though the surgery at Royaumont was excellent, the hygiene was not. This is not very surprising when one remembers the rapid flow of desperately wounded patients in May, June and July of that year. The shortage of linen became acute, and she remembers having to put new arrivals in the bloodstained sheets of the previous occupant.[4] However, in quieter periods Royaumont was famous for its cleanliness and order.

Training of the staff was taken seriously. It was particularly successful in the x-ray department. Vera Collum, a freelance journalist on her arrival, only had experience as an amateur photographer to offer, but became a highly skilled technician, especially in the localization of foreign bodies. G.L. Buckley was an undergraduate at Cambridge and had partially completed her medical training when she came to Royaumont and worked in the x-ray department. After the war and completion of her training she became a distinguished radiologist, and during the Second World War served in the RAMC as a consultant. Her experience at Royaumont probably determined her future career. Other x-ray orderlies were singled out for praise by Dr Savill and Miss Stoney as 'excellent', and in the laboratory Dr Dalyell had a high opinion of Maud Smieton, her orderly assistant.

⁂

Probably the most important contribution to the treatment of battle casualties made by the women doctors at Royaumont was in the field of gas gangrene. They showed how cooperation between physician, surgeon, bacteriologist and radiologist, combined with the use of specific anti-gas gangrene sera, could combat wound infection of this type with success. They could not have done this without the enthusiastic cooperation of Professor Weinberg of the Pasteur Institute in Paris, who was widely recognized as the leading authority on the bacteriology of gas-gangrene infections. Royaumont first came to the attention of Professor Weinberg in 1915, and he was so impressed with the efficiency of the hospital, and in particular the laboratory work, that he selected it as one of the hospitals in which his new sera were to be tried out as they were developed. He had, he said, 'seen hundreds and hundreds [an exaggeration, surely!] of military hospitals, but none, the organization and direction of which won his admiration so completely'.

From the outbreak of the war, Professor Weinberg had devoted himself to the study of the anaerobic organisms of gas gangrene. His researches threw new light on the complicated bacteriology of these organisms. The next step was to prepare specific anti-gas gangrene sera appropriate to the different organisms and to evolve a suitable mixture for use in the field. This work occupied him for the next twenty years. He had great confidence in the ability of women doctors, a confidence that was fully justified. On their part they were alert to the fact that they were privileged to receive supplies of specific sera, and they recognized they had an obligation to record carefully the results of treatment. Miss Ivens herself published two papers in the medical press.[5,6]

As has been mentioned, infection of wounds by gas gangrene was particularly common in France, where the heavily manured soil of the battlefields contained high concentrations of the organisms responsible. In addition, the nature of the injuries (from high-explosive shells and multiple injuries from machine-gun fire) resulted in soil and clothing, as well as metallic fragments, being driven deep into the tissues, where they formed a focus of infection. Soon after the outbreak of hostilities the British GHQ issued a circular alerting the medical services to the condition, as it became clear that gas-gangrene infection was going to be a serious problem, and one with which few medical officers would be familiar.[7]

The infection spreads rapidly after injury, and symptoms include crepitation (crackling or popping sounds) in the tissues indicating gas formation, discolouration of muscle, bronzing of the skin, oedema (swelling), and exudation of a foul-smelling fluid. Death of the tissues (gangrene) follows. The patient suffers vomiting, often severe, and collapse. Death follows rapidly once the infection is established. One of the most distressing features is that the mind remains perfectly clear until near the end. Dr Henry described the mood of the victim as 'often one of abnormal cheerfulness'.[8] Writing in 1916, Dr Savill commented:

> The most terrible of all the horrors which come under the care of the surgeon in this war is undoubtedly gas gangrene. Dramatic in the suddenness of its onset, the rapidity of its advance, and the repulsiveness of its too frequently fatal outcome, it has reaped a cruel harvest of our young and vigorous manhood.[9]

A procedure was gradually developed at Royaumont whereby, on admission, cases were examined by one of the assistant medical officers, and case sheets started, with records of temperature and pulse. Clothes were removed or cut off, wounds cleaned, and cases graded according to their apparent severity. Smears were taken from every wound and sent immediately to the laboratory for examination. The presence of gram-positive bacteria was reported back to the receiving ward as this indicated the presence of anaerobic, and possibly gas-gangrene, infection. Final identification of the organism took longer, but treatment could not wait for a final identification. If gas gangrene was evident on admission but there was delay in getting the patient to the theatre, serum was administered in the receiving ward. Otherwise it was given via intramuscular or subcutaneous injection in the theatre once the patient was anaesthetized. Cardiac stimulants were also given, and sometimes rectal or intravenous saline (blood was not available). The wounds were fully opened up, foreign bodies removed (shell fragments, pieces of cloth, loose pieces of bone, damaged muscle and blood clots) and drainage established using Carrell's tubes.

Smears were taken from all the material removed and sent to the laboratory. Subsequently films and cultures were sent to the Pasteur Institute in Paris. To reduce cross-infection as far as possible, one theatre was reserved for the most severely infected cases, another for the less severe, and a third for those in whom gas gangrene was only a possibility.

The choice of serum depended partly on what was available at the time. The serum produced by Weinberg and his colleague Séguin (W and S) was active against *Clostridium perfringens* (*C. welchii*), *C. septicum* and *C. novyi* (*C. oedematiens*). The alternative serum, that of Leclanche and Vallée (L and V) was effective for the first two of these, but not for *C. novyi*. It had the advantage, however, of having some anti-streptococcal effect. Streptococcal infection was an extremely serious complication, and on occasions death was due to a streptococcal septicaemia after gas gangrene had been brought under control. Sometimes both sera were used. If a follow-up operation was necessary, it was always preceded by a repeat injection of serum, and repeat doses as long as necessary.

The x-ray appearances were described by the chief radiologist, Dr Agnes Savill.[10] She analysed 100 plates of gas-gangrene cases all taken during the summer of 1916 at Royaumont. By the end of July (the Somme rush having started at the beginning of the month) she was able to conclude that the presence of gas, its extent and situation as seen on the x-ray, was of great value to the surgeon. By September she was able to report on the probable variety of gas infection by x-ray appearances alone – information that could be of value before bacteriological examinations were complete. This was significant, as often at this stage the presence of gas was not detected clinically.

In 1916 Miss Ivens published her first report, already mentioned, in which she analysed her cases from 1915 to October 1916. She described clearly the different types of gas infection she had observed and the operative and post-operative techniques she used, which must have been of great value to new doctors joining the forces. Anti-sera were then very scarce, but she obtained sufficient to treat ten very seriously infected cases, all of whom might be expected to be fatal. Of these, five died, one from a septicaemia after the gas infection had subsided.

By 1918 the development of specific anti-sera had advanced, and Miss Ivens was able to test her belief in the value of the preventive use of sera.[11] Between 21 March and 6 September 1918, 3660 wounded were operated on, and 433 cases of gas infection, all severe, were treated. These 433 seriously infected cases were treated with different combinations of sera. There were 38 deaths, only seven of which were due to gas gangrene. Of these seven, three also had a streptococcal septicaemia, in itself a fatal condition.

In her MD thesis on the serum treatment of gas gangrene infections[12], Dr Henry compared the period 1915 to 1917, when serum treatment was in its infancy, with 1918, by which time it had become much more developed. Comparing similar cases – fractured tibia and fibula – there were 40 cases in the earlier period with three deaths and 12 amputations. In 1918, out of 107 similar cases, there were five deaths, only one of which was due to gas gangrene; there were 10 amputations, six of which were due to gas gangrene.

A third series of patients from Royaumont were reported to a French medical society in 1918.[13] Out of 1666 severely wounded patients admitted in June and July 1918, 155 were treated with anti-gas gangrene serum; 16 of these died, but not one of these was attributable to gas gangrene. During the same period there were eight deaths from gas infection, all of which occurred in patients who had not received serum owing to shortage of supplies.

From all this data one can conclude that the results of serum treatment reported from Royaumont compare favourably with others reported from French hospitals. Royaumont also had a great advantage over the British medical services, who only obtained sera towards the end of the war, and their sera were of far lower efficiency.

❦

If the hospital at Royaumont had an advantage over British hospitals in the treatment of gas gangrene, it was at a disadvantage regarding blood transfusion. By 1917 blood-transfusion services were slowly becoming organized in the RAMC, but not by the

French medical services, and it was on the French that the hospital had to rely. They were forced to use less effective forms of fluid replacement, though they did seem to have realized its importance.

Apart from the purely medical and surgical treatment, some of the good results that were obtained at Royaumont could have been due, in part, to the generally happy atmosphere, the beauty and peace of that lovely building and the woods surrounding it. Navarro wrote, 'and when evening has come, a night of silence and of stars – the soothing babble of the fountain lulling the nerveracked sufferers to sleep'.[14] (Navarro, of course, was writing in 1917, before the nightly visits of the Gothas in 1918 rendered the abbey less peaceful.)

Open-air treatment was a feature of Royaumont. Another factor that probably contributed to the recovery of the patients was the excellence of the food. There were shortages, of course, from time to time, but overall the patients were probably far better fed than in almost any other hospital. Some, at least, of the credit, must go to Michelet, who was not only an excellent chef, but also a bit of a genius at finding supplies.

On the outbreak of war French services for the collection, transport and treatment of the wounded were very defective. The French had envisaged a short war and were totally unprepared for the scale of the casualties. Compared with the British and German armies, over the whole period of the war the French experienced the highest ratio of deaths among the wounded. In addition to 895,000 men killed in action, almost half as many again died from wounds or sickness.

In France public concern rose steadily over the appallingly bad facilities for treating the wounded. This reached a climax in August 1915 when a debate took place in the Chamber of Deputies, a debate that almost precipitated a political crisis. The arrangements for dealing with the casualties from the Battle of the Marne in 1914 were described as 'most casual'. An example was given where 1200 wounded men were sent to a place where there was not a single bed to receive them. There were no hospital trains, only cattle trucks, and journeys could take days. Hospital equipment was hopelessly inadequate. Linen, clothing, instruments and appliances were all in short – very short – supply. Hospital orderlies had no training, and no effort was made to heat the wards. Medical officers were desperate. They were totally dependent on the Medical Department of the War Office. One senior officer received a reply from a lay official in the department – 'Your demands are justified in principle, but they are too numerous, and will end by trying the patience of the minister.' The debate continued the following week when the minister claimed that improvements had been made. The deputies seem to have been unconvinced and endorsed the principle that 'the less non-medical ministers meddled with professional details, the better'. The debate was clearly becoming uncomfortable for the government. It was continued the following week, but this time was held in camera.[15]

After this disastrous beginning, as the war progressed many improvements did occur in the French medical services. The story of Royaumont shows how greatly it was valued by the French doctors administering the services in the field, not only for the work it did but also for the example it set.

It was fortunate for Royaumont that it had a determined, effective and conscientious committee behind it to keep the supplies flowing, often with great difficulty. Naturally there were some shortages from time to time, but the records do not suggest that these were ever as desperate as those suffered by the French military hospitals.

The committee at home learned to appreciate the valuable work being carried out on their behalf at Royaumont. In September 1916 Dr Erskine, a medical member of the committee, wrote:

To begin with, we would emphasize to the Committee the magnificent quality of the work that is being done at the Hospital. On all sides we found that this was cordially recognized by the French authorities. Over and over again, the Officers of the Service de Santé have expressed their pleased surprise at the number of limbs that have been saved from amputation – and at the numbers of men who recover. They show their appreciation by sending into the hospital the very serious cases that it would be dangerous to send further.

During the recent advance of the French all the severe cases of gas gangrene were sent in to Royaumont somewhat to the astonishment of some of the Paris hospitals. Many of these cases were saved by the prompt and skilful treatment they received, the percentage of recovery being wonderfully high considering the severity of the condition.[16]

One of the objects of Dr Erskine's visit was to investigate if there was needless extravagance. She reported that in this supposition, which she had shared, she was mistaken:

... I think the Committee can discount the prevalent rumours of extravagance as being without foundation. That the hospital is expensive to run is, unfortunately, true, but the conditions render this inevitable. The initial error lay in fixing on such a building which, though beautiful in the extreme, has certain disadvantages when considered as a hospital. The following are instances:

1. The fact that no hot water is laid on throughout the house – that ward utensils etc have to be carried sometimes considerable distances to be emptied and cleansed, thus entailing much labour and a much larger staff than would otherwise be required.
2. That there are no lifts of any sort, so that all food has to be carried from the kitchens by hand, and all patients carried on stretchers up and down stairs when required for operation or for x-ray examination.
3. That to keep the place tolerably warm a large expenditure of fuel is necessary.
4. That the distance from a railway station and the fact that the hospital is situated in a military zone, further enhances the price of supplies which are even dearer than in the country.

On the other hand the advantages of the place must not be forgotten. The extreme beauty of the surroundings – the spacious airiness of the wards – the facilities for open-air treatment, are points of great value and are in strong contrast to the conditions prevailing in other hospitals in the vicinity. No doubt all of these contribute to the success that has attended the work of the staff.

She saw no way to reduce expenditure – in fact she expected it to rise:

I had to revolutionize my ideas as to the amount of dressings required. I have to admit that I was quite mistaken in my estimate. I went round the wards of the various doctors and saw the majority of the cases being dressed and certainly could discover no waste . . . But the amount of dressings required by these extremely septic cases was certainly a revelation to me. The conditions I found were not at all comparable to anything in this country . . . The Committee have to bear in mind that the work done is probably on a much larger scale and of greater value than that done in any of the other SWH Units. This arises from the circumstances and must in no way be taken as implying any disparagement of the other units.[17]

Reflecting on the hospital in 1928, one member of the unit wrote:

Women's work will be judged, not by the bravery of the women and their readiness to face danger and death, but by its economic results – by the number of men their hospitals were able to restore to the effective forces, whether in the army or in the militarized industry, for a given number of days of hospitalization and for a given expenditure of money and personnel. We do not boast when we claim that Royaumont, from this point of view, is in a unique position of having functioned uninterruptedly from 1914 to 1919, and hence of providing the only data that will be of any value to posterity as an example of consistent evolution and well-tested efficiency during an entire campaign.[18]

꒰

The Women

Although many of the staff of the hospital have been encountered as the narrative has unfolded, it has not always been possible to fill in all the details of their personal histories. It is fitting to end the book by remedying some of these omissions.

Miss Frances Ivens,
CBE, MS (Lond), ChM (Liverp), FRCOG (1870–1944)

'*Quels yeux, quel esprit, quelle femme*' – 'What eyes, what spirit, what a woman.' These words, spoken by a French general at the end of a visit to Royaumont, sum up the very remarkable woman at the head of a very remarkable hospital.[1] But what of her life before Royaumont, and her career afterwards? What kind of woman was she? And what did her friends and colleagues think of her?

Mary Hannah Frances Ivens was born in 1870, the fifth and youngest surviving child of William Ivens and his wife Elizabeth (née Ashmole). Her father was a successful timber merchant, while her mother was 'beautiful, lively and gay, and full of go', but sadly died of consumption when Frances was only seven. A close and lifelong friend wrote of Frances when she was 13 as 'heavily built, large and unattractive in appearance'.[2] As a young woman she was reckoned to be less good-looking than her sisters, but 'very attractive, interested, keen and intelligent'.[3] Photographs taken during the First World War show her to be a very handsome woman – her sisters must have been really exceptional.

As a girl, Frances attended a number of undistinguished schools and showed no special distinction except for French, in which she passed second in all England in the Oxford Senior Certificate. At the age of 20 she was living at home with her father, to whom she was closely attached, when he suddenly 'announced to the family at the mid-day meal his intention to marry again. They were eating bread-and-butter pudding (he evidently let them enjoy their first course happily), a pudding Frances could not bear to touch again. The shock was terribly severe.'[4] William Ivens settled his first family in a house nearby while he, his new wife and, in due course, their two little girls continued in the original home.

Frances was a witness of her sister's unhappy marriage, and her close friend Lillie Robinson believed that this influenced her 'to put aside all idea of marriage for herself'. There was said to be 'a young man, a lawyer and brainy ... who evidently fell for her' whom she met at some relative's, but 'it came to nothing'.[5]

The family seemed to have been very happy at Pailton, the new house, just 'pottering about'. There was tennis, horse-riding and other country amusements, and Frances apparently excelled herself at a women's cricket match. Her friend Margaret Joyce described her at that time as 'a healthy girl with lovely brown eyes and beautiful teeth – I do not think she ever spent an idle moment. She was a keen gardener, played the organ at church, ran the village tennis club and other local enterprises, and entered eagerly into all the pursuits of the countryside – she drove a high-stepping Arab horse in a tall dog cart.'[6]

Frances did not seem to have had any idea of working until she met Margaret Joyce, who was a student at the London School of Medicine for Women. This seemed to have fired her with the idea of making a career for herself in medicine. 'When she told her family they all laughed aloud at the idea of her doing *anything*, but she did.'[7] She took her London Matriculation Examination and entered the London School of Medicine for Women (LSMW) in 1894 at the age of 24. During term-time she lived in College Hall, where she made some lifelong friends including Elizabeth Courtauld and the Lewin sisters, Octavia and Jessie Augusta (later Mrs Berry); both Berry and Courtauld served for long periods at Royaumont. In vacations Frances lived with her father's second family with whom she was on good terms. Her stepsisters Dora and Clare remember 'when she came home at Christmas or Easter or, indeed any time, she seemed to bring a strong breeze from outside. Frances always did energetic things, swept us out for long walks or "turned out" the attic. On one occasion they saw her rushing about saying "Where are my eyes?" Clare and I could not understand this but heard the butcher being blamed. Later we peeped through the dairy window and saw Frances standing at the sink, examining something in a bowl. She told us to run away. She was wearing a white surgical overall.' Dora sums up: 'She was very bright, lively, vivacious, ready to laugh and talk with anyone. So she was generally very popular.'[8]

At medical school she was 'a very happy student. Her brilliant examination results, and the important posts she was given show how hard she worked but then – as throughout her life – she entered with zest into the various activities and diversions of College life. She was elected "student representative", which office she filled with dignity on all formal occasions, and was a successful advocate when controversies arose between the authorities and the students.'[9]

Her fellow-student, Elizabeth Courtauld, remembered Frances as 'a fine student, never content till she had got to the bottom of any job she was doing. I remember watching her in the dissecting room one day and being so impressed by her patience and perseverance as she searched for a small nerve and not satisfied until she had traced it out from its origin to its end. She was a fine worker and determined to get on.'[10]

She qualified in 1900 with the London University gold medal in obstetrics, and honours in medicine and forensic medicine, and graduated MBBS with honours in 1902. In 1903 she became master of surgery – the third woman to achieve this degree. She furthered her experience in obstetrics and gynaecology in Vienna and Dublin. After early training posts in London she was appointed as consultant in gynaecology to the Liverpool Stanley Hospital, the first woman to hold an honorary post in Liverpool. Later she held another honorary post in the Liverpool Samaritan Hospital, and, after the war, at the Liverpool Maternity Hospital. She took a house where she held clinics for the babies of the poor – this was before infant welfare clinics were general.

After her arrival in Liverpool she became, as Dr Catherine Chisholm remembered, a 'protagonist in all our feminist struggles. She was the leader of our younger medical women whom she never ceased to spur on to further achievements. Much fighting for hospital posts was necessary then and Miss Ivens proved a magnificent leader. Manchester and Liverpool met and formed the North of England Medical Women's Society. Miss Ivens was always ready to go almost anywhere in the North ... to read papers for us or to help politically with advice – her social experience was a valuable asset for she took part in everything going on in Liverpool.'[11]

This was her life until the outbreak of war. She was then a woman of 44, highly respected in her profession, and playing a notable role in Liverpool and the women's movement.

On the outbreak of war she volunteered at once for service in Belgium, but had to return without landing because of the rapid German advance. Still determined to serve overseas, she volunteered for Dr Elsie Inglis's Scottish Women's Hospital then preparing for France. A medical woman wrote at the time, 'Elsie Inglis makes a habit of biting off more than any human being can chew – and then of finding other people to go and do the chewing for her.' Vera Collum later wrote:

> That, I think, sums up the history of the Royaumont Unit. No one but the founder could have bitten off such a big piece of military prejudice against the work of women in war. That is just her unique title to fame. The second magnificent thing she did was to find and send Miss Ivens to France to 'chew' this particular war project for her. 'More than any human being can chew.' It was. But – the Chief did it! Had there been no Elsie Inglis there would have been no Scottish Women's Hospitals. Had there been no Miss Ivens there would never have been a Royaumont. Royaumont – we are proud of it – was a success from start to finish and all through the four and a half years of its existence it was the Chief who made Royaumont. We only held up her hands.[12]

Preparations went on apace, but it was a measure of the quality of the woman that amid all the uncertainties of her immediate future she did not shirk her commitment to deliver the inaugural address to the LSMW students on 1 October 1914 on 'Some of the Essential Attributes of an Ideal Practitioner'. 'I am hoping,' she said, 'and I think it is not a forlorn hope, that it will not be long before there is a very decided public opinion formed, that it is not right for an able-bodied young woman, in whatever station of life, to eat the bread of idleness or to allow her brains to atrophy for lack of use.'[13] She placed high on her list the gift of imagination – 'it will enable the fortunate possessor to place herself in the position of those with whom she is brought in contact, and so to realize the facts of life as they affect another'. There were other attributes she commended to the students, but her final advice was 'to concentrate on work when you are working – unwearying sustained effort will be necessary. But above all do not neglect outside interests or limit your horizon, for one of your most difficult tasks is to learn how to deal with people.' And for the weaker students she had a word of encouragement: 'if unsuccessful be patient and persevering. There is a niche for you somewhere.'

How did Miss Ivens prepare herself for the great task ahead? Probably first and foremost in her mind would have been the very different surgery she would be called upon to undertake if, as these pioneers all fervently hoped, they would be called on to treat battle casualties. There was much reading to be done – and we know from the books she later donated to the Liverpool Medical Institution that she read widely on different types of injury. She would know, however, that experience would bring more knowledge, and the learning process would have to continue. She kept up with the new developments in the treatment of battle casualties as the war progressed and contributed to this herself, becoming a recognized authority on the treatment of gas gangrene (as discussed in Appendix One).

Miss Ivens was already an experienced administrator, and probably had little difficulty in that aspect of her work. She seems to have had considerable skills in problem-solving, as the history of Royaumont shows.

Miss Nicholson, her second in command, recalled her first
meeting with Miss Ivens, in December 1914, just before they
crossed over to France in that terrible storm:

My first impressions were of a retiring feeble woman, but I
was quite wrong and I found that she was suffering from
sinus trouble and a temperature. This was not improved by
the crossing, the worst known for years ... Very quickly I
found I had misjudged Miss Ivens' character when I saw how
she tackled the rather depressing situation which awaited us in
Paris. Starting as an unwanted unit under the French Red
Cross with a beautiful old abbey as hospital, but without heat,
light or sanitation, and equipment still on the seas, she set to
work to move all the possible influential powers, French and
English. Before long the hospital was ready for inspection by
high officials of the Red Cross. Never shall I forget our
disappointment when our two top wards were condemned ...
and we all, including our Médecin-Chef, had to move huge
pieces of furniture belonging to the owners from two large
rooms downstairs. Even then, before any soldiers arrived,
Miss Ivens had to tour the Casualty Clearing Stations in the
neighbourhood, and by persuasion of her powers of fascina-
tion she induced the commanding officers to send us cases.
The one hundred beds were soon filled and the hospital never
again lacked work.[14]

The chauffeur Edith Prance recalled Miss Ivens in the early days of
the hospital, when those who were there

... admired perhaps most of all her quiet courage and
persistence in overcoming the somewhat understandable
hesitation of the high French authorities, who would not
at first send high-skilled work to Royaumont. These women
surgeons, women doctors, were an innovation, they had still
to prove their technical and practical ability in a sphere which
they entered as total strangers. With infinite patience Miss
Ivens gave herself up to this wearying work. She went round

French war hospitals, speaking with her fellow professors, gradually permeating their minds with growing recognition of her high ability. Without her patient victory and winning of this trust, the Scottish Women's Hospital at Royaumont would never have made its way, and in this, very specially, she was the creator of what was to become a by-word all over France and far beyond, as one of the finest war hospitals on all the fronts.[15]

After the final closure of the hospital at Royaumont in March 1919 and a well-earned holiday, Miss Ivens returned to Liverpool and resumed her posts at the Stanley and Samaritan Hospitals, and also became a university lecturer in obstetrics and gynaecology. She was said to be a good teacher with an emphasis on the practical, and with the ability to draw the best out from those she taught. One of her students, Dr Hilda Cantrell, remembers her as 'a very charming person. She was very good-looking and carried herself well and wore beautiful clothes. She tried to remember everybody's name and particulars and if she didn't she worked round it until she found her way.'[16] She was involved in the planning of the new maternity hospital and helped to found the Crofton Recovery Hospital for Women (no longer existing) and the Liverpool Women's Radium League. She was already a member of the Liverpool Medical Institution, one of the oldest medical societies in the country, and in 1926 she became vice-president, the first woman to hold that position.[17]

Miss Ivens also played a leading role in the Medical Women's Federation (MWF), serving on the executive committee from 1921, and as president from 1924 to 1926. During this period the MWF was engaged in the battle for the status of women doctors and ensuring better medical services for women, particularly maternity services. In 1929 Liverpool University awarded Miss Ivens an honorary degree of Master of Surgery (ChM), and in the same year she was made a Commander of the British Empire.

After this double recognition she astonished all her friends by announcing her decision to marry. She was almost 60 years of age, but was ready to begin a new life. Her intended husband, Charles Matthew Knowles, was a barrister and widower, whom she had known since student days. Former members of the unit were thrilled. There must have been many of that generation who were unable to marry following the enormous loss of young men during the war years, and they revelled in the romance of their beloved chief. Fifteen Royaumont veterans flocked to Liverpool to form a guard of honour and shout 'Vive la Colonelle' as she came out:

> Every now and then we stole a glance at one another to make sure it was not all a dream. We are such creatures of habit. La Colonelle seemed to belong so exclusively to Royaumont, to sit so much apart, to be so entirely the supreme and unique head. And now, after two decades of professional work, at a time when she was beginning to toy with the idea of retiring from her honorary posts and her strenuous life in Liverpool, we had heard her, that very day, making solemn vows to obey...! And we had watched her go out on a new adventure, to start a new life, with as much zest as she had gone off to Royaumont in 1914.[18]

After her marriage, she lived in London for a few years, working, but probably less intensively than in Liverpool, until her husband's retirement, when they moved to Killagordon, near Truro, which had been the family home of his first wife and was now theirs. Here Mrs Ivens-Knowles, as she was now known, became a great gardener, devoting as much thoroughness to her garden as to all her other activities. She also took part in many public activities in her adopted county. She was a county medical officer for the Red Cross, head of the women's section of the Truro British Legion, and a governor of the High School. When war came in 1939 she became chairman of the Cornwall Committee of the Friends of the Fighting French, and played a leading role in initiating the Second World War activities of the Royaumont and Villers-Cotterêts Association both in Britain and in Canada with her old ally Dr Henry. She was active to the end, and died after a short illness in 1944 at the age of 73.

Such was the life of this remarkable woman. But what was she really like? There are many stories that could be told, but perhaps an overall impression can be gained from Vera Collum's speech at the first reunion dinner on 28 November 1919, when almost 100 members of the unit met to honour 'the Chief':

However did she achieve this superhuman success? Not by courting popularity. She never cared a tinker's curse whether we liked her or not. She did it always by putting the hospital first. She was ready to sacrifice us all to it. She was ready to work us to death for it. And when the call came we quite contentedly fell in with her views – and just let her! Why was it? Because we all knew our Chief never asked any of her staff to do anything or face anything that she would not do, endure or face herself. She beat us all into a cocked hat in endurance, in fortitude, in singleness of aim. The certainty, the ruthlessness, with which she went straight to her objective was the certainty, the ruthlessness of a tank. But now that the war is all over, we know that the objective was worth it – all France knows it, and pays her homage. I think no woman and few men in the Allied Medical Services worked so hard and so unremittingly as our Chief – or got so much work out of her staff! Few lived so simply. Very few preserved through those long four and a half years that extraordinarily sensitive human sympathy with the wounded men themselves. They all had implicit confidence not merely in her skill, but in her human understanding of their personal pains and fears. And yet, some of you who did not know the Chief very well, used to think her hard. She was – hard as Aberdeen granite on the outside, and it was a pretty thick outside. It had to be. How could she have gone on getting us to do impossibilities by simply ordering us to do them and then expecting them to happen, if she had not wrapped herself in a coat of steel? What I would like to make clear tonight is that some of those who knew her better – most of us who had known her in the beginning before the hospital got so big and unwieldy – had discovered that there was a very *human* human being inside.

Afterwards – well, her isolation was the isolation of a captain of a great battleship. The Chief, I grant you, could be a hard-hitting enemy. But – I can tell you that she can also be a very staunch friend ...[19]

Collum picked out several facets of her character that others who knew her enlarged upon. First, there was her very human understanding towards her patients. 'They were not so astonished at their own particular "doctoresse" being interested in them,' wrote an unnamed orderly, 'but that "La Colonelle" should know and name them ... always amazed them.' She continues:

It was small wonder they loved her. During one of the worst rushes of 1918, a boy was brought in with a dreadful leg, and as gas gangrene had set in, amputation was necessary. The poor lad, however, was too far gone, and there was no hope. He knew he was dying, and kept asking for 'la Colonelle'. Sister eventually went down to see if Miss Ivens could spare time to come and see the boy. Miss Ivens had been operating night and day for days past and, as it happened, was just going to rest for half an hour. But she came to the ward and sat with the boy, doing everything for him herself till he died.[20]

Dr Henry recalls how she would get up in the middle of the night to bestow a medal on a dying *blessé*.[21]

Miss Ivens was always eager to supply amusements for the men – for this she had the enthusiastic support of her unit, which always seemed to include a number of extremely gifted people. With Cicely Hamilton and the willing assistance of the two cooks she organized splendid Christmas festivities. She also made a point, whenever she could, of attending the parties that were such a feature of life at Royaumont. Her care for the morale of her staff was constant. Right at the beginning, in December 1914, she helped them get over their deep discouragement when the hospital failed the first inspection by the Service de Santé.

Inevitably there were problems that sometimes arose between the different nationalities under her care, and she handled these with great diplomacy. Navarro relates how on one occasion she was summoned to the top of a cold staircase where a proud Algerian had stubbornly installed himself because a Frenchman in the next bed had called him a pig. She never scolded, but sorted out the problem quietly, with tact, and to everyone's satisfaction.[22] Her second-in-command Ruth Nicholson wrote of her 'social charm and tact, as well as her indomitable character and boundless energy which carried her through all obstructions'.[23]

We saw some evidence of Miss Ivens's 'hardness' in her annoyance and impatience with those sisters who in 1917 protested to the committee about advertising for nurses who were not fully trained. She perhaps saw their dissatisfaction as a threat to the smooth working of her beloved hospital; nevertheless, her attitude does seem unsympathetic to a body of women who had not yet achieved even the limited measure of security in their profession that medical women were just beginning to win for themselves.

According to her (non-Royaumont) friend Dr Chisholm, Miss Ivens had a 'forceful personality, refused to have any fools around her and had a unique power of stimulation'.[24] Some thought she lacked a sense of humour – others strongly denied this. According to Norah Mackay, who was a clerk at Royaumont, 'what endeared her so much to us all, and especially to the orderlies, was her sense of humour, for she would laugh wholeheartedly at all our vagaries'.[25] She had a gift for friendship, and after the war she spent many holidays, chiefly in France, in the company of old Royaumont colleagues, and she maintained links with her French friends.

Her generosity was great, much of it known only to the committee at home. She repeatedly refused the increases of salary offered her and was prepared to dip into her own pocket to retain the services of the two chauffeurs who could no longer afford to work as volunteers. She was generous in providing champagne and splendid food (when possible) for special occasions. After the war, in 1922, she attended the unveiling of the monumant at Royaumont to commemorate those who had died in the hospital. When she discovered that the young Belgian sculptor who had created the monument had given his services free, she asked the committee to send him the amount they had budgeted for her personal expenses.[26]

The admiration of her staff has been described in many different ways. 'She made it her business to know everyone in the hospital from the oldest hand to the latest inarticulate new-comer.'[27] She knew which of them was working well, but she could also detect the slacker. A few she sent home as unsuitable, but she fought hard to retain the chauffeurs in whom she had great confidence, and did not hesitate to voice strongly her differences with the committee. To the orderlies she was 'Auntie' or sometimes 'Fanny', but we may be sure this was behind her back. As we have seen, the French – for whom she represented a totally new kind of woman – admired her greatly. For example, the French *directeur* stationed in the abbey described her as '*une femme tout-à-fait supérieure*' ('an altogether superior sort of woman').

Vera Collum was speaking for the whole unit when she described Miss Ivens at the first reunion dinner as 'so entirely the supreme and unique head'. She had, Collum maintained, 'a genius for scrounging talent and holding on to it'. 'Our Chief led gallantly and greatly,' she said, concluding, 'Her lexicon knew no such word as fail.'[28]

Dr Elizabeth Courtauld,
LSA (1901), MD Brux. (1903) (1867–1947)

As the oldest member of the staff at Royaumont, Dr Elizabeth Courtauld was one of those pioneers who at the close of the 19th century began to realize the possibility that there could be careers in medicine for women. She thus represents an important part of medical history.

Elizabeth Courtauld came from a well-known Huguenot family who had settled in Essex, where they founded a large and successful silk business. Her family had a strong tradition of social responsibility. In 1858, for example, one member of the family (a woman) founded a day nursery, a hostel and a night school for women working in the local silk factory.[1] Elizabeth's father, George Courtauld, founded the Halstead General Hospital in

1884. Elizabeth herself was a generous benefactor of the hospital and to many good causes locally and nationally.

The third child in a family of nine, Elizabeth was born on 2 December 1867. When she began her diary at the age of 16 her mother was dead. She had completed her formal education at a school in Wimbledon and was then living at home, where she had some private tuition. She refers to lessons in botany, music, drawing, geography, French, German, geology, 'sums' and Euclid. Apart from her occasional lessons she led a life that must have been very common for girls living in well-off families in rural communities, and one that was not dissimilar to that led by Frances Ivens before she considered a career in medicine. Social events, gardening, 'doing the flowers', tennis, reading and card games filled her time, but a certain rather endearing enthusiasm lightens the earnestness of many of her diary entries. She was 16 when she wrote: 'I ran nine times round the garden without stopping', and 'went on the common and jumped'.[2]

Three years later, when she was 19, she took up her diary again. She still had music and drawing lessons, but now she was also housekeeping and teaching the younger children. Sometimes, however, she just 'muddled about'. Visits to London for concerts and theatres were highlights in her life.

The pattern was broken when she was 21. Her father suddenly announced his intention to marry again. She said little, but for the next few weeks the diary entries were brief or absent altogether. 'Did not go out' or 'in bed all day'. Soon after the wedding, which she did not attend, she went off to friends in Germany for a month.

On her return home she began classes in nursing, physiology and 'ambulance' (but 'forgot to go'). She bought a clinical thermometer, learned bandaging, heard lectures on digestion and psychology, and went up to St Thomas's Hospital to 'discuss nursing plans'. Nothing seems to have come of this. Instead she went back to Germany on a prolonged visit. There she had a merry time skating, snowballing, sledging ('many tumbles but very exciting'). There was also plenty of dancing – 'Had plenty of partners – not in bed till four.' Then after Christmas she began serious nursing studies at the Deaconess's Institute of Kaiserswerth (now part of Düsseldorf), where Florence Nightingale had gone many years earlier on a similar search for practical nursing experience. She worked hard, improved her German and enjoyed life.

After a year on the Continent she returned home. A diary entry records: 'Talk about my being a doctor. Ways and means.'[3] Dr Courtauld later told Dr Henry that her father had strongly disapproved.[4] She seems to have renounced the idea (this was in 1890) and instead began to attend the local hospital regularly, helping where she could, and finally came to a decision to follow a career in nursing. In January 1891 she began work in Cheltenham Hospital, where she remained for the next four and a half years.

The next we hear of Elizabeth Courtauld is on her entering the London School of Medicine for Women (LSMW) in the autumn of 1895. She was now 28 years old – but she had finally reached her goal of committing herself to a medical career.

At the LSMW Frances Ivens and Augusta Lewin (known at Royaumont as Mrs Berry) were her fellow students. Elizabeth and Frances had adjoining rooms in the student hostel and shared their cocoa in the evenings after the day's work.[5] They had much in common – similar backgrounds, a search for a more fulfilling life that had led them towards a career in medicine, and a shared experience of a dearly loved father's second marriage.

Elizabeth Courtauld qualified in 1901 by sitting for the licentiate of the Society of Apothecaries, which entitled her to be entered on the Medical Register. She followed this with a Brussels MD in 1903 (she did not have the necessary qualifications to sit for the London University degree.) After qualification she worked as a junior doctor in the New Hospital for Women (later known as the Elizabeth Garrett Anderson Hospital), and as an assistant anaesthetist at the Royal Free Hospital. Her experience in anaesthetics later proved invaluable at Royaumont. Her next move was to southern India, where she worked at the Church of England Zenana Mission Hospital in Bangalore. Apart from her war service she spent the remainder of her professional life there. She described herself as 'an independent worker, not a missionary'.

She loved her work in India, where there was greater scope for medical women to use their training and talents than was often possible at home. In 1909, after a difficult night's work, she wrote of the satisfaction she experienced: 'A successful maternity case, followed by an Indian sunrise, makes life very well worth living.'[6] In 1924 she was still urging young women to go out to India: 'Until the coming of the English lady doctor millions of women living under the purdah system "just suffered".'[7] She was on leave from India when Miss Ivens invited her to join the unit at Royaumont, where she worked from January 1916 to March 1919.

A devout Anglican, at Royaumont she conducted the daily morning service for staff in the St Louis Chapel until this had to be abandoned in the rush of work in 1918.[8] It was she who conducted the funeral services in the local cemetery when a Protestant clergyman could not be found.

'With her white hair and gold eyeglasses,'[9] she became one of the members of the unit best loved by the staff and by the patients. She was affectionately teased by the younger members, as recounted by Orderly Minchin, who had the task of doing the make-up for those participating in the Armistice festivities:

When Miss Courtauld was told that make-up was necessary for the plays she refused point-blank. I told the others to 'talk her round'. Finally she consented, and I went to her room to do the deed *in private*. I explained that under powerful lights, if she had none on, she would look very ill indeed. So, with a mirror firmly grasped in her hand, I started. When I got to the rouge and the lipstick my impatient protegee kept backing her head away and shuddering at the very idea – but – *I got it on.*[10]

Ruth Nicholson remembered Dr Courtauld's first appearance at Royaumont in January 1916:

A quiet little grey woman with spectacles half way down her nose. Soon she made her way into all our hearts by her kindness, her understanding, her unselfishness, her sense of humour, and, above all, her simplicity, and had bestowed on her the well-loved name of 'Mammie'. Whenever there was any work, unspectacular, rather dull but necessary, of the nature of filling the breach, she volunteered to do it and did it well. And yet she was shrewd and practical and full of common sense and so respected she was never imposed upon. ... I remember her thoughtfulness when I first settled in practice in Birkenhead and was trying to make ends meet and she insisted on coming as a (very profitable) paying guest for some weeks. It is not everyone who knows how to use riches in the unostentatious way which she had mastered.[11]

Dr Potter, one of the surgeons, knew her work at first hand. She wrote:

> ... although frail physically she was always at work and took practically no time off – she did not object to other medical officers taking time off but was merely mildly surprised that they should want to do so.[12]

Dr Henry remembered her as 'that sweet woman'. 'E.C. was amazing – looking so frail yet a tower of strength. In times of stress when a convoy of badly wounded arrived we had to work in the operating theatre without let-up until all was done. E.C. was our chief anaesthetist and she could outstrip many of the younger colleagues when they were visibly tiring after long hours.'[13]

After leaving Royaumont and working for a time in the devastated areas of northern France, Dr Courtauld returned to her beloved hospital in Bangalore until her retirement in 1927. She died on 26 December 1947, shortly after her 80th birthday.

Dr (Mrs) Agnes Savill,
MA, MD (Glasgow), FRCPI (1875–1964)

Dr Agnes Savill was one of the original group of women doctors who went out to Royaumont at the beginning of December 1914, and shared in its many vicissitudes throughout the war. A woman of great intellectual brilliance, charm and vitality, she contributed much in the way of professional expertise, often at great personal sacrifice, and her colourful personality enriched the community at Royaumont.

She was born Agnes Forbes Blackadder in 1875, the daughter of an architect. She soon showed her intellectual calibre by graduating MA at St Andrews University in 1895 at the early age of 20. She then went to Glasgow and enrolled in Queen Margaret College for Women, graduating in medicine in 1898, and gaining her MD in 1901. In 1904 she became a member of the Royal College of Physicians of Ireland, only the sixth woman to achieve this distinction. Her clinical experience followed what was a common pattern for women doctors at that time – resident house appointments in a maternity hospital and a children's hospital, and medical officer in a workhouse infirmary – all posts for which there was not much competition from the men. After her marriage in 1901 to Dr Thomas Savill she moved to London, where she began to develop her interest in skin diseases, electrotherapy and radiology. At some stage she went abroad to gain further training in her specialties. By now she was among the most highly qualified women in the country, and in 1907 she had the rare (possibly unique) distinction at that time of being appointed to a consultancy at a hospital that was not exclusively for women. This was at St John's Hospital for Skin Diseases. In addition she was a consultant to the South London Hospital for Women. After her husband died in 1910, she not only continued her own work but also undertook the editing of her husband's standard textbook, *Savill's System of Clinical Medicine*, and continued editing this right up to 1942.

Her strength of character is shown by an episode that led to her dismissal from St John's Hospital. A member of staff had complained about the actions of the senior physician, and many other members of the staff, including Dr Savill, endorsed the complaints. They were all called upon to resign, and when they refused 'were given imperative notice of dismissal'.[1] This unhappy episode did not, however, appear to have damaged Dr Savill's subsequent career.

She was very much in sympathy with the suffrage movement, and in 1912 published papers in the medical journals on the forcible feeding of suffrage prisoners on hunger strike,[2] based on an investigation carried out by herself in association with two of the leading surgeons of the day – Mr Mansell Moullin and Sir Victor Horsley. They concluded that the many case studies they undertook themselves, or obtained from physicians who had attended the women, 'give the direct negative to the Home Secretary's assertion that forcible feeding as practised in Her Majesty's prisons is neither dangerous nor painful. We are confident that were the details of the statements we have read, and cases we have examined, fully known to the profession, this practice, which consists in fact of a severe physical and mental torture, could no longer be carried out in prisons of the twentieth century.'[3]

On the day war was declared on 4 August 1914, Dr Savill held in her hands a ticket for a holiday in Germany. 'With hourly news of doom the first terrible weeks crept past – long months of black depression followed.'[4] Her response to this depression was to volunteer for the Scottish Women's Hospital unit that was preparing to go to Royaumont. She was to be responsible for the installation and operation of the radiological equipment and for the training of the radiographers, which she did to a high standard of efficiency. Her pioneering studies of the x-ray appearances of gas gangrene are described in Appendix One.

Dr Savill did not remain continuously at Royaumont. During the winter months when there was a lull in the fighting, the corresponding slackening of hospital work enabled her to return to her practice in London; but as spring approached, she recalls her sense of eager anticipation:

Every return to Royaumont from 'home leave' was accompanied also by profound gratitude that once more one was safe within these lovely stones, once more privileged to live among beauty so rich that the early waking thought would acclaim it as a dream too fine for reality. Royaumont was beautiful at all times of the day and night; that one never ceased to be aware of and grateful for this beauty was one of the strange facts of the situation.[5]

Her eyes were not closed, however, to more unglamorous aspects of the old abbey. She commented in August 1915: 'Royaumont drainage smells worse than ever.'[6]

Her dedication to her work was demonstrated by her rapid response to the request to return from home leave to oversee the introduction of the new x-ray car in 1915. She installed the x-ray equipment at Villers-Cotterêts in 1917 with her usual efficiency and enthusiasm. Again in July 1918, in response to the then desperate need for a radiologist, she came back. She had been ill, and on her return Dr Courtauld commented: 'She does look ill, absolutely cadaverous.'[7]

Dr Savill was also active in the cultural life at Royaumont, and her great love of music led her to install a pianola in the great refectory. After the war she helped a number of young musicians to get established, often through musical soirées held in her own house. She was also a pioneer in the use of music as therapy. Her book, *Music, Health and Character*, published in 1923, caused a stir in the musical world, and later led to the foundation of the Council for Music in Hospitals.

In 1944 Dr Savill was elected a fellow of the Royal College of Physicians of Ireland – the sixth woman to receive this honour. She continued with a distinguished professional career into old age, still seeing patients at the age of 83, but recouping her strength by spending weekends in a nursing home.[8] In her late 70s she published *Alexander the Great and his Time*.[9] This was an immediate success, went into three editions, and led to a request from the publishers of the *Encyclopaedia Britannica* for an article on Alexander. She died in 1964 – truly an indomitable woman.

Dr (Mrs) Berry,
MB (Lond) 1904 (died 1956)

Apart from Miss Ivens and Miss Nicholson, Mrs Berry served at Royaumont longer than any other doctor. She arrived on 30 November 1914 and remained until August 1918. There were many new – and often homesick – orderlies who had reason to be grateful for Mrs Berry's sympathy and kindness, earning her the affectionate nickname of 'Mother'. Although some of the medical women might give a first impression of 'hardness', this was never the case with Mrs Berry. An unidentified orderly, writing home in January 1915, remembered:

> Last night I waited on the doctors and staff, all indifferent to anything save food, except for one doctor, Mrs Berry, who beckoned me to sit down, pointing to a chair by the door. She has such a sweet face and is so different from the others.[1]

Vera Collum remembered her as 'always a kind friend of the orderlies, ready to overlook their occasional unprofessional conduct and to sympathize with their troubles'. She was equally sensitive to the unspoken needs of the patients. One example is told by Mrs. Hacon, technically the housekeeper, but who liked to describe herself as the 'Head Char'. '"Mother Hacon," Mrs Berry said, "make something to amuse that poor boy in Jeanne." The result was a rag doll, "Tommy", a complete success for the lonely wounded boy. With a handkerchief tucked under his chin, "Tommy" shared all his foster-father's meals.'[2]

Mrs Berry was born Jessie Augusta Lewin. She entered the London School of Medicine for Women in 1894. As we have seen, with her older sister Octavia she was a fellow-student of Miss Ivens and Dr Courtauld, though she herself did not qualify until 1904. Little is known of her career after graduation, though Miss Ivens referred to work in public health. In 1911 she married Mr Grosvenor Berry, a Norfolk farmer. It was probably at the personal request of Miss Ivens that she joined the unit in November 1914. Miss Ivens later described her (together with Drs Nicholson, Ross and Savill) as 'a prop of the hospital from the beginning'.[3] Ruth Nicholson remembered her as 'one of our most loved members. She was a woman who put her hand to everything from ward dressings and toe-nail cutting to cleaning out drains and cutting wood. She also had a fine brain and a very tender heart.'[4] Collum remembered her as an enthusiastic and hard-working doctor as they laboured together getting the clothing department into some sort of order.[5] She also concerned herself with the hospital hygiene – an uphill task considering the primitive nature of the sanitary installations. 'I can see her now,' wrote Dr Martland, 'in her white coat and gum boots, up to her ankles in water, endeavouring to "débouche" [unblock] the choked drains.'[6] Although she did no surgical work, she had a gift for restoring function to wasted limbs and fingers after surgery.[7]

Mrs Robertson, visiting on behalf of the committee in the autumn of 1916, wrote that she was 'the funniest thing on earth', but:

> ... she is very sweet and unselfish and would do anything on earth for the patients, and a very skilful and devoted doctor, but utterly unpractical. One man in her ward told me he owed his life to her spending whole nights attending to him when he had frightful haemorrhages, and the men in 'Mary' simple adore her.[8]

She also looked after the health of the staff, a task she carried out with great devotion. Mrs Robertson saw her in action when a number of staff were suffering from 'chills':

> The funniest thing was Mrs Berry, or Mother as we call her, being 'dévouée' [devoted] to the invalids. In our sitting room was a scene of wild confusion. The fire raked till it was half out, an enormous saucepan with a huge iron spoon in the embers, the spoon having on the end of it one speck of Oxo, another sticky cube on the mantelpiece among Dr Ivens' notes on gas gangrene. Each chair had a piece of burnt toast, and a plate, cup and spoon. Some burnt milk was in another saucepan, and Mother was found coming upstairs with a loaf of bread under one arm, and a third saucepan with an excessively greasy soup in it – and a raw egg in the other. ... Whenever anything in the house is missing – medical papers, things from the wards or x-ray room, a book that one is reading, a pet hot water can, the one bottle of red ink in the establishment which belongs to the lab etc, etc, it is found in Mrs Berry's room, after she has denied all knowledge of it.[9]

She cared little for her appearance – 'a frail, unprofessional-looking figure, uniform worn anyhow and hat askew'.[10]

Mrs Berry was noted for her wit, gaiety and fun. Dr Martland recalled her first sight of her when she arrived, 'young and bewildered', in June 1916. She came into the cloisters while they were at supper,

> ... having been in Paris on business for the Médecin-Chef. Suddenly the whole sombre atmosphere changed, and in a moment the doctor's table was rocking with laughter with her fantastic tales of the day's adventures told with rare and delicate wit. But someone said 'Mrs Berry will have a head-ache tomorrow,' and sure enough she paid for her brilliance with a formidable migraine next day. That was a characteristic episode. Hers was a spirit too intense and sensitive for the tragedy of war. But she threw herself into the life of Royaumont with passionate energy, sparing herself nothing.[11]

Besides her gaiety she also had a 'driving sense of duty that could on occasion be puritanical. She could not rest while anything remained to be done – so she never rested'.[12]

Perhaps it was this driving sense of duty, combined with her highly strung and sensitive nature and the terrific pressures of the spring and summer of 1918, that led to her collapse. She had to return home in August. Her illness seems to have been a serious one. In April 1919 her husband asked the committee to write to her as warmly as possible about her work. The chief cause of her depression, he said, was the feeling that she had been of no use to Royaumont.[13]

Perhaps the wounds healed eventually – one can but wish that this very lovable woman found some happiness in later life, and realized that her work at Royaumont was, if not spectacular, of real value to the total well-being of the unit.

Miss Ruth Nicholson,

MB BS (Durham) 1909, MS (Liverp), FRCOG (1884–1963)

Ruth Nicholson was an important member of the unit from its arrival in December 1914 to final closure in March 1919. She was second-in-command, and the principal surgeon after Miss Ivens herself.

The eldest of a large clerical family in the north of England, she had made her decision to study medicine at a very early age when her father took her to an exhibition of medical missionary work in Newcastle. At medical college in Newcastle she was the only woman in her year (though there were a few in other years). She graduated in 1909, and after work in a dispensary in Newcastle she went to Edinburgh, where she became an assistant to Dr Elsie Inglis in the Bruntsfield Hospital. Like many women of her generation, she saw the mission field as an opportunity to gain wider experience than was easily available at home. Until the outbreak of war she worked in Gaza in Palestine. Wishing to participate in the war effort, she returned home and joined a voluntary unit. Standing on Victoria Station about to depart, she had the bitter experience of being turned down by the doctor in charge; he refused to have a woman on his staff. 'Imagine the feelings of a strong feminist,' her sister commented.[1] This rebuff, however, was a fortunate one for Miss Ivens, who gained a second-in-command on whom she could, and did, utterly rely. She also proved a popular member of staff at Royaumont, known for her liveliness and sense of fun. Many were impressed by her 'scarf dances', and her role as a 'dancing dervish' was remembered with pleasure.

Work at Royaumont certainly gave her a great opportunity to develop her surgical skills. After the war, and with the strong encouragement of Miss Ivens, she determined on a career in obstetrics and gynaecology. 'She gave me all my chances,' she wrote later in a tribute to Miss Ivens.[2] After a period in general practice in Birkenhead while she prepared herself, she gained her own consultancy appointments in the same Liverpool hospitals as Miss Ivens and successfully developed her own practice. She inspired confidence in her patients, and was well-known for her sympathy and dedication. Perhaps more unusually, she was 'a great favourite with the nurses. Her visits to the ward always gave pleasure, and the mornings in the theatre left no nervous wrecks behind.'[3]

Dr Nicholson succeeded Miss Ivens in her university appointments when Miss Ivens left to get married in 1930, and in 1933 she became one of the earliest fellows of the new Royal College of Obstetrics and Gynaecology. She became the first woman president of the North of England Society of Obstetrics and Gynaecology, and earned the respect of her male colleagues, one of them commenting, 'I think we have picked a winner.'[4] As might be expected, she played a prominent part in the Medical Women's Federation. She died in 1963 at the age of 79.

Dr Elsie Jean Dalyell,
OBE, MB (Sydney), ChM (1881–1948)

Elsie Dalyell was one of the most distinguished of the Royaumont 'doctoresses'. She was born in Sydney, Australia, in 1881, and first intended a career in teaching, but the 'shattering blow' of a hysterectomy, with the interruption of an incipient romance, led to her decision to study medicine.[1] As a student she was said to be an extremely attractive girl with corn-yellow hair, a fair (some said 'apricot') complexion and blue eyes. The combination of her personal attractiveness, her general charm and her brilliant intellect led the young male graduates to dub her 'the Yellow Peril'. Her fame as a fast rider on a motorbike may also have contributed to the sobriquet.[2] She graduated with first-class honours in 1909, and in the following year graduated ChM.

She became the first woman resident in the Royal Prince Alfred Hospital, and later the first woman to be appointed to a full-time post in the medical school. She was described as a 'superb teacher with tremendous enthusiasm'.[3] In 1912 she became the first woman in Australia to be appointed to a Beit research fellowship at the Lister Institute in London.[4] She was then well-set on a promising career.

On the outbreak of war Dr Dalyell offered her services to the War Office. Not unexpectedly, as she was a woman, she was refused. Instead she joined the Serbian Relief Fund unit that was leaving for Skopje, where an epidemic of typhus was raging. Her appointment was as bacteriologist, but with only two doctors available she had to turn her hand to much other work.[5] After the typhus epidemic had subsided there was a continuous inflow of all types of infectious diseases. The hospital was finally overrun by the Bulgarian army in October 1915.

In May 1916 Dr Dalyell went to Royaumont to take charge of the bacteriological laboratory, remaining until October. The focus of her work was on the complicated bacteriology of gas gangrene and other infections of war wounds. Her own brief account of her work at Royaumont is given in Chapter Four. After the rush resulting from the Somme battles was over she volunteered for the RAMC. Being a woman, she was only 'attached' to the RAMC, with no real status in the male-dominated British army. She served as a bacteriologist in Malta and Salonika, and after the end of the war went to Constantinople (as it was then called) to deal with an outbreak of cholera. Her work with the RAMC was recognized with two 'mentions in despatches' and the award of the OBE in 1919.[6]

She returned to the Lister Institute in London and then embarked on her most important contribution to medical science. With Dr (later Dame) Harriet Chick, Dr Helen Mackay and an experienced hospital nurse, Miss Henderson-Smith, and with the support of the Lister Institute and the Medical Research Council, she went to Vienna. Vienna at that time was experiencing extreme conditions of poverty and deprivation, and Dalyell and her team were trying to establish whether rickets – widespread among the debilitated children of the city – was due to a vitamin deficiency or to a low-grade infection. Over a period of two years they were able to demonstrate conclusively not only that the addition of cod liver oil to the diet could prevent the development of rickets and promote healing when rickets had already occurred, but also that sunlight and ultraviolet light could also have a beneficial effect. This led to an important leap forward in public health policy.[7,8]

Her deep compassion for the suffering children of Vienna was illustrated by her action on returning from home leave. She discarded all her equipment in her surgical suitcase and took it back filled with butter.[9] On completion of her rickets research she returned to Australia.

One might speculate how Dr Dalyell's career might have developed had she been a man. Probably she would have reached great heights in academic medicine. As G.D. Richardson comments, 'she was still too far ahead of her time and suffered a regrettable lack of scope for her talents'. In 1924 she was appointed senior assistant microbiologist in the Department of Public Health, where she remained until her retirement in 1946. But, Richardson continues, 'it was inadequate use of a splendid mind and a forceful and most engaging personality'.[10] Her nephew reported that she herself felt frustrated and that the work did not give her the satisfaction she could have wished.[11] This is in no way to denigrate her work, but emphasizes that career possibilities for women were different from those available to men. She developed a clinic and laboratory service for the treatment of venereal disease in the Rachel Foster Women's Hospital, work that could only effectively be done by a woman. She did this with her customary skill and dedication so that her clinic, and the methods she employed, were copied all over Australia. When the Second World War broke out, in addition to her routine work, she organized the Red Cross Blood Transfusion Service.[12] She died in 1948 at the age of 67.

Dr Dalyell was a very popular member of the Royaumont Unit and was remembered with great affection. Dr Martland wrote of her:

Whatever time she may have spent in that remote attic up the spiral stair, she certainly became a ubiquitous and beneficent presence throughout Royaumont. If a medical officer was wanted to give an anaesthetic or evacuate a batch of blessés, there was Dalyell, a calm, fair, massive figure, always available, utterly efficient, never in a 'flap'. She had a genius for appearing in any place where trouble was; that soft Australian voice murmuring, 'Can do, honeyeee?' in a tight spot, is one of my most blessed memories of Royaumont. Another good memory is of her diverting a bunch of depressed 'doctoresses' by quick-change impersonations of Scottish Women in the incredible variety of tartan-trimmed garments which Edinburgh considered suitable as uniform. Her gaiety was one of her best gifts to Royaumont. I never saw her gloomy, though sometimes saddened by the waste and muddle of war. Just to speak of Dr Dalyell brings a sense of healing to the spirit – that is the kind of woman she was.[13]

Dr Lydia Manley Henry,
MB ChB, MD (Sheffield), DSc (Hon) (Sheffield) (1891–1985)

'I have never lost the spell it had on me,' Dr Henry wrote of Royaumont later in her life. The years she spent there, she said, were 'the happiest years of my life'. Dr Henry arrived at Royaumont on 25 July 1917, aged just 27, and having only graduated the previous year. She was then the youngest doctor on the staff – a fact that may have owed something to her winning personality and the impression she conveyed to a somewhat reluctant committee of her unusual ability. Her future career demonstrated that their judgement had been sound.

Dr Lydia Manley Henry (or Leila as she liked to call herself) was the fourth and youngest child of William Patterson Henry and his wife Lysbeth. She was born on 30 June 1891 in Macduff, Banffshire, Scotland. Her father had been a tea planter in Ceylon (Sri Lanka), but had returned to Scotland with tuberculosis and died when Leila was only two and a half years old. The older children went to public schools while 'Little Leila' stayed on in Macduff with her aunt, who was the local postmistress and a widow with children of her own. Leila attended the local school until she was 14 years old, then went down to Sheffield to join her mother. Here she attended the Sheffield High School for Girls.

As Leila was leaving school, the medical school in Sheffield was just opening its doors to women. Apart from the first two years' slog in physics and chemistry she thoroughly enjoyed her training, though she was amused that she had to have separate instruction from the men in pathology, obstetrics, gynaecology and urology. Her period at medical school did not pass entirely smoothly. One of the bodies provided for dissection had not been properly prepared. A fellow student developed an acute dermatitis, and she an acute streptococcal infection – a very dangerous condition at that time, before antibiotics or anti-streptococcal sera. Her brother, who was a bacteriologist, treated her with an autogenous vaccine. She recovered but had to miss a year of her studies.

On returning to college she found that many of her fellow students and a large number of junior staff had gone to serve in France. This gave her a great opportunity, as it was now much easier for her to gain practical experience than it had been for earlier women medical students. The hospitals in which she worked, the Sheffield Royal Infirmary and the Sheffield General Hospital, were close to a munitions works; there were many serious casualties, so providing her with invaluable training for her later work at Royaumont.

Dr Henry graduated on her birthday, 30 June 1916, the first woman in Sheffield to do so, and next day became the city's first woman intern. Her intern year was an exceptionally heavy one owing to wartime conditions and shortages of staff. Zeppelin raids and accidents in the munitions works resulted in a strenuous workload, and as a woman she was required to live out, apart from her night shifts on casualty, and had to walk several miles after her day's work – 'Not very pleasant,' she later commented. But it proved her stamina.

During 1916 it became clear that venereal disease was rampant. The Royal Infirmary responded by setting up free clinics for men and women, and Dr Henry became the first woman assistant in the female clinic. Looking back on this experience in the 1960s she wrote, 'I doubt if we ever see now such horrible lesions as we had to treat.' She learnt the current methods of drug treatment, knowledge which served her well after the war in her work in Blackburn.

The day after she completed her one-year internship she responded to the appeal of the Scottish Women's Hospitals committee for women doctors to serve in France. At first she was refused on account of her age. Nothing daunted, she travelled up to Edinburgh to plead her cause in person – and was accepted.

At Royaumont she was an assistant surgeon and, with Sister Rose-Morris, had charge of the Blanche de Castille Ward. She immediately found her place in the unit. Of Dr Courtauld and Dr Savill she said that 'although twice my age they gathered me into their group'.[1] She played a full part in the work of the unit, both at Villers-Cotterêts and at Royaumont, during the rushes of 1918. In later life she recalled one incident from her days at Villers-Cotterêts that shows the affection the patients had for the 'doctoresses':

> A few nights before we retreated I was called to one of the wooden huts: a patient was haemorrhaging. It was moonlight and as I was walking along the duckboards between the huts, a tall figure appeared: as I got closer I recognized him as a French sergeant we had as our patient in Royaumont. I asked him how he had got to our CCS and he told me the trenches all round us were filled with French soldiers. 'I came to see if my Royaumont doctoresses were all safe.' He left as suddenly as he came and I walked into the hut – but I had not realized until then that we were right in their midst.

After the war she obtained several offers of employment, but decided to pursue her academic studies, and to this end applied for a Beit fellowship. There was only one dissenting voice, that of Sir Edward Mellanby, who grumbled that 'she would only get married'. In 1920 she submitted her MD thesis on gas gangrene to Sheffield University, becoming one of the first two to receive a Sheffield MD and the first woman to do so. She later switched her interest to the fast-growing area of public health, and became assistant medical officer of health in Blackburn, Lancashire, an industrial town with many problems. This was a new and important post – 'I had a free hand in virgin soil ' – and she was the only woman doctor in the area. In addition to organizing clinics in preventive medicine, she did a great deal of public lecturing to women and girls. She saw the dreadful consequences of numerous backstreet abortions, and had to use most of her allotted number of hospital beds to restore the damage. Many midwives were untrained, some almost illiterate, though fortunately trained midwives were beginning to make their appearance. As far as public health was concerned she was amused – and dismayed – to see the dustcarts going up and down the old cobbled High Street while the milk was being delivered into the open jugs and basins waiting to receive it on the window-sills. She was able to organize a (limited) supply of pasteurized milk before she left.

Dr Henry made such a success of this post that in 1923 she was invited to head the Social Services Department at the King's College for Women in the University of London, and became a lecturer and a member of Senate. In 1925 she went out to Canada, married and spent the remainder of her life there. Until then she had always maintained that being a woman had never stopped her from doing what she wanted. But this changed when she went to Canada, a move that put an end to her medical career – her daughter describes this as a period of some frustration for her. Nevertheless she had a happy life. In 1978 Sheffield University Medical School celebrated its 150th anniversary, and to mark the occasion awarded Dr Henry – their first woman graduate and first woman MD – an honorary DSc degree.

In World War Two she busied herself in providing warm clothing and other comforts for the British minesweeping crews and Free French sailors in northeast Scotland. She lectured extensively on the war effort at the request of the Canadian government, and raised Canadian support for the Scottish Women's Hospitals canteens in France in 1940. Her health gradually declined, and her last year was somewhat disturbed by her memories of the Villers-Cotterêts evacuation, which seemed to haunt her. She died in 1985 at the age of 93.

Dr Edith Marjorie Martland,
MB BS (London) (1888–1962)

Dr Martland was another of the Royaumont doctors who achieved consultant status after the war. She was born in 1888 in Oldham, Lancashire, where she was the eldest child of a medical family. In

1906 she went to Newnham College, Cambridge, where she obtained her natural science tripos in 1909. From Cambridge she went to the London (Royal Free Hospital) School of Medicine for Women, graduating in 1915. In July 1916, after a year as an intern, she went to Royaumont as an assistant surgeon. The hospital was then extremely busy as a result of the enormous influx of patients from the Somme battlefields. She proved to be a very competent surgeon, and enjoyed the work so much that she toyed with the idea of making her career in surgery. It became clear to her, however, when she broke down in the late summer of 1918, that her physique was too frail for the rigours of such a life. Instead she switched her interests to biochemistry and pathology, joined the Elizabeth Garrett Anderson Hospital for Women, and in addition worked at the Lister Institute. She soon rose to be consultant pathologist. On the outbreak of World War Two, when the hospital was evacuated to Barnet, she organized a highly efficient and widely admired pathology service under very difficult conditions. After the war she moved to Salisbury, again as consultant pathologist, until her retirement in 1954. She moved back to Cambridge where she had been so happy during her student days. She died in 1962 at the age of 73.

At Royaumont, Orderly Proctor regarded her as 'a brilliantly clever little thing and one of the nicest people you could meet anywhere, and a clever surgeon'.[1] One American officer, Lieutenant Hickman, never forgot his 'doctor with the red hair who wouldn't let anyone take his leg off'. Their enthusiastic judgements were endorsed by her more knowledgable peers:

... an excellent brain, clear and accurate and her intellectual honesty and capacity for going to the root of the matter made her a most stimulating professional colleague and friend ... she had a shining integrity which made her loved and respected by all who knew her ... She loved music, painting, and literature, especially poetry ... Her gaiety and love of life made her the best of friends. She moved through life a little aloof, yet warm and loving, poised and clear-cut, yet warm and compassionate.[2]

Vera Collum,
Chronicler and X-Ray Technician (1885–1957)

It could be said that it was due to Vera Collum more than to any other single member of the Royaumont and Villers-Cotterêts units that, apart from the official archives, so much information about the women who worked in them has come down to us. It is therefore only fitting to add some notes about Collum herself.

Her articles in *Blackwood's Magazine* under the pseudonym 'Skia' and her contributions to the *Common Cause*, the magazine of the National Union of Women's Suffrage Societies, record some of the story as (or shortly after) it occurred. She was also one of the moving spirits who set up the Royaumont and Villers-Cotterêts Association after the war 'to maintain and strengthen our war-time comradeship'. This resulted in regular newsletters, which continued almost uninterruptedly until 1973, almost 60 years after the opening of the hospital.

Collum was an only child. Her childhood was not a happy one. The remarriage of her widowed mother was a shock and she never managed to get over her dislike of her stepfather.[1] Throughout her life she threw herself into one enthusiasm after another: for Japan, where she seems to have become interested in Eastern religions; for the suffrage movement; and then for Royaumont. This last enthusiasm, fortunately for us, stayed with her for the rest of her life. After the war other enthusiasms followed, but never displaced her love for Royaumont.

On the outbreak of war Collum was earning her living as a freelance journalist, and was also working in the press department of the London office of the National Union of Women's Suffrage Societies (NUWSS). There she fell under the spell of Dr Elsie Inglis, and arranged the newspaper coverage and other publicity to help her get the Scottish Women's Hospital project off the ground. She persuaded her friend Cicely Hamilton (a friendship rooted firmly in the women's suffrage movement) to volunteer for the first unit departing for Royaumont in November 1914. She looked on rather enviously as other recruits left for Royaumont, but on 28 February 1915 she was able to follow them and realize her ambition. She was then 30 years of age.

Her first assignment was to the clothing department and then, when her interest in photography became known, Miss Ivens moved her into the x-ray department. She was enthusiastic, devoted to her work and to her patients, and became a highly skilled technician. She developed a very strong empathy with the French – *poilus* and officers alike. She felt deeply the suffering she sometimes had to cause them as she positioned them on the table so that she could take her pictures to reveal and localize the shell fragments and other foreign bodies in their wounds.

Collum's strong sense of duty brought her back to Royaumont as soon as possible after suffering serious injuries in March 1916, when the *Sussex*, the ship in which she was returning from leave across the Channel, was torpedoed.

Two months later she described her experience in *Blackwood's Magazine*:

In a moment the whole earth and heaven seemed to explode in one head-splitting roar. In the thousandth part of a second my mind told me 'Torpedo-forward – on my right' – and then the sensation of falling, with my limbs spreadeagled, through blind space. When I came to myself again I was groping among a tangle of broken wires, with an agonizing pain in my back and the fiercest headache I had ever known. My hair was down and plastered to my chin with blood that seemed to be coming from my mouth. There was more blood on my coat-sleeve. I was conscious that I was bleeding freely internally with every movement. My first definite thought was 'If only it is all a ghastly nightmare!' But I remembered. My next thought was a passionately strong desire not to die by drowning. I crawled free of the wires that were coiled about me and stood up. In one unsteady glance I took in a number of things. Near me a horrible piece of something, and a dead woman. I never heard a sound – I had been deafened. So I had been blown up to the top deck, to the other end of the ship. I swayed to and fro and looked for a stairway, but could find none, and began to be aware that I had only a few moments of consciousness left me. – I found I could not speak.[2]

A boat was lowered and men were climbing down into it. She took hold of a loose davit rope and, making a mighty effort, managed to slide down until she was just above the water. She waited till the roll of the ship brought her near enough to the boat to catch hold of another rope and so lower herself into the boat:

> Men were pouring into her. I saw a man's knee hooked over the side of the boat where I sat. I could not see his body, but it was in the water between us and the side of the Sussex. As in a dream I held on to his knee with all the grip I had left. I could do nothing to help him in, but so long as I remained conscious, his knee-hold should not be allowed to slip. No one took any notice of either of us.

The man whose knee she was holding was eventually pulled into the boat, which was now dangerously overcrowded. Three oars were produced – they had to get away from the steamer before it went down, and pulled them down with it. Their boat was taking in water; it was now up to her knees. Between cries of '*Ramez!*' (row) and '*Mais non! Videz l'eau! Videz l'eau!*' (bale out the water), she tried to guide the oars of a young Frenchman who had no idea what to do and was gazing vacantly before him. The balers could keep the water from rising further, but they could not lower it. And then:

> I saw our steamer riding quite happily on the water with her bows clean gone. Afterwards I learnt that the torpedo had cut off her fore part, to within an inch or two to where I had been standing, and that it had sunk.

In her boat hysteria broke out. Some wanted to row and get away; others, including Collum and a Belgian who seemed to have been the only effective one in the boat, thought they should return to the *Sussex* before they were swamped. The sight of another boat returning to the *Sussex* decided the cooler heads to go back to the steamer and get the captain's advice. The boat had to be turned. No one knew how. '*Ramez au sens contraire*', Collum cried, this being the nearest she could get to 'backwater'. Her Frenchman was too dazed to understand:

> So I simply set my teeth and pulled against him. With my injured back and inside I could only just compass what I did. A mutinous mood came on the boat. Every few minutes they wavered and prepared to flee again. It was like a political meeting. The boat followed the wishes of those who shouted loudest. When the oars ceased dipping I called out as encouragingly as I could 'Courage, mes amis! Ramez! Ramez! Courage mes enfants!'

Later she realized, with some amusement, she had been following French newspaper accounts of how sergeants encouraged their men in battle. But it worked: 'No one thought it odd. The dazed ears heard, the nerveless arms worked again.' They drew alongside the *Sussex*. The Frenchwomen in the boat appealed for Collum to be taken off first as she was the only one who was injured. In spite of that she was left behind alone apart from the one Belgian. The boat was floating away. She could not stand. The water came over the gunwale, poured over her legs to her waist, soaked through her thick greatcoat and chilled her to the bone. Help came from the same Belgian who had done more than anyone to control the boat, and, with the help of sailors from the *Sussex*, he hauled her up by the arms 'like a sack' and propped her against a wall.

The Belgian gave her what help he could. A man with a wounded head sat patiently in a corner; a girl, in great pain, struggled down the stairs, lay on a couch, and never moved or spoke again: 'She died bravely and silently, quite alone.' There followed long hours of waiting:

> It is nerve-racking work lying helpless in a damaged vessel wondering whether the rescue ship or another enemy submarine will appear first on the scene.

A French fishing vessel drew alongside. Her Belgian friend, with the help of a young Chinese, carried her up to the rail, but they were too late. The boat had already sailed. Half an hour later a destroyer was on the scene and this time she was lucky. The crew got her on her back as far as the ship's rail: 'British sailors grasped my arms and pulled me over. For one sickening second my legs dangled between the two ships, but the sailors hauled me in before the impact came.'

She was now safe in the hands of the Royal Navy. Early next morning she was transferred to a hospital ship: 'I was in very great pain and suffering physically more than I have ever suffered in my life, but my memory of those hours between dark and daylight is one, not of personal misery, but of the beautiful tenderness of those Nursing Sisters.'[3]

She spent a few days in a local hospital after landing in England and then went by ambulance train to 'one of the great London Hospitals'. She had a smashed foot, a fractured lumbar process on her spine, strained muscles in back and thigh, and some internal injuries.

Three months later she was back at Royaumont – 'going back to a life I loved, to a Chief I delighted to work with, to comrades proven in long months of alternating stress and monotony and to a little group of friends'. She was back in time to play a heroic part in the tremendous rush of work which commenced on 2 July in the first Battle of the Somme (Chapter Four). She also performed magnificently during the crises of 1918 (Chapter Seven), until injuries from exposure to x-rays forced her to leave in July.

After the war, she pursued a great range of interests, from ancient religions to social Darwinism. Her passion for archaeology led to some rather cranky theories, and her attempts to harmonize the philosophies of East and West resulted in books such as *The Music of Growth* (1933) and *Manifold Unity* (1940). She was no pacifist. She strongly criticized Vera Brittain's *Testament of Youth* in 1934 for its emphasis on the 'exquisitely painful experiences she and her circle had suffered', but she had forgotten 'the unfortunate peasant soldier who stolidly fought as though obedient to destiny and died of wounds'. 'Royaumont,' she maintained, 'saw war through the less sentimental, not at all hysterical, and more realistic eyes of French youth. ...We who saw that comradeship and knew it among ourselves during the war, let us at all events keep it untarnished – the "Testament of Maturity".[4] During World War Two her great energies were diverted to soil fertility research – she was indeed a woman of many achievements. After the war her health deteriorated seriously and she died after much pain in 1957 at the age of 72. In a typical gesture, she left her body to the Royal College of Surgeons of England.

Cicely Hamilton,

Playwright, Actress, Writer, Suffragist, Administrator (1872–1952)

Cicely Hamilton, who worked at Royaumont for two and a half years from December 1914 to May 1917, is one of the outstanding personalities among the many striking and interesting women who brought their talents and dedication to the unit at Royaumont. Cicely's life is well documented both in her own writings, such as her autobiography, *Life Errant*[1], and in those of others, such as Lis Whitelaw's biography, *The Life and Rebellious Times of Cicely Hamilton*.[2]

On the outbreak of war Cicely was 42, and had already achieved fame as an actress, a playwright and a leading character in the suffrage movement. In August 1914 she found herself caught up in the general upsurge of patriotic feeling. She felt the need to assist the war effort and show in a practical way what women could do.

Her friend Vera Collum, who was then working in the press office of the NUWSS, suggested to her that she might consider volunteering for one of the SWH units that Dr Inglis was then planning. Cicely leapt at the opportunity and promptly offered her skills – an adequate knowledge of French and, curiously enough, book-keeping. The offer was accepted and she was engaged as a clerk at the princely salary of ten shillings a week.

How did this strongly individualistic woman fit into the life of a community such as Royaumont? Cicely had, for years, been accustomed to associating with women who were talented, intellectual and professional. At Royaumont she clearly enjoyed the companionship of the medical women, all of whom had come up the hard way and had had to struggle to a greater or lesser extent for their qualifications and experience in a man's world. They, in turn, appreciated her as an efficient member of the team, first as clerk, later as administrator, and as a lively and entertaining colleague. The rather rigid hierarchy that required the orderlies, the sisters and the doctors each to have their separate sitting rooms and dining tables was waived for Cicely, who shared with the doctors. Miss Ivens in particular relied enormously on Cicely for her meticulous keeping of accounts (Dr Inglis considered this was not Miss Ivens's strong point), and for her knowledge of French, especially before Miss Ivens became fluent herself.

Miss Ivens expressed her appreciation in August 1916 when she requested the committee to raise Cicely's salary to the same level as that of the doctors – £200 per annum. She wrote:

> Her work has been so invaluable I think it would be disastrous for the hospital if her services could not be retained for pecuniary reasons. We all use her brain so much that even a temporary absence on leave makes us feel extremely helpless. I should like the Committee to realize how much the hospital is indebted to her, not only for the accurate and scrupulous accounts, but for the tactful and clever letters she writes for me to many of the French officials with whom I have to conduct negotiations.[3]

Cicely was also the perfect morale booster, first showing her mettle in what might have been a very gloomy Christmas in 1914 when their Herculean efforts had been rebuffed by the French authorities. In an effort to dispel the general despondency, she laid on a pageant of the history of the abbey enlivened by her own humorous comments. Thereafter she was the prime mover and inspiration of many other shows during the slacker periods of the hospital.

There must have been moments when the restrictions of communal life proved too irksome for Cicely. She disliked wearing uniform, and whenever she could wore a working man's 'blouse', which puzzled Miss Tod, the first matron (Chapter Three). She rode her bicycle in the woods, which was not allowed by the

French authorities. (Later this regulation was quietly ignored.) Mrs Owen, the first administrator, who had difficulties with Miss Ivens and with her job, recorded an 'extraordinary exhibition of temper from Miss Hamilton'.[4] Mrs Owen's successor, Mrs Harley, however, wrote to the committee in March that she was 'a delightful person to work with and so helpful to us all'.[5] Dorothy Littlejohn, one of the somewhat disgruntled cooks in the kitchen in 1914, wrote home of

A Miss Cicely Hamilton, a thorough Bohemian ... a most understanding person and fortunately sees the funny parts. Certainly if you could see Miss Swanston and me simply weak with laughter you would be able to comfort yourself that I am not taking life too seriously, but if we did not laugh we would probably do the other thing.[6]

One of Cicely's saddest duties was attendance at funerals in the local cemetery when doctors and nurses were too busy to spare the time. 'It was a duty I never got hardened to.'[7] She felt deeply the suffering of ordinary people caught up in the horrible wastage of war. She describes in her autobiography a scene she witnessed when medals were being bestowed by the French military authorities:

Among the soldiers there was an elderly man in a clean and tidied workman's suit. That meant a dead son whose cross he was that day receiving. – When the ribbon was pinned on the workman's coat, a woman beside me stirred and drew a breath – a young woman dressed all in black; then, the ceremony over, she slipped under the rail, and went forward to meet the old man. I remember a thin fine rain was falling and they said not a word as they met; but the woman took out a square of white handkerchief, unfolded it, spread it on her hands, and stood waiting. The father unfastened the cross from his coat and laid it on the linen, and they stood in the rain and looked down on it – all they had received for the life of a man! Then slowly, she folded the handkerchief and covered it, and they

271

walked away together, still without a word; she carrying the medal as a priest might carry the Host.[8]

Her bicycle rides led to an extraordinary experience, which she recorded in her autobiography. Riding home one evening she saw

> ... a woman, some yards ahead, walking in the same direction as myself – walking swiftly at the side of the road. She wore no hat, her dress was dark and, in the dusky light, looked black. I took her for some young woman of the village to whom, as I overtook her, I should call the customary greeting. I was just drawing level with her, when – she cut across the bend diagonally by darting out into the road and right in the path of my bicycle; I saw we must collide, shouted something, took my foot off the pedal and put my brake hard on. And then – nothing happened. The blackness of her dress was against my front wheel – but the wheel went on without impact! My impression – my belief – was that I and my bicycle had passed through the figure. ... I believe wholeheartedly that I saw a ghost and rode through that ghost but I don't expect those who read of my adventure to share my personal belief![9]

She had other strange experiences in the autumn of 1916, this time in the abbey itself. Night after night the handle of her door was rattled – and there was no one there. She tried leaving the door open, but taps and knocks around the room took the place of the handle-turning. She never spoke of these events, but one day, as she was going through the housekeeping accounts with a member of the staff, 'there came the familiar twist of the handle; I tried to ignore it but my companion, when it was repeated, rose to open the door'. As usual there was no one there. Finally there was 'a final and violent wind-up of the manifestations'. She went to bed early and Orderly Margaret Davidson, who was accustomed to putting a hot water bottle in her bed, came in and started chatting:

> Suddenly the door of my room was rattled as I had never heard it rattle before – with an energy suggestive of anger or

desperate haste. D. jumped up promptly and made for the door; from the inner side it opened easily enough, and she had it wide in an instant. This time I had not recognized my visitor – his furious way of making himself known was new – but I wasn't so surprised as D. when the open door revealed nothing but an open door. She looked up and down the corridor and turned and looked at me; and I think I said something rather lamely about wondering who it was, and why they had run off like that – knowing all the time it was quite impossible for anyone to vanish so quickly. Whether she accepted my attempt at an explanation I don't know, but she shut the door, came back to my bed, and sat down again; but hardly had she done so than my visitor came back, and more thunderously. This time he left the handle alone; his assault was on the door itself. Judging by the sound a man, and a heavy man, was hurling himself against the door which (this I will swear to) actually cracked on its hinges. For a second or two I think we were both of us staggered; then D. naturally was the quicker of the two. Before I was out of bed she was back at the door, and once again flinging it open – with the same result as before – I don't know what we said about it but I know it wasn't much – D. respecting my obvious desire to avoid discussion and after a few minutes taking herself off to her own quarters. When she had gone I got up – the new developments had made me uneasy [she had had bad news that morning about the health of her old aunt], and stood outside my door. A nurse came out into the corridor and as she walked away I called after her 'Sister, did you hear someone banging on my door a few minutes ago?' 'No, I didn't hear anyone,' and departed down the corridor ...[10]

(Cicely was not the only one to suffer such visitations. One night in July 1916, while on duty in Canada Ward, Madge Ramsay-Smith, then an orderly and later the administrator, heard the door into the passage 'suddenly shaken violently as if someone were endeavouring to get in'. When she opened the door, there was no one there.

273

A few moments later, the rattling resumed. Again, there was no one. After that she was left in peace.)

In the spring of 1917 Cicely Hamilton was feeling the need for a change. She had served two and a half years, and the hospital was going through a quiet period. She joined Lena Ashwell's Players, returning to her old love of acting. They performed in Abbeville and Amiens till the end of the war and then, in 1919, in Cologne and the devastated areas. In 1920 she went to Austria on behalf of the Save the Children Fund, and in Vienna observed 'the children stunted for lack of nourishment, the shabbiness and beggary and the queues at the soup kitchens'.[11] Throughout the 1920 and 1930s she campaigned tirelessly on women's issues, and became one of the most respected feminists of the day. On her death at the age of 80 in 1952, Ruth Nicholson spoke of her as 'the person who kept us sane'. 'So lovable, so interesting and entertaining, so erudite, always friendly and so brave. She was the one who really understood the French and guided us on the right path.'[12]

The Orderlies

Miss Ivens regarded her orderlies as the mainstay of the hospital. She formed this opinion when she witnessed the enormously heavy work they carried out in the initial period of preparation and, in spite of the occasional misfit, had no reason to change this opinion throughout the subsequent history of the hospital.

Vera Collum wrote of them:

The orderlies were untrained, raw material, most of them lacking even the personal discipline that comes from going down into the world's arena and competing there for a living. Even in the matter of physical strength they came up to a male standard. Throughout the rush of work that came to the hospital during the Somme battle, when the convalescents who usually give a hand had been evacuated, and the wounded poured in all day and all night long in a steady stream, every stretcher had to be carried upstairs to the wards, the x-ray rooms and the operating theatre, by women.[1]

These opinions were in stark contrast to those of John Masefield (later poet laureate) when he worked as a volunteer orderly in the spring of 1915 in a hospital in Arc-en-Barrois, Haute Marne:

> We have a lot of catty young minxes here and they have catty ways of wheedling when it is a question of carrying stinking blood in a bucket ... There were a lot of lady probationers who have lived idly and luxuriously and who are now, in the main, useless nuisances.[2]

The Royaumont orderlies, for the most part, came from similar backgrounds. So what made them so different?

Perhaps it was partly due to the fact that the hospital was so unusual in employing only women, and the orderlies were as keen as the doctors to prove what women could do on their own. There were no men to fall back upon to do the unpleasant tasks – they had to get on with them and they did. They also knew that those in charge were observing the work and determining where their particular talents lay. It was possible for an orderly to train as a radiographer or a laboratory technician, or to take overall charge of different departments – clothing, stores, linen, housekeeping, pharmacy and so on. Those who proved themselves particularly valuable in the wards could be upgraded to the rank of auxiliary nurse with a salary and a defined status. These auxiliary nurses did not have the knowledge that a fully trained nurse might have had, but they knew what was required for the military nursing at Royaumont.

Orderlies had to be sufficiently well-off to give their services voluntarily; only uniforms, travel expenses and board and lodging were supplied. They came from a variety of backgrounds, and some already had their own profession. Margaret Davidson was teaching modern languages at Dornoch Academy; Norah Neilson-Gray was well-embarked on her successful artistic career (she was one of the famous 'Glasgow Girls'); G.L. Buckley and Charlotte Almond were medical students; and Doris Woodall and Margaret Freeman interrupted their studies at Girton College, Cambridge; Irma Minchin was in the Margaret Morris School of Dancing; and

Mrs Hacon had been at the centre of a cultured circle of writers and artists. There were a few widows, some of them widowed as a result of the war. Evelyn Proctor had lost her fiancé in the Royal Flying Corps, and there may well have been others in a similar situation. Some had had previous VAD experience in military or voluntary hospitals in Britain; some no experience at all. A few, in the later stages of the war, came from other SWH hospitals in Serbia or Corsica. As a very old lady Una Moffat, speaking of Royaumont where her sister Florence was an orderly and later a physiotherapist, said it was a very popular place.[3]

In spite of the then current French view that the women at Royaumont must have been among the most ardent of feminists, the facts do not bear this out. Cicely Hamilton, Vera Collum, Mrs Hacon and Miss Loudon – among others – were involved in the suffrage movement. Norah Neilson-Gray certainly held strong feminist views: when she was commissioned after the war by the Imperial War Museum to paint a picture of life at Royaumont, she was adamant that her painting should not be included in the 'Women's Work' section of the proposed exhibition.* Some, like Dorothy Littlejohn, were heartily opposed to women's suffrage. Marjorie Starr's fears that some of the more outspoken and unconventional orderlies might be 'militant suffragettes' seem to have been without foundation. Grace Summerhayes was actually ashamed to have an aunt who chained herself to railings (though on later reflection she thought she ought to have been proud!). On the whole it was not women's rights that drew women to work at Royaumont. It was rather the opportunity to spread their wings, to escape from the restrictions of life at home, to answer the call of freedom and adventure with the added attraction of serving overseas. The

---

* She described her picture as 'a view of soldier patients ... (seen by a woman if you like) – It was painted from within and absolutely true to fact. The scene would be unfamiliar to anyone who has not worked in a first-line hospital in France. It was unlike the pictures of rows of tidy beds which usually are the subject of hospital pictures.' She believed the Imperial War Museum should have a record of 'what was done by the British for the French Army in the way of hospitals'. This picture, *Hôpital Auxiliaire d'Armée 30, Abbaye de Royaumont*, is now in the Dumbarton District Library. Her other big picture, *The Scottish Women's Hospital*, was commissioned by the Imperial War Museum and painted after the war. It can still be seen there.

Gamwell twins, who arrived in 1914, were 'very anxious to get to business and have a go at the Germans'.[4] Summerhayes tells us how the war relieved her of a rather uncongenial job at home:

> I was teaching in a little school up in the north. ... I taught everything. And praise be, the war came, and I got called up and I was able to leave without dishonour. I didn't let the school down.[5]

For Hilda Smeal, a Scot living in California, it was the sinking of the *Lusitania* that persuaded her to volunteer.[6]

Discipline was slack, but disciplinary problems were few. Having worked in a British military hospital before coming to Royaumont, Summerhayes found the lack of discipline strange, and considered it could not have worked with a 'less-committed set of orderlies'. Mrs Manson (Orderly Starr) agreed:

> An enthusiastic band – some very knowledgeable, others, like myself, willing but inexperienced. There was a fine feeling of camaraderie but always a helping hand in a difficulty. We were not surrounded by red tape. There was mutual trust and respect, and there was never any thought of abusing this.[7]

They had little idea when they arrived at Royaumont what might lie ahead of them. On landing in France for the first time, Evelyn Proctor 'felt alone and homesick, far from England and home and safety. I was on a great adventure – the greatest of my life.'[8] She was not the only one to feel a pang. Jean Berry, an early arrival in January 1915, was 'awfully homesick and shocked by the unconventionality and extreme discomfort at that time and said she wouldn't stay'.[9] Nevertheless stay she did, going on to become an expert radiographer.

They could smile later at their naïveté. Another of the first arrivals in December 1914 wrote:

> Do you recall our youthful enthusiasm in those early days, our keenness starting out for France with vague ideas of rescuing

soldiers in the trenches (otherwise why take wellington boots?) and finding ourselves not on a battle field but in a lovely old Abbey with other strange women and a few chronic cases of bronchitis. You had, perhaps, pictured yourself wearing your wellington boots and tartan-trimmed coat, bringing comfort and relief to some poor poilu, instead, at first, it seemed rather problematical whether you would ever see a poilu, let alone look after one. Certainly you wore your wellington boots, but in the scullery where, ankle deep in water, you washed dishes and wondered why the cooks were so disagreeable. They too, no doubt, had dreamed of other sorts of kitchens in or near the front line, run by trained men orderlies.[10]

Looking back, it was the fun they remembered most clearly – possibly the more painful memories were suppressed. The orderlies were indefatigable at devising amusements for themselves and for their patients – and with the variety of talents among them these could be of a very high order. Millicent Armstrong produced some 'stirring dramas' – a skill she later developed in Australia. Christian Warren was a brilliant pianist ('Mees Piano' to the patients), and several of the orderlies had very good voices – Margaret Don, for one, had been training to be an opera singer. Perhaps it was a little disappointing for Mabel Watt ('*le miss qui rit*' – 'the miss who smiles') to be told by a French officer that although her voice was beautiful her French accent was dreadful and she should stick to singing in English.[11] Irma Minchin, a pupil of Margaret Morris, was well-versed in all the details of stage management and was, in addition, a beautiful dancer. Susan Richmond had already embarked on her acting career under Sir Henry Beerbohm Tree when she came to Royaumont, and later went on to great successes in London and Australia, and at the BBC, becoming co-director of a drama school and writing a popular *Textbook of Stagecraft*. She was remembered by her Royaumont friends as the 'personification of gaiety and happiness', and for her rendering of Irish folk songs.[12] Evelyn Moore's acting experience at Royaumont would have prepared her for her eleven years in *The Mousetrap*.

Cicely Hamilton's dramatic productions have already been described.

From time to time some of the orderlies got themselves into scrapes. Grace Summerhayes remembers a spot of trouble shared with her friend Florence Simms over the huge *marmite* in the bathroom in which water was heated. On night duty:

> We used to have to clear it out, it was really rather an awful task, and the only thing to do was to laugh because if not you'd have cried, really, digging out all these ashes. And then we used to put them in a bucket, and then we left them, and one day the bucket set on fire and we found the fire brigade rushing madly round the abbey saying 'Where is the fire coming from?' I said, 'Quickly, Simms, quickly, put it outside in the cloisters, we can't be had up for this! 'So just in time we were able to get rid of our incriminating ashes which were burning through the bottom of the bucket. It was a good thing to have a good pal there. We had great times.[13]

They coped in varying ways with the suffering they saw. For many there was no gentle introduction. Mabel Watt found her first night in the ward 'terrifying', with a soldier lying there dying. Summerhayes's first task was to carry the body of a young village woman with a ruptured uterus to the chapel used temporarily as a mortuary. She had never before seen a corpse. Marjorie Starr was deeply distressed, and almost overwhelmed, by the sights and sounds of men in agony, and was only saved from breakdown by the understanding and sympathy of some of the senior staff. Evelyn Proctor felt being young helped her to cope. Summerhayes 'took it perhaps for granted and knew that was what one had gone out for'.

Keeping pets was one area where authority was flouted – or perhaps authority turned a blind eye. The story of Jimmy the canary (whose adventures have been recounted in Chapter Seven) was only one of a number of birds bred by Sister Everingham. Another was Dinkie, who was housed in a little wooden cage on top of the pulpit in the chapel, 'and how he sang! I think he felt he was in the right place to sing'.[14] Yvonne Barclay also kept birds, and when one of these died in the dead of winter, a colleague remembered 'her pretty tear-stained face as she rushed through the passages with the dead bird in her hand' on her way to the incinerator.[15] 'Everyone knew La Colonelle's efforts to suppress surreptitious livestock that *would* find its way into the wards but they suffered a severe setback when Butler's condemned bitch was not only living long after the date of her supposed execution but had brought up a flourishing family – one of whom rode in her lap driving up to Villers-Cotterêts.'[16] Spot the mongrel, left behind at Villers-Cotterêts by retreating British troops, became the hospital mascot and so held almost an official position. A study of Royaumont photographs reveals other items of livestock, such as Jack the rabbit, Tranche the cat, and a number of other dogs.

There was some slight shortening of the skirts as the years rolled on, in line with general fashion. Miss Ivens was adamant about keeping hair short, as obtaining sufficient water for washing was always a problem. Some tried to keep their long hair, and there were probably others besides Agnes Rolt who betrayed themselves when their hair fell down in moments of crisis. Florence Simms recorded that at Villers-Cotterêts, 'I had to have my hair cut off again yesterday, it was getting so untidy. A Frenchwoman sat watching the operation with her mouth open. There are three others here with cropped heads, one a sister, so I'm not lonely.'[17]

Two orderlies, apart from Mary Peter (see Chapter Five), found their future husbands at Royaumont. In 1914 A.M. Percival came over with her car, and, in case the authorities would not allow her to drive it, she brought along her brother for a short period. But this was long enough for him to fall in love, and later marry, her fellow-orderly, Dorothy Allan. Towards the end, a relative of Mary Anderson, who was ill, asked a young French officer to visit her. She became Madame Petitpierre and settled permanently in France.

For a few of the orderlies their experiences at Royaumont set the pattern of their future careers. Lucy Cranage, Netta Stein and Grace Summerhayes qualified in medicine, and G.L. Buckley and Charlotte Almond completed their interrupted medical studies. A few, having gained considerable competence in nursing in the hospital, embarked on full training after the war. Marjorie Miller became sister-tutor at the Stanley Hospital in Liverpool, and later held the same position at the Edinburgh Royal Infirmary. Agnes Anderson, 'Big Andy', trained in midwifery, worked in India and Ceylon and had a distinguished nursing service in World War Two with the British Red Cross. Anna Merrilees was a 'masseuse' (physiotherapist) in St Bartholemew's Hospital for 20 years, and Rachel Middleton became an almoner at St Thomas's Hospital. Angela Carter (later Lady Hills) became an economics don at Cambridge; Margaret Davidson went back to teaching; and Margaret Freeman and Eveline Martin were both, in turn, headmistress of Westonbirt School for Girls.

There was a wide scattering over the globe after the end of the war. Some followed their husbands, but a considerable number who remained unmarried seem to have sought more experience and adventure abroad. For others the return from a life of adventure and achievement was less exciting. Some went back to the traditional role of caring for the family. Chapman brought up her motherless nephews and nieces; others cared for aging parents. Many did useful work in World War Two. They kept up their wartime friendships to a remarkable degree.

Looking back, Lucy Bruce found it was 'an amazing and unforgettable experience – that widened one's outlook and enriched one's life',[18] and for Irma Minchin it was 'an enchanting memory'. When she visited Royaumont much later Norah Mackay wrote:

> But isn't it curious today, twenty years after the war, that little and tragicomic part of our lives which we spent at Royaumont should stand out so clearly amongst much that is blurred and half-remembered? Quite apart from the fact that many of us were then in what is called an impressionable age, none of the other war work some of us did before or after our time at Royaumont left the same clear-cut imprint on our memories. Yet those of us who have visited Royaumont and its surroundings find that few if any of the inhabitants remember

the strange badly-dressed foreign ladies who worked there during the war.[19]

The Sisters

The work of nurses in World War One was a crucial milestone in the long evolution of the nursing profession. In the pre-Nightingale days the standards of so-called 'nurses' were abysmally low, but by the turn of the century the Nightingale reforms had already achieved great changes and standards were rising. The need for training was fully recognized, but there was not as yet any agreement as to what that training should be. The Nightingale reforms required that 'ladies' of higher social class and education who were destined for positions of authority should undertake one year's training in hospital. 'Probationers', on the other hand, on whom the basic work of the hospital depended, and who were generally recruited from a lower and less well-educated class, were required to have three years' training. In the later decades of the 19th century and up to the beginning of the war the demand for nurses had been increasing. More patients were being treated in hospitals; there were more patients in the workhouses; and the demand for home nursing was rising – by the rich in their own homes and by the poor since the introduction of the District Nursing Service in 1900.

The new 'lady nurses' now leading the profession wanted to make a clear distinction between 'trained' and 'untrained', both to protect the public and to enhance the prestige of the profession. This was part of the wider feminist movement that came increasingly to the fore in the years preceding the war. On the outbreak of war the movement towards the registration of nurses, based on recognized standards of training, was gathering strength, though there was still considerable opposition both in the country at large and also among some leaders of the profession. How, they asked, could they ever, given the general state of girls' education at the time, provide the very large numbers required? This question was still unresolved when war broke out, and, as with so many issues, active campaigning died down and energies were directed towards the war effort. It was not until 1919 that the registration of nurses was finally introduced.

The war produced an enormous escalation in the demand for nurses. Nursing the wounded was a popular goal for many women, both for trained and experienced nurses as well as for members of Voluntary Aid Detachments. However, the success of the armed forces and the voluntary hospitals abroad in attracting nurses was unfortunate for the civilian population at home. Throughout the war it was the chronic sick, the sick in the workhouse infirmaries and in the mental institutions, as well as the 'ordinary' patient in the civilian hospitals, who suffered most from the shortages. By the final year of the war even recruiting nurses for the armed forces and voluntary hospitals such as Royaumont was becoming difficult.

In all, 184 nurses served at Royaumont. Of these, almost all completed their six-month contract: 37 extended their service, presumably an arrangement satisfactory for both sides; three returned for further service after a spell at home or elsewhere; 18 did not complete their contracted service of six months, but of these, 11 left because the war had come to an end and the hospital was closing. Three were dismissed: one for insubordination, one for 'bad behaviour', and one for reasons unspecified. Miss Ivens asked the committee not to renew the contract of a fourth as she was the cause of much friction with the other sisters. It was only to be expected that there should be some variation in the quality of the sisters sent to Royaumont – some indifferent, but others of top quality. The orderlies were well-placed to judge the quality and character of the sisters. One was known as 'God Almighty'; another was deemed 'lazy' but obeyed her orderly when told it was time to make the beds! Orderly Starr provides clear evidence of the variable quality in her diary during the 'rushes' of autumn 1915:

> I have had the most trying sister to train me. Now I have another and what a difference – the other used to lose her head in a rush ... now it is heaven in comparison.[1]

The replacement was probably Sister Gertrude Lindsay from Glasgow Royal Infirmary – 'A first-rate surgical nurse – she gets all the difficult dressings to do'. She was a very popular member of the unit, and was later promoted to matron, proving to be one of the most successful of the Royaumont appointments. 'She had patience and understanding,' one orderly remembered, 'when dealing with inexperienced young women.'[2]

Isabella Duncan, the second matron, had a difficult time with some of her staff, as Starr noted when she was nursing her during a short illness. She was 'a nice old soul' but 'the sisters are always squabbling among themselves and tattling to her and she has to please them all and it is no joke as she hasn't the authority she should have'.[3]

The sisters have left very little record of their own views and experiences of their time at Royaumont, but for the 38 who joined the Royaumont Association after the war one can assume that it was a positive experience. This was certainly the case for Sister Mary Douglas. She wrote from the Royal Naval Hospital Haslar in Gosport in July and August 1917:

I gave my name to the Navy a short time ago not expecting to be called up for a long time. Unfortunately they have called me up so soon. It was a terrible wrench to leave Royaumont. I would go straight back now if I could. I don't know why I ever thought of leaving it ... Haslar is very nice, and we have a very nice time, picnics, tennis, bathing, cycling etc. Yet I believe if it were possible I'd start back to Villers-Cotterêts tomorrow ... The life in France suited me better than all the conventional civilization here. Then the cases are less interesting, and the treatment – much the same as was done in the days of Nelson!!! – I keep wanting to tell them how things were done at Royaumont, but of course it wouldn't do, and also like everything else the treatment must be carried out according to routine and as it has always been done. All the time is taken up with rules and regulations.[4]

Sister Catherine O'Rorke was another who regretted leaving Royaumont, but, unlike Sister Douglas, she did manage to return.

Writing from the enormous 4000-bedded Policlinico in Rome in May 1916, she wrote:

> I am very lonely over leaving Royaumont but had to do so, having unhappily signed on for service in Italy during the early days of the war, however I do not like the work here as the patients are not at all nicely treated, so I am resigning and will write to 2 St Andrew Square [the HQ of the SWH committee] to ask if they will put me on their list.[5]

The case of Sister O'Rorke illustrates the pragmatic attitude taken by Miss Ivens, for which she had the support of the committee. Technically Sister O'Rorke did not fulfil the War Office definition of 'trained' nurse because she had received her training from Nurse Edith Cavell* in the Belgian Institute of Nursing and not in a recognized British hospital. Nevertheless Miss Ivens promoted her to be 'sister-in-charge' to succeed Sister MacKnight – who had been in the forefront of the campaign to bar 'not fully trained' nurses (see Chapter Seven). She was now to take charge of Sister MacKnight's ward. Miss Ivens wrote:

> Sister O'Rorke has taken on a very difficult post owing to the agitation created by Sister MacKnight . . . she is doing extremely well and is one of the few nurses who is always prepared to do her utmost without argument and I think it would be treating her with base ingratitude not to appoint her.[6]

O'Rorke stayed at Royaumont until the end, was awarded the Croix de Guerre, and then transferred to the Scottish Women's Hospitals in Serbia to help with a typhus epidemic. In 1921 she joined the staff of the Anglo-Serbian Children's Hospital and remained in Serbia until her final illness in 1931. She was awarded the Order of St Sava, and on her death her obituary in *The Times* noted:

---

* Executed in Brussels by the Germans in 1915 for her part in assisting in the escape of Allied prisoners of war.

Her life was an example of rare devotion to others and of true charity, and her name will not soon be forgotten among the peasants of Serbia who entrusted their children to her care.[7]

Other sisters also served Royaumont well: Sister (later Matron) Winstanley, 'an excellent organizer' who was remembered for her 'quickness, brightness and willingness to take on any amount of work'; Sister Grey, whose death so saddened the unit and called forth the tribute of a *poilu* – 'our good friend Miss Grey who has always something gentle to do to us'; Sister Inkson, 'hardworking and efficient throughout those terrible months'; Sister Whitworth, 'one of our favourite and most efficient sisters'; Sister Rose Morris of Blanche de Castille Ward, loved by her orderlies; Sister MacGregor, admired by Dr Courtauld and her patients in 'Mary'; Sister Williams, who drew the admiration of Mrs Robertson for her devotion to her Senegalese and North African patients; Sister Everingham, chief theatre sister through the stresses of the evacuation of Villers-Cotterêts and subsequently at Royaumont in 1918; and Sister Goodwin, who was surgical nurse through the bombardments when, as she wrote to Miss Ivens:

> ... we stayed for hours in the darkness and that ammunition train was bombed, and we had so much work to do, and the shrapnel was flying in all directions. That indeed was a dreadful night but you were like the Rock of Gibraltar and inspired us all.[8]

Miss Ivens paid tribute in turn to Sister Goodwin, and recommended her (successfully) for the Croix de Guerre. After the war Goodwin went to Serbia with the Scottish Women's Hospitals, then to the American Red Cross, and finally to the Belgrade Nursing Training School. For all of these the experience of working at Royaumont must have been very significant. What a loss it is that they said so little about it themselves.

Notes and References

Abbreviations used in the references:

CC   *Common Cause.* Journal of the National Union of Women's Suffrage Societies, 1914–1919

IWM   Imperial War Museum, London. Collection of Documents. SWH Collection

ML   Mitchell Library, Glasgow. Department of Rare Books and Manuscripts. Scottish Women's Hospitals Collection. Held in numbered tins and boxes, approximately in date order, but not further catalogued.

NL   Newsletters of the Royaumont and Villers-Cotterêts Association, 1923–1973. Held in Liddle Archive of First World War, University of Leeds, Scottish Women's Hospitals Collection. Box Miss Miller.

Preface

1. Antonio de Navarro *The Scottish Women's Hospital at the French Abbey of Royaumont* (Geo Allen and Unwin, 1917) and Mrs Eva Shaw MacLaren, *A History of the Scottish Women's Hospitals* (Hodder and Stoughton, 1919).
2. Dr Leah Leneman, *In the Service of Life: The Story of Dr Elsie Inglis and the Scottish Women's Hospitals* (Mercat Press, 1994).

Chapter One

1. NL 1973, p. 7, Mrs Falconer (née Manson).
2. Mrs Robertson. Letter 10 Nov 1916, by kind permission of Mrs Ailsa Tanner.
3. Navarro, *The Scottish Women's Hospital at the French Abbey of Royaumont*, p. 171.
4. Personal communication, Dr Grace MacRae (née Summerhayes).

5. NL 1950, p. 3. Mrs Haydon (née Richmond).
6. Information drawn from Henry Goüin and Claude-Jacques Damme, *Royaumont. Mons Regalis.* Editions Valhermeil 1990.
7. Royal Free Hospital Press Cuttings, Book 5 p. 86.
8. McLaren, *A History of the Scottish Women's Hospitals*, pp. 4–7.
9. ML Tin 49, Inglis to French ambassador, 15.10.14.
10. Leneman, *In the Service of Life.*

Chapter Two

1. Personal communication from Miss Rachel Hedderwick, daughter of Dorothy Littlejohn.
2. IWM. Letters of Dorothy Littlejohn to her fiancé, H.J. Hedderwick, 11.12.14.
3. Mrs Withell's Diary, 1914–1915, unpublished, p. 39, kindly communicated by Mr Charles Clark.
4. NL 1946.
5. IWM, *loc. cit.*
6. *CC*, Cicely Hamilton, 11.12.14, p. 599.
7. *CC*, CH, 24.12.14, p. 622.
8. IWM, *loc. cit.*
9. *CC*, CH *loc. cit.*
10. NL 1955, p. 8.
11. ML. Tin 12, Loose leaf file, F. Ivens to committee, 14.12.14.
12. ML. Tin 12, FI to E. Inglis 31.12.14.
13. ML. Tin 12 FI to Compton, 3.1.15.
14. MHF Ivens *Brit. Med. J.*, Aug. 18 1917, p. 203.
15. ML. Tin 12, EI to Compton, 26.12.14.
16. ML. Tin 12, Report of Sanitary Department of Military Government of Paris, 24.12.14.
17. IWM. DL 26.12.14.
18. 'Skia' (V.C.C. Collum), *Blackwood's Magazine*, November 1918, p. 614.
19. ML. Tin 12, FI to EI, 2.1.15.
20. IWM. DL, *loc. cit.*
21. Miss Rachel Hedderwick. Personal communication.
22. ML. Tin 12, FI to EI, 31.12.14.
23. IWM. DL, 20.12.14.
24. IWM. DL, 26.12.14.
25. *Auntie Mabel's War: an account of her part in the hostilities, 1914–1918*, p. 31.
26. ML. Tin 12, FI to EI, 2.1.15.
27. ML, Tin 12, FI to EI, 7.1.15.
28. ML. Tin 12, FI to Crompton, 6.1.15.
29. ML, Tin 12, FI to EI, 10.1.15.
30. ML. Tin 12, FI to EI, 15.1.15.
31. FL. Box 304/2, Loudon 1.7.15.

32. NL 1961, p. 5, extracts from orderlies' letters home.
33. IWM. DL 7.1.15.
34. 'Skia', *op. cit.*, p. 620.
35. NL 1936, p. 11, E. Prance, 'Education of a Well-loved Chief'.
36. NL 1941, p. 37.
37. NL 1966, p. 2.
38. IWM. Diary of M.L. Starr, 18.10.15.
39. ML. Tin 12, FI to Laurie, 1.8.15.
40. ML. Tin 13, EI to Crompton, 26.12.14.
41. ML. Tin 49, FI to EI, 31.12.14.
42. Dr Leila Henry. Reminiscences, kindly made available by Miss Helen Lowe.
43. ML. Uniform Committee Minutes, 4.12.17.
44. FL., Box 304/3, Kinnel to Gosse, 28.7.16.
45. NL 1968, p. 6.
46. ML. Tin 2, Loudon to Mair, Sept. 1915.
47. *Livre d'Or des Oeuvres de Guerre 1915*, by Lucie Berillon, 'Une Visite à l'Hôpital de Royaumont', pp. 4–5. (Our translation.)
48. IWM. Starr Diary, 7.12.15.
49. NL 1964, p. 9.
50. NL 1939, p. 8.
51. Mrs A.M. Robertson, letters transcribed by her granddaughter, Mrs Ailsa Tanner and kindly made available.
52. ML. Tin 12, FI to EI, 6.4.15.
53. NL 1966, p. 6.
54. F.B. Simms, letter to her governess 1.9.18, kindly supplied by her niece Miss M.P. Simms.
55. Dr Grace MacRae, née Summerhayes. Personal communication 12.7.93.
56. NL 1968, p. 6.
57. NL 1937, p. 9.
58. ML, Tin 12, FI to Russell, 12.3.16.
59. IWM. Starr Diary, 18.10.15.
60. ML. Tin 42, Loudon to Maris, 26.9.15.

Chapter Three

1. 'Skia' (V.C.C. Collum), *Blackwood's Magazine*, Nov. 1918, p. 615.
2. ML. Tin 12, F. Ivens to E. Inglis, 10.1.15.
3. ML. Tin 12, FI to EI, 15.1.15.
4. ML. Tin 12, FI to Mrs Laurie, 1.2.15.
5. ML. Tin 49, C. Hamilton to Crompton, 20.2.15.
6. ML. Tin 12, Harley to EI, 26.2.15.
7. ML. Tin 12, FI to EI, 11.3.15.
8. ML. Tin 12, FI to EI, 27.3.15.
9. ML. Tin 12, FI to Laurie, 26.3.15.

10. 'Skia', *op. cit.*, p. 617.
11. ML. Tin 42, FI to EI, 6.4.15.
12. ML. Tin 13, EI to FI, 30.3.15.
13. ML. Tin 13, EI to Laurie, 30.3.15.
14. ML. Tin 13, EI to Mair, 25.4.15.
15. ML. Tin 13, EI to Laurie, 25.4.15.
16. ML. Tin 12 (loose leaf file), FI to EI, 6.4.15.
17. ML. Tin 12, Mrs Harley to EI, 10.2.15.
18. Leneman, *In the Service of Life*.
19. Hamilton, *Life Errant*, p. 117.
20. NL 1931, p. 1.
21. ML. Tin 13, EI to Miss Mair, 25.4.15.
22. ML. Tin 12, FI to EI, 6.4.15.
23. NL January 1929.
24. ML. Tin 49, C. Hamilton to Miss Crompton, 20.2.15.
25. 'Skia', *op. cit.*, p. 616.
26. *Ibid.*
27. *Ibid.*
28. *Ibid.*
29. *CC*, C. Hamilton, July 15 1915.
30. Dr L.M. Henry. Reminiscences presented by her to Miss Helen Lowe who kindly made them available to me.
31. NL 1970, p. 2.
32. Liddle Archive in Leeds University. Taped interview with Miss Margaret Ainslie Stewart, chauffeur, 5.5.17 to 7.11.17.
33. ML. Tin 42, C. Hamilton, 2.8.15.
34. ML. Tin 1, Report to Personnel Committee, 5.6.15.
35. ML. Tin 12, FI to Miss Marris, 17.9.15.
36. Navarro, *The Scottish Women's Hospital*, p. 171.
37. Wellcome Institute for the History of Medicine. Dr Elizabeth Butler to secretary, Lister Institute, 31.8.14.
38. ML. Tin 12, FI to Miss Marris, June 1915.
39. ML. Tin 42, 3.3.16.
40. ML. Tin 12, Miss Loudon to Mrs Laurie, 26.6.15.
41. *CC*, July 2 1915.
42. *CC*, July 9 1915.
43. *CC*, Cicely Hamilton, July 30 1915.
44. *CC*, V. Collum, July 30 1915, p. 219.
45. *CC*, C. Hamilton, August 27 1915, p. 261.
46. *CC*, December 3 1915, p. 450.
47. ML. Tin 42, Miss Loudon to Marris, 6.8.15.
48. ML. *loc. cit.*, 29.9.15.
49. FL. Box 304/3, C. Hamilton to Dr Savill.
50. ML. Tin 42, FI to Marris, 29.9.15.

51. IWM. Diary of Marjorie Starr (Orderly 30.8.15 to 26.2.16). Dates of entries as given in text.
52. ML. Tin 6, Rutherford to Russell, 23.10.15.
53. ML. Tin 41, Mrs Hunter's Report to the Hospital Committee, 27.11.15.
54. ML. Tin 42, Loudon to Marris, undated.
55. Frances Ivens. Newsletter Medical Women's Federation 1926, p. 19–20.
56. Louisa Martindale, *A Woman Surgeon* (Gollancz, 1951), pp. 166–8.
57. ML. Tin 41, Hospital Committee Minutes, 15.10.15.
58. NL 1937, p. 10.

Chapter Four

1. ML. Tin 12, 'Impressions of Hospital at Abbaye de Royaumont' (source not stated).
2. *CC*, 21.1.16. Reported by Miss Loudon.
3. ML. Tin 42, C. Hamilton to Kemp, 17.2.16.
4. ML. Tin 42, Mrs Laurie and Mrs Robertson. Report, April 1916.
5. ML. Tin 42, F. Ivens to Kemp, 28.2.16.
6. ML. *ibid.*
7. ML. Tin 42, FI to Russell, 2.4.16.
8. ML. Tin 42, Loudon to Kemp, 13.3.16.
9. *Leven Advertiser.* Obituary notice, Jan. 1916.
10. ML. Tin 42, FI to Russell, 2.4.16.
11. ML. Tin 42, 7.4.16.
12. *CC*, C. Hamilton, 18.8.16.
13. ML. Tin 42, FI to Hunter, 21.6.16.
14. ML. Tin 42, FI to Russell, 21.5.16.
15. ML. Tin 42, FI to Russell, 18.6.16.
16. ML. Tin 42, 16.6.16.
17. ML. Tin 42, FI to Kemp, 12.3.16.
18. ML. Tin 12, 4.7.16.
19. 'Skia', *Blackwood's Magazine*, March 1917, pp. 339–40.
20. 'Skia', *ibid.*, pp. 340–342.
21. 'Skia', *op. cit.*, November 1918, p. 622.
22. 'Skia', *op. cit.*, March 1917, p. 346.
23. *Ibid.*
24. ML. Tin 42, Savill to Russell, 4.7.16.
25. Dr Elsie Dalyell, letter *Sydney and NSW Daily Telegraph*, 22.1.18.
26. Navarro, *The Scottish Women's Hospital*, p. 165.
27. ML. Tin 42, FI to Kemp, 3.7.16.
28. ML. Tin 42, FI to Kemp, 16.7.16.
29. 'Skia', *op. cit.*, March 1917, p. 342–343.
30. *CC*, C. Hamilton 4.8.16. p. 215.
31. ML. Tin 41, 9.8.16.
32. ML. Tin 42, 30.8.16.

33. ML. Tin 42, FI to Kemp, 13.8.16.
34. Dora Pym, 'Patchwork from the Past'. Unpublished memoirs by kind permission of her daughter, Mary Pym.
35. NL 1936, pp. 5–6.
36. NL 1964, p. 9.
37. ML. Tin 42, FI to Kemp, 19.8.16 and Tin 12, FI to Laurie, 12.8.16.
38. ML. Tin 42, Erskine to May, 19.8.16.
39. ML. Tin 42, *ibid.*
40. ML. Tin 12, FI to Laurie.
41. ML. Tin 42, FI to Kemp, 19.8.16.
42. ML. Tin 42, Erskine to May, 16.9.16.
43. ML. Tin 42, *ibid.*
44. *Ibid.*
45. ML. Tin 41, Executive Committee Minutes, 20.12.16.
46. Mrs A.M. Robertson. Letters home, 3.11.16. By kind permission of her granddaughter, Mrs Ailsa Tanner.
47. Ibid., 14.11.16.
48. *CC*, 25.8.16, p. 248.
49. McLaren, *A History of the Scottish Women's Hospitals*, p. 40.
50. ML. Tin 42, FI to Kemp, 27.8.16.
51. Mrs A.M. Robertson, *op. cit.*, 25.10.16.
52. Mrs A.M. Robertson, *op. cit.*, 14.11.16.
53. Mrs A.M. Robertson, *op. cit.*, 12.11.16.
54. Mrs A.M. Robertson, *op. cit.*, 1.11.16.
55. Mrs A.M. Robertson, *op. cit.*, 29.10.16.
56. Mrs A.M. Robertson, *op. cit.*, 29.10.16.
57. Mrs A.M. Robertson, *op. cit.*, 31.10.16.
58. Mrs A.M. Robertson, *op. cit.*, 2.11.16.
59. Mrs A.M. Robertson, *op. cit.*, 19.11.16.
60. Mrs A.M. Robertson, *op. cit.*, 4.11.16.
61. 'The Call of our Allies and the Response of the Scottish Women's Hospitals for Foreign Service', June 1915, p. 14.
62. ML. Tin 42, Loudon to Marris, 6.8.15.
63. ML. Tin 42, Mrs Robertson to Marris, 23.11.16.
64. Dr L.M. Henry. Reminiscences, by kind permission of her daughter, Mrs Anne Murdoch.
65. NL 1970, p. 6.
66. NL 1961, p. 2.
67. Dr Grace MacRae (née Summerhayes). Personal communication.
68. ML. Tin 42, Russell to FI, 3.7.18.
69. ML. Tin 42, FI to Russell. No date but probably 15 or 16.7.18.
70. *CC.*, 19.1.17, p. 536.
71. F. Ivens, *Proc. Roy. Soc. Med. 1916–1917 Part 3. Surgical Section*, pp. 29–110.
72. 'Skia', *Blackwood's Magazine*, November 1918, p. 621.

Chapter Five

1. Ducasse, Meyer & Perreux, *Vie et Mort des Français, 1914–1918*, p. 78.
2. Horne, *The Price of Glory*, p. 71.
3. Navarro, *The Scottish Women's Hospital*, p. 210.
4. Horne, *op. cit.*, p. 71.
5. Ducasse *et al, op. cit.*, p. 81.
6. Ducasse, *et al, op. cit.*, p. 79.
7. Ducasse *et al, op. cit.*, p. 99.
8. Horne, *op. cit.*, p. 74.
9. F.M. Ivens, 'Clinical Study of Anaerobic Wound Infections. Analysis of 107 cases of gas gangrene', *Proc. Roy. Soc. Med. 1916–1917, part 3. Surgical Section*, pp. 29–110.
10. Horne, *op. cit.*, p. 75.
11. IWM. Georgina Cowan Collection, Pte Breuil to GC January 1918.
12. IWM. GC Collection, Cpl Matthieu to GC January 1918.
13. FL. Box 309, 9.4.18.
14. *CC*, 15.2.18.
15. Personal communication from Miss Heather Mackay (niece).
16. 'Skia' (V.C.C. Collum) *Blackwood's Magazine*, March 1917, p. 346.
17. NL 1965, p. 10.
18. NL 1970, p. 8.
19. 'Skia', *op. cit.*, November 1918, p. 624.
20. Personal communication from Dr Grace MacRae (née Summerhayes).
21. 'Skia', *op. cit.*, March 1917, p. 34.
22. *Ibid.*
23. Navarro, *op. cit.*, p. 189.
24. *Ibid.*
25. 'Skia', *op. cit.*, March 1917, p. 345.
26. Dr L.M. Henry, *loc. cit.*
27. NL 1936, p. 9.
28. NL 1967, p. 11.
29. NL 1973, p. 7.
30. IWM. Letters of E.H. Proctor transcribed by Dr Leah Leneman and made available to me and used by permission of her nephew, Mr David Proctor.
31. Personal communication, Dr Grace MacRae (née Summerhayes).
32. Dr E. Courtauld, *loc. cit.*, 27.6.18.
33. Dr L.M. Henry, *loc. cit.*
34. 'Skia', *op. cit.*, November 1918, p. 637.
35. Dr Grace MacRae. Interview recorded by Dr Leah Leneman and kindly made available to me, June 1993.
36. Mrs A.M. Robertson. Letters home, by kind permission of her granddaughter Mrs Ailsa Tanner.
37. NL 1968, p. 1.
38. NL November, 1928, p. 5.

39. *Ibid.*
40. *Ibid.*, p. 4
41. NL 1965, p. 10.
42. NL 1964, p. 9.
43. Navarro, *The Scottish Women's Hospital*, p. 209. Navarro's translation.
44. ML. Tin 42, Ramsay-Smith to Committee, August 1918.
45. NL November, 1928, p. 4

Chapter Six

1. Horne, *The Price of Glory*, p. 71.
2. *Ibid.*
3. Fl. Box 305, 'Extract of letter from Royaumont', undated.
4. NL 1935, p. 5.
5. 'Skia' (V.C.C. Collum), *Blackwood's Magazine*, November 1918, p. 623.
6. ML. Tin 42, *loc. cit.*, 19.1.17.
7. ML. Tin 42, FI to May, 24.2.17.
8. ML. Tin 31, 6.7.17.
9. ML. Tin 42, FI to Russell, 18.3.17.
10. ML. Tin 42, telegram FI to committee, 2.5.17.
11. ML. Tin 42, FI to Hunter, 17.5.17.
12. ML. Tin 42, Hamilton to May, 7.5.17.
13. ML. Tin 42, FI to May, 26.6.17.
14. *Ibid.*
15. Binyon, *For Dauntless France*, pp. 243–6.
16. ML. Tin 42, 'From the Sisters at Royaumont', 11.6.17.
17. *Ibid.*, 31.7.17.
18. *CC*, V.C.C. Collum, 13.7.17.
19. ML. Tin 41, telegram, 6.6.17.
20. ML. Tin 42, FI to May, 10.8.17.
21. McLaren, *A History of the Scottish Women's Hospitals*, p. 60.
22. ML. Tin 42, Robertson to Russell, 8.6.17.
23. Robertson to Russell, *loc. cit.*, ?date.
24. ML. Tin 42, Erskine ?date.
25. NL 1965, p. 6.
26. 'Skia', *Blackwood's Magazine*, November 1918, p. 624.
27. ML. Tin 42, FI to Craigie, 25.7.17.
28. ML. Tin 42, FI to May, 8.8.17.
29. ML. Tin 42, Winstanley to May, 12.8.17.
30. ML. Tin 42, Savill to Willis, 16.8.17.
31. ML. Tin 42, Savill to Russell, 3.9.17.
32. ML. Tin 42, Ramsay-Smith to Russell, 6.10.17.
33. ML. Tin 42, FI to Russell, 15.10.17.
34. ML. Tin 42, Ramsay-Smith to May, 7.11.17.

35. ML. Tin 42, FI to Laurie, 14.11.17.

36. Hutton, *Memoirs of a Doctor in War and Peace*, p. 134.

37. Information kindly supplied by Dr Jean Guy.

38. Liddell Archives, Leeds University, file of Dr L.M. Henry.

39. ML. Tin 12, Dr Louisa McIlroy, 8.8.16.

40. Tin 42, Erskine to Kemp, 22.11.17.

41. ML. Tin 12, Stoney to Laurie, 21.11.17.

42. Frances Ivens, obituary notice in *Brit. Med. J.*, 18.8.17, p. 237 and *Lancet*, 18.8.17, p. 259.

43. *The Englishwoman*, November 1917. Quoted in NL November 1934.

44. Dora Pym, 'Patchwork from the Past'. Unpublished memoirs, by kind permission of her daughter, Miss Mary Pym.

45. IWM. Evelyn Hope Proctor. Letters to her mother, 27.7.17. By kind permission of her nephew, Mr David Proctor.

46. *Loc. cit.*, 8.8.17.

47. *Loc. cit.*, 29.8.17.

48. *Loc. cit.*, 16.9.17.

49. *Loc. cit.*, 1.10.17.

50. *Loc. cit.*, 30.10.17.

51. *Loc. cit.*

52. *Loc. cit.*, 11.10.17.

53. *Loc. cit.*, 30.10.17.

54. *Loc. cit.*, 25.10.17.

55. *Loc. cit.*, 18.12.17.

56. *Loc. cit.*, 29.12.17.

57. *Loc. cit.*, 18.12.17.

58. Personal communication from Dr Grace McRae, July 1993.

59. IWM. Proctor 10.1.18.

60. NL November 1928.

61. ML. Tin 42, FI to Russell, undated, probably 15 or 16.7.17.

62. IWM. Proctor 29.12.17.

63. Dr L.M. Henry. By kind permission of her daughter, Mrs Anne Murdoch.

Chapter Seven

1. B.H. Liddell Hart, *History of the World War (1914–1918)* (1934).

2. IWM. E.H. Proctor, letters to her mother, 1.1.18. By kind permission of her nephew, Mr David Proctor.

3. McLaren, *A History of the Scottish Women's Hospitals*, p. 44.

4. Decassé et al., *Vie et Mort des Français, 1914–1918*, p. 310.

5. McLaren, *op. cit.*, p. 44.

6. ML. Tin 42, Robertson to Laurie, 16.1.18.

7. *Ibid.*, 8.1.18.

8. ML. Tin 42, Frances Ivens to Kemp, 7.2.18.

9. ML. Personnel Committee File, Dr Bennet to Russell, 7.6.17.
10. ML. Tin 42, FI to Kemp, 15.3.18.
11. ML. Tin 42, Collum to Committee, 11.4.18.
12. ML. Tin 42, FI to Kemp, 15.3.18.
13. 'K.S.B.', 'Through the War with a Motor Car', *The Englishwoman*, Oct. 1919, p. 35.
14. ML. Tin 42, FI to Kemp, 25.4.18.
15. *Ibid.*
16. ML. Tin 49, FI to Hon. Sec., 20.5.18.
17. Dr E. Courtauld, letter to her sister Ruth, 25.4.18, by kind permission of her great-nephew, Mr Samuel Courtauld.
18. ML. Tin 49, FI to Hon. Sec., 20.5.18.
19. Dr Grace MacRae (née Summerhayes). Personal communication.
20. Liddle Archive, Leeds University, Dr L.M. Henry papers.
21. 'Skia' (V.C.C. Collum), *Blackwood's Magazine*, November 1918, p. 62.
22. ML. Tin 42, FI to Kemp, 30.6.18.
23. *Ibid.*
24. Dr E. Courtauld, letter to her father, 31.5.18, by kind permission of Mr S. Courtauld.
25. Dr L.M. Henry. Reminiscences. By kind permission of her daughter Mrs Anne Murdoch.
26. *Ibid.*
27. Personal communication from Mrs Anne Murdoch.
28. 'Skia', *op. cit.*, p. 629.
29. NL 1968, p. 5.
30. ML. Tin 42, Georgina Cowan to Committee, 30.5.18.
31. NL 1938, p. 14.
32. ML. Tin 42, Florence Anderson to Committee, 1.6.18.
33. ML. Tin 49, unnamed and undated.
34. NL 1968, p. 6.
35. ML. Tin 49, *loc. cit.*
36. NL 1947, p. 9.
37. ML. Tin 49, *loc. cit.*
38. ML. Tin 42, Edith Stoney to Mrs Walker, 30.6.18.
39. NL 1968, p. 6.
40. NL 1928, p. 9.
41. ML. Tin 42, E. Stoney to Mrs Walker, 30.6.18.
42. ML. Tin 12, ES to Laurie, 17.7.18.
43. *Ibid.*
44. Dr E. Courtauld, letter to her father, 31.5.18, by kind permission of Mr Samuel Courtauld.
45. 'Skia', *op. cit.*, p. 628.
46. *Ibid.*
47. 'K.S.B.', *The Englishwoman*, Oct. 1919, pp. 35–36.
48. FL. SWH Collection, Collum to Committee, 5.6.18.

49. 'Skia', *op. cit.*, p. 630.
50. 'Skia', *ibid.*, p. 631.
51. ML. Tin 42, Georgina Cowan to Committee, 30.5.18.
52. F.B. Simms, letter to her governess, Miss Grignells, 10.6.18, by kind permission of her niece, Miss M.P. Simms.
53. Dr Grace MacRae. Personal communication.
54. ML. Tin 42, FI to Russell, undated, probably 15 or 16.7.18.
55. *Ibid.*
56. 'Skia', *op. cit.*, p. 632.
57. ML. Tin 42, Ramsay-Smith to Laurie, 4.6.18.
58. ML. Tin 42, ES To Walker, 30.6.18.
59. NL 1938, p. 13.
60. ML. Tin 42, ES to Walker, 30.6.18.
61. *Ibid.*
62. ML. Tin 42, Dr Florence Stoney to Laurie, 17.6.18.
63. Dr Leah Leneman, *Brit. Med. J.*, 1993, Vol. 307, 18–25, 'Medical Women in the First World War – Ranking Nowhere'.
64. ML. Tin 42, Dr Guest to Russell, undated.
65. ML. Tin 42, Dr Guest to Russell, 21.6.18.
66. ML. Personnel Committee Minutes, 25.6.18.
67. ML. Tin 42, FI to Russell, undated, probably 15 or 16.7.18.
68. ML. Tin 42, D.H.K. Stevenson to Russell, 29.5.18.
69. *Ibid.*
70. ML. Tin 42, Stevenson to Ivens, 8.6.18.
71. ML. Tin 42, Ramsay-Smith to Russell, 13.6.18.
72. ML. Tin 42, Stevenson to Russell, 12.6.18.
73. *Ibid.*
74. ML. Tin 42, FI to Russell, 26.6.18.
75. ML. Tin 42, FI to Russell, undated.
76. ML. Tin 42, Agnes Anderson to Russell, 25.6.18.
77. *Ibid.*
78. *Ibid.*
79. ML. Tin 42, statement by Sister Thom, enclosed in letter FI to Russell, 26.6.18.
80. Statement by Miss Lindsay, *loc. cit.*
81. ML. Tin 42, FI to Committee, 6.6.18, 13.6.18 and 25.6.18.
82. ML. Tin 42, undated telegram.
83. ML. Tin 42, FI to Russell, undated.
84. *Ibid.*
85. ML. Tin 42, Miss Simpson to Committee, 5.12.18.
86. *Ibid.*
87. ML. Tin 42, FI to Russell, undated.
88. ML. Tin 42, FI to Kemp, 30.6.18.
89. 'Skia', *op. cit.*, p. 637.
90. Dr Grace MacRae. Personal communication.

91. Dr E. Courtauld, *loc. cit.*, 27.6.18, by kind permission of Mr Samuel Courtauld.
92. *Ibid.*
93. *Ibid.*
94. ML. Tin 42, Dr A. Savill to Russell, 15.7.18.
95. Miss F.B. Simms, letter to governess, 30.7.18, by kind permission of Miss M.P. Simms.
96. *Ibid.*
97. ML. Tin 42, FI to Committee, telegram 7.8.18.
98. IWM. E.H. Proctor, letters to her mother, undated, by kind permission of Mr David Proctor.
99. *Ibid.*
100. *Ibid.*
101. *Ibid.*
102. Dr. E. Courtauld, *loc. cit.*, 28.8.18, by kind permission of Mr Samuel Courtauld.
103. ML. Tin 42, E. Stoney to Laurie, 7.10.18.
104. Dr E. Courtauld, *loc. cit.*, 8.10.18.
105. Account of ceremony kindly supplied by Mr Samuel Courtauld.
106. Dr E. Courtauld, *loc. cit.*, 14.11.18, by kind permission of Mr Samuel Courtauld.
107. *Ibid.*
108. *Ibid.*

Chapter Eight

1. Dr E. Courtauld, letter to her sister, 13.12.18, by kind permission of Mr Samuel Courtauld.
2. *Ibid.*
3. *CC,* January 7 1919.
4. Dr E. Courtauld, *loc. cit.*
5. Dr E. Courtauld, *loc. cit.*
6. *Ibid.*
7. ML. Tin 42, Report to Committee from Yeats, December 1918.
8. *Ibid.*
9. Dr E. Courtauld, letter to her sister, 12.1.19, by kind permission of Mr Samuel Courtauld.
10. Dr L. Henry. Reminiscences, by kind permission of her daughter, Mrs Anne Murdoch.
11. Dr E. Courtauld, *loc. cit.*
12. Dr L. Henry, *loc. cit.*
13. ML. Tin 42, Laurie to FI, 30.11.18.
14. ML. Tin 42, FI to Laurie, 13.12.18.
15. ML. Tin 12, Laurie to FI, 30.11.18.
16. ML. Tin 41, Hospital Committee Minutes, 1.2.19.
17. IWM. Proctor letters to her mother, undated, by kind permission of Mr David Proctor.

18. *Ibid.*
19. *Ibid.*
20. ML. Tin 12, ES to Laurie, 7.10.18.
21. ML. Tin 12, ES to Laurie, 2.5.19.
22. *Ibid.*
23. ML. Tin, 12, Dr F. Stoney to Laurie, 23.4.19.
24. NL 1965, p. 10.
25. NL 1937, p. 10.
26. ML. Tin 42, E. Courtauld to Russell, 24.2.19.
27. IWM. Proctor letters, undated, by kind permission of Mr David Proctor.
28. ML. Tin 49, Descoings to Laurie, January 1919.
29. ML. Tin 12, Laurie, undated.
30. ML. Tin 49, 1.1.19.

Appendix One

1. *Official History of the War. Medical Services, Vol 2*, pp. 49–50.
2. Frances Ivens-Knowles, *Brit. Med. J.*, Nov. 25 1939, p. 1058.
3. L.M. Henry, 'The Treatment of War Wounds by Serum Therapy'. MD thesis, University of Sheffield, 1920.
4. Dr Grace MacRae. Personal communication.
5. Ivens, F.M. 'A Clinical Study of Anaerobic Wound Infection. Analysis of 107 Cases of Gas Gangrene', *Proc. Roy. Soc. Med. 1916–1917*, X Part 3, Surgical Section, 29–110.
6. Ivens, F.M., 'The Prevention and Curative Treatment of Gas Gangrene by Mixed Serums', *Brit. Med. J.* Oct 19, 1918, 425–427.
7. Bowlby, A.A. and Rowland, S., Field Laboratory GHQ, Nov 11th 1914.
8. Henry, *op. cit.*
9. Savill, A., *Archives of Radiology and Electrotherapy*, Vol XXI No. 7, December 1916.
10. *Ibid.*
11. Henry, *op. cit.*
12. Henry, *op. cit.*
13. Delbet, P., *Presse Médicale*, Aug 29, 1918 (verbal communication).
14. Navarro, *The Scottish Women's Hospital.*
15. *Brit. Med. J.*, Aug. 21 1915, p. 301 and Aug. 28 1915, p. 334.
16. ML. Tin 42, Erskine and Low, Report to Committee, 16.9.16.
17. *Ibid.*
18. NL 1928, November, p. 3.

Appendix Two

Frances Ivens

1. *J. Medical Women's Federation*, 1945, p. 198.
2. Mrs Lillie Robinson to Mrs Dora Pym, August 7 ?year. By permission of Miss Mary Pym.

3. Writer unknown – footnote to above letter.
4. Dora Pym, Unpublished memoirs, 'Patchwork from the Past', by kind permission of Miss Mary Pym.
5. Robinson, *loc. cit.*
6. NL 1945, p. 3.
7. Dr Hilda Cantrell, taped recording kindly sent by Dr James Carmichael.
8. Dora Pym, *loc. cit.*
9. NL 1945, p. 3.
10. *Ibid*, p. 4.
11. Dr Catherine Chisholm, *Journal Medical Women's Federation*, 1945, p. 41.
12. V.C.C. Collum, speech at First Royaumont dinner, 28.11.1919, transcribed and kindly made available to me by Miss Mary Pym.
13. Royal Free Hospital School of Medicine Press Cuttings Book 4.
14. *J. Med. Women's Fed.*, 1945, p. 42.
15. NL 1936, p. 12.
16. Dr Hilda Cantrell, *loc. cit.*
17. Information kindly supplied by Mr D.M. Crook, librarian, Liverpool Medical Institution.
18. NL 1930, p. 6.
19. V.C.C. Collum, *loc. cit.*
20. McLaren, *A History of the Scottish Women's Hospitals*, p. 53.
21. L.M. Henry, tape recording kindly supplied by her daughter, Mrs Anne Murdoch.
22. Navarro, *The Scottish Women's Hospital*, p. 53.
23. NL 1945, p. 2.
24. *Ibid.*, p. 3.
25. *Ibid.*, p. 1.
26. ML. Tin 49, 1922.
27. NL 1945, p.1
28. V.C.C. Collum, *loc. cit.*

Elizabeth Courtauld
1. Moberley Bell, *Storming the Citadel*, p. 18.
2. Elizabeth Courtauld, unpublished diaries, 1883, by permission of Mr Samuel Courtauld.
3. E. Courtauld, diaries, 1886, 1888, 1889 and 1890.
4. Dr L. Henry to Mr Samuel Courtauld, 15.3.79, by permission of Mr Courtauld.
5. NL 1945, p. 4.
6. E. Courtauld, Session Papers, RFHSMW (Royal Free Hospital School of Medicine for Women) 1908–1909, p. 25, 'Sketches from a South Indian Hospital'.
7. Courtauld, Edinburgh *Evening News*, 25.7.24
8. Dr L. Henry to Mr Samuel Courtauld, 15.3.79, *loc. cit.*
9. Mrs A.M. Robertson, letter 29.10.16, by kind permission of Mrs Ailsa Tanner.
10. NL 1964, p. 7.
11. NL 1948, p. 2.

12. 'L.M.P.', *Brit. Med. J.* 1948, Jan 17th, p. 129.
13. Dr L. Henry to Mr Samuel Courtauld, 15.3.79.

Agnes Savill
1. St John's Hospital for Diseases of the Skin, 1863 to 1963, pp 31, 32. By courtesy of Dr I.R. White, honorary archivist.
2. A.F. Savill, C.W. Mansell Moullin and Sir Victor Horsley, *Lancet* 13 July 1912, p. 119; and *Lancet* 24 August 1912, p. 549, 'Preliminary Report on the Forcible Feeding of Suffrage Prisoners'.
3. *Ibid.*
4. Savill, *Music, Health and Character* p. 48 *et seq.*
5. *Ibid.*
6. ML. Tin 12, AS to Committee, 6.8.15.
7. Dr E. Courtauld, letter to Ruth, 16.7.18, by kind permission of Mr Samuel Courtauld.
8. Dr L. Henry, memoir on Dr Savill written in April 1964, by kind permission of Mrs Anne Murdoch.
9. Agnes Savill, *Alexander the Great and his Time*. Rockcliffe Publishing Corporation, 1955.

Dr (Mrs) Berry
1. NL 1956, p. 5.
2. NL 1961, p. 5.
3. McLaren, *A History of the Scottish Women's Hospitals*, p. 39.
4. NL 1956, p. 2.
5. NL 1931, p. 2.
6. NL 1956, p. 5.
7. *Ibid.*, p. 2.
8. Mrs A.M. Robertson, letter 14.11.16, by kind permission of Mrs Ailsa Tanner.
9. *Ibid.*
10. NL 1956, p. 5.
11. *Ibid.*, p. 5.
12. *Ibid.*
13. ML. Tin 30, Mr Grosvenor Berry to Mrs Laurie, April 1919.

Ruth Nicholson
1. NL 1964, p. 4.
2. NL 1945, p. 2.
3. NL 1964, p. 4.
4. *Ibid.*

Elsie Jean Dalyell
1. *Australian Dictionary of Biography. Vol 8. 1891–1939*. Melbourne University Press, pp. 201–202.
2. G.D. Richardson, 'The Dalyells and their Kin'. 1988. By kind permission of the author.

3. *Ibid.*
4. *Australian Dictionary of Biography, op. cit.*
5. E.J. Dalyell, letter to Professor Welsh, University of Sydney. 31 May 1915.
6. *Australian Dictionary of Biography, op. cit.*
7. Post-graduate Bulletin, University of Sydney, May 1958, p. 48.
8. Harriet Chick, Margaret Hume and Marjorie McFarlane, *War and Disease: A History of the Lister Institute.* Andre Deutsch, 1971, Ch. 15.
9. Mr William Dalyell. Personal communication.
10. G.D. Richardson, *op. cit.*
11. Mr William Dalyell. Personal communication.
12. University of Sydney. Centenary Book, Faculty of Medicine, 1984, p. 234.
13. NL 1950, p. 5.

Lydia Manley Henry

Information from Dr Henry's own papers and tape recordings very kindly supplied to me by her daughter Mrs Anne Murdoch, who has also added some further information about her mother. I am indebted also to Dr Harold Swan, Honorary Lecturer in the History of Medicine in Sheffield University, for the citation for her honorary degree and information about her mother's career in Sheffield.

1. L. Henry to Mr Samuel Courtauld, 15.3.79, by kind permission of Mr Samuel Courtauld.

Edith Marjorie Martland

1. IWM. E.H. Proctor, letters to her mother, 1.1.18.
2. *Lancet,* April 7 1962; *Brit. Med. J.,* March 24 1962, pp. 885–886.

Vera Collum

1. NL 1958, p. 2.
2. 'Ski' (*sic*), 'Torpedoed!', *Blackwood's Magazine,* May 1916, pp. 690–698.
3. *Times,* 25.3.16 to 30.3.16.
4. NL 1934, February, p. 3.

Cicely Hamilton

1. Hamilton, *Life Errant,* J.M. Dent & Co, London 1935.
2. Whitelaw, *The Life and Rebellious Times of Cicely Hamilton,* The Women's Press, London 1990.
3. ML. Tin 12, FI to Laurie, 12.8.16.
4. ML. Tin 12, Mrs Owen 2.2.15.
5. ML. Tin 12, Mrs Harley to Committee, March 1915.
6. IWM. D.H. Littlejohn, letter to fiancé, 11.12.14, by permission of her daughter, Miss Rachel Hedderwick.
7. Hamilton, *Life Errant,* p. 106.
8. *Op. cit.,* pp. 110–111.
9. *Op. cit.,* p. 230.

10. *Op. cit.*, pp. 233–236.
11. *Op. cit.*, p. 201.
12. NL 1953, p. 2.

The Orderlies

1. 'Skia' (V.C.C. Collum), *Blackwood's Magazine*, Nov. 1918, p. 620.
2. *John Masefield's Letters from the Front, 1915–1917*. Ed. Peter Vansittart. Constable 1984, pp. 57 and 84.
3. Interview with Miss Una Moffat (aged 98), 1.7.93, by courtesy of Dr Leah Leneman.
4. Antonia Marian Gamwell, IWM SR 502/11.
5. Interview with Dr Grace MacRae (née Summerhayes) 10.6.93, by courtesy of Dr Leah Leneman.
6. Personal communication from Mrs Fairlie (niece).
7. NL 1973, p. 7.
8. IWM. E.H. Proctor, 'On landing in France'. An essay.
9. NL 1956, p. 5 and NL 1961, p. 5.
10. NL 1950, p. 1.
11. Personal communication from Mrs Mona Calder (daughter).
12. NL 1959, p. 2.
13. Interview Dr MacRae (née Summerhayes).
14. NL 1955, p.7.
15. NL 1957, p.7.
16. NL 1928, April, p. 9.
17. F.B. Simms, *loc. cit.*, 27.3.18.
18. NL 1962, p. 4.
19. NL 1934, p. 1.

The Sisters

1. IWM. Starr Diary, 27.9.15.
2. NL 1967, p. 3.
3. IWM. Starr Diary, 2.12.15.
4. ML. Tin 30, Douglas to Laurie, 28.7.17.
5. ML. Tin 36, O'Rorke to Laurie, 7.7.16.
6. ML. Tin 42, Ivens to May, 30.8.17.
7. *Times*, 13.1.32.
8. NL 1938, p. 14.

Bibliography

Brian Abel-Smith, *History of the Nursing Profession*. Heinemann 1960.

W. Alexander, *First Ladies of Medicine*. Wellcome Unit for the History of Medicine. University of Glasgow 1987.

Auntie Mabel's War: An account of her part in the hostilities, 1914–1918. Compiled by Marion Wengel and John Cornish. Allan Lane 1980.

Henri Barbusse, *Le Feu*. Flammarion 1965.

E. Moberly Bell, *Storming the Citadel. The Rise of the Woman Doctor*. Constable 1953.

Lawrence Binyon, *For Dauntless France. An Account of Britain's Aid to the Wounded and Victims of War*. Hodder and Stoughton 1918.

Catriona Blake, *The Charge of the Parasols. Women's Entry to the Medical Profession*. Women's Press 1990.

Gail Braybon, *Women Workers in the First World War. The British Experience*. Croom Helm 1981.

Roland Dorgeles, *Les Croix des Bois*. Albin Michel 1919.

André Ducasse, Jaques Meyer, Gabriel Perieux. *Vie et Mort des Français, 1914–1918*. Hachette 1962.

Cicely Hamilton, *Life Errant*. Dent 1935.

B.H. Liddell Hart, *History of the First World War*. Cassell 1970.

Alastair Horne, *The Price of Glory: Verdun 1916*. Penguin Books 1964.

Alastair Horne, *Death of a Generation. Neuve Chapelle to Verdun and the Somme*. McDonald Library of the Twentieth Century 1970.

Isabel Hutton, *Memoirs of a Doctor in War and Peace*. Heinemann 1960.

M. Hutton-Neve, *This Mad Folly. The History of Australian Pioneer Women Doctors*. Library of Australian History 1980.

Imperial War Museum (Malcolm Brown), *The First World War* 1991.

Monica Krippner, *The Quality of Mercy*. David and Charles 1980.

Margot Lawrence, *Shadow of Swords. A Biography of Elsie Inglis*. Michael Joseph 1971.

Leah Leneman, *In the Service of Life: The Story of Dr Elsie Inglis and the Scottish Women's Hospitals.* Mercat Press 1994.

Leah Leneman, *The Guid Cause: The Women's Suffrage Movement in Scotland.* Mercat Press 1995.

Leah Leneman, 'Medical Women of the First World War – Ranking Nowhere.' 1993, *British Medical Journal, 307*, 1592–1594.

Leah Leneman, 'Medical Women at War, 1914–1918.' 1994, *Medical History, 38*, 160–177.

Andro Linklater, *An Unhusbanded Life. Charlotte Despard, Suffragette, Socialist and Sinn Feiner.* Hutchinson 1980.

Lyn Macdonald, *Roses of No Man's Land.* Michael Joseph 1980.

Lyn Macdonald, *Somme.* Michael Joseph 1983.

Lyn Macdonald, *They Called it Passchendaele.* Penguin 1993.

Lyn Macdonald, *1915: The Death of Innocence.* Headline 1993.

Eva Shaw McLaren, *A History of the Scottish Women's Hospitals.* Hodder and Stoughton 1918.

Redmond McLaughlan, *The RAMC.* Leo Cooper 1972.

Jessie Main, chapter on 'Nursing' in *Improving the Common Weal. Aspects of the Scottish Health Service, 1900 to 1984*, ed. Gordon McLaughlan. Edinburgh University Press 1987.

Louisa Martindale, *A Woman Surgeon.* Gollancz 1951.

Arthur Marwick. *The Deluge: British Society in the First World War.* Bodley Head 1965.

Arthur Marwick, *Women at War, 1914–18.* Croom Helm 1977.

John Masefield's Letters from the Front, 1915–1917, ed. Peter Vansittart. Constable 1984.

David Mitchell, *Women on the War Path: The Story of Women in the First World War.* Jonathan Cape 1966.

Flora Murray, *Women as Army Surgeons.* Hodder and Stoughton 1920.

Antonio de Navarro, *The Scottish Women's Hospital at the French Abbey of Royaumont.* Geo. Allan and Unwin 1917.

Official History of the War. Medical Services. 12 vols, ed. Major-General Sir W.G. Macpherson. HMSO 1923.

A.F. Savill, *Music, Health and Character.* John Lane 1923.

Denis Stuart, *Dear Duchess: Millicent, Duchess of Sutherland, 1867–1955.* Constable 1953.

John Terraine, *The Road to Passchendaele.* Leo Cooper 1984.

Lis Whitelaw, *The Life and Rebellious Times of Cicely Hamilton.* Women's Press 1990.

Leslie M. Williams, *No Easy Path: The Life and Times of Lilian Violet Cooper.* Brisbane 1991.

Index

Abbey of Royaumont 1–7, 11, 17–24 and *passim*

Adams, Annie K.B. (Mrs Buckby) (sister) 97

Adams, Dr Mary 158

Aldrich-Blake, Dame Louisa 62, 154

Allan, Dorothy (Mrs Percival) (orderly) 280

Almond, Charlotte K. J. (Mrs Johnson) (orderly) 275, 280

Anderson, Agnes Lang (auxiliary nurse, 26.4.15 to 11.8.18) 187, 281

Anderson, Alison Fairlie (Lady Blood) (orderly, 10.2.18 to 11.8.18) 181

Anderson, Elizabeth Garrett *see* Garrett Anderson, Elizabeth

Anderson, Florence Amy (Mrs Longrigg) (x-ray orderly, 15.8.15 to 27.9.16 and 25.4.18 to 25.10.18) 167, 170–1

Anderson, Mary Mack (Mme Petitpierre) (dispenser) 181, 280

Arabs *see* North Africans

Armistice 115, 199–202

Armstrong, Grace E.H. (Mrs Woodhouse) (orderly) 204

Armstrong, Millicent (clerk) 30, 278

Ashton, Eva Margaret (cook, 5.9.17 to 18.3.19) 168, 181

Banks, Isabel (Mrs Simmonds) (chauffeur) *See illustrations*

Barclay, Yvonne (Mrs Golding) (orderly, 25.5.16 to 28.5.17) 32, 280

Berry, Dr (Mrs) J. Augusta 14–15, 25, 71, 133, 144, 147, 162, 194, 204, 215, 223, 234, 251–4

Berry, Jean E. P. (x-ray) 71, 122, 277

Binyon, Lawrence 126–7

Birks, Constance (Mrs Dunsmore) (orderly, 17.2.16 to 22.8.17) 83

Bossières, Dr 66

Boutet, Eugène 69

Bruce, Lucy H.M. (masseuse) 281

Buckley, G.L. (x-ray) 71, 77, 82–3, 224, 275, 280

Butler, Dr (Mrs) Elizabeth 47–8

Butler, Marian Ada (x-ray orderly, 18.10.17 to 3.6.18) 156, 170–1

Campora, Lucien 106

Canteens 129–131

Cardew, (Mr) Sydney (chauffeur) 82–3, 85, 88

Carey-Morgan, *see* Morgan

Carter, Angela (Lady Hills) (orderly) 281

307

Celebrations, entertainments and
parties 23, 49–50, 64, 90–5, 122,
193, 200–1, 211–12, 242, 247, 270
Ceremonies 89–90, 203–5
Chapman, Marjorie (auxiliary nurse,
6.5.15 to 22.3.19) 105, 130–1,
204, 211–12, 281
Chauffeurs 26–8, 84–5, 123–5,
155–6, 161–3,175, 204, 205–7
Christmas 23, 64, 98–9, 147–8,
211–12, 242, 270
Clothing department *see* Vêtements
Collum, V(era) C.C. (x-ray, 28.2.15
to 7.18) 11, 22, 27, 38–9, 41, 43,
48–9, 64, 71, 72–7, 80–1, 106–9,
110, 113–114, 122, 129–30, 134,
154, 155, 166, 174–6, 178–9,
180, 192, 224, 236, 241–2, 244,
252, 264–9, 269, 274
Courtauld, Dr Elizabeth 71, 92, 94,
107, 111, 131–2, 157–8, 159,
163–5, 173, 190, 192–3, 196–7,
198–202, 204, 205, 207–9, 213,
215, 216, 234, 235, 244–8, 252, 261
Coussergues, Dr 24, 60, 66–7, 70
Cowan, Georgina (orderly, 23.11.17
to 8.6.18) 167, 177
Cranage, Lucy Margaret (Dr (Mrs)
Costa) (orderly, 22.9.17 to
22.6.18) 216, 280
Crawshay-Williams, *see* Williams
Creil 1, 20, 24, 27, 36–7, 44, 80,
119, 120, 155, 177
Curé, M. l'Abbé Rousselle 4, 113–
116, 200
Curie, Mme Marie 51

Dalyell, Dr Elsie Jean
(bacteriologist, 5.16 to 10.16) 47,
71, 78, 224, 256–9

Daunt, Dorothea O'Neill (orderly,
18.8.17 to 25.2.19) 204
Davidson, Margaret (orderly,
auxiliary nurse 23.5.15 to
29.8.17) 272–3, 275, 281
Delacoste, M. 86
Descoings, General 135–6, 200
Descoings, Marie (orderly, 2.8.18 to
26.1.19) 200, 217
Dobbin, Dr Dorothy 158
Doctors 233–63, and *passim*
Don, Margaret (orderly) 278
Douglas, Mary (sister) 284
Doumergues, M. (minister for
colonial affairs) 87
Duncan, Isabella (matron, 6.15 to
15.12.16) 49, 57, 70, 284

Entertainments *see* Celebrations
Erskine, Dr (committee member)
84–6, 132, 139, 230–2
Estcourt-Oswald, Dr 71
Everingham, Winifred (sister,
18.8.17 to 30.12.18) 163, 172,
177, 279, 286

Fawcett, Millicent 8, 13
Figgis, Ella Margaret (dispenser,
5.5.17 to 2.1.19) 33, 111
Food 18–19, 56, 86–7, 95–8, 142,
153, 168
Fox, Mme Marie (orderly) 31, 43,
134, 136
Freeman, Margaret (orderly) 275,
281
French Red Cross (Rouge Croix),
Service de Santé 10, 11, 21, 24,
31, 79, 121, 126, 155, 178, 188,
209–10, 230

Index

Fulton, Katherine (chauffeur, 10.2.18 to 10.11.18) 155–6, 204

Funerals 57–8, 115, 197, 247, 271

Gamwell, H. (orderly) 277

Gamwell, J. M. (orderly) 277

Garrett Anderson, Elizabeth 8, 9

Gas gangrene 48, 61, 75, 80, 99, 104, 121, 224–8

Gas poisoning 146

Ghosts 272–4

Goodwin, Harriet Elizabeth (sister, 29.9.17 to 15.1.19) 167, 204, 286

Goüin, M. Edouard 5, 7, 19–20, 24, 40, 92, 178, 209–10

Grandage, Katherine (orderly, 27.11.15 to 31.5.17 and 9.3.18 to 1.12.18) 181

Grant, Dr Jessie (doctor, 6.6.18 to ?) 181, 195

Gray, Margaret 'Disorderly' (auxiliary nurse), 67–8, 200

Grey, Mary (sister) 67, 90, 286

Guest, Dr Edna Mary (doctor, 16.6.18 to 5.8.18) 182–3

Hacon, Mrs (Mrs Rubislaw) (kitchen superintendent) 44, 68, 69, 70, 88, 92, 252, 276

Hamilton, Cicely (clerk-administrator, 12.14 to 5.17) 15, 16, 17, 18, 23, 26, 33, 37, 41–2, 44, 49–50, 51–2, 64, 81, 85, 88, 90, 93, 122–5, 216, 242, 264, 269–74

Hancock, Dr M.D. (Mrs Barfett) 15

Harley, Mrs (administrator) 41, 42, 271

Hawthorne, Dr L. 48

Hendrick, Dr Rhoda Grace 195

Henry, Dr Lydia Manley (Leila) (Mrs Henry) (doctor, 25.7.17 to ?) 29–30, 44–5, 97, 110, 111–112, 115, 132, 136, 139, 148, 158–9, 165–6, 204, 207–9, 215, 224, 226, 228, 240, 246, 248, 259–62

Heyworth, Dr W. (Mrs Hinds) 15

Hodson, Dr Eleanor 81

Howard-Smith, Irene (orderly) 211–12

Hunter Mrs (chair, hospital committee) 60

Influenza 198–9

Inglis, Dr Elsie Helen Maud (founder) 7–10, 29, 39–40, 41, 195, 236, 255, 264, 269, 270

Inglis, Etta Helen Maud (auxiliary nurse, January to March 1915 and 30.11.15 to 22.3.19) 40, 130–1, 144, 152, 166, 204, 211–12

Inglis, Dr Florence 132, 144

Inglis, Violet A.H. (orderly, 28.7.16 to 18.10.16 and 22.9.17 to 22.3.19) 144

Inkson, Kathleen (sister) 286

Ivens, Miss (Dr) Mary Hannah Frances (chief medical officer). References to Miss Ivens appear so frequently throughout chapters One to Eight that they have not been listed separately. There is a short biography in Appendix Two, pp. 233–244.

Jamieson, Anna Louisa (cook, 5.10.16 to 5.1.19) 144, 153

Jeffrey, Mabel (sister) 24

Jex-Blake, Sophia 8, 13
Joyce, Dr Margaret 234

Kemp, Miss (SWH committee member) 64

Laboratory 45, 47–8, 71, 78, 204, 225–7, 257
Language 31–4
Large, Mrs Ruby (Mrs Wilson) (x-ray orderly, 11.7.18 to 9.11.18) 194
Laurie, Mrs (treasurer, SWH committee) 68, 173, 209–10, 213, 214, 217
Lillie, Dr Helen 154
Lindsay, Gertrude (sister, then matron, 22.3.15 to 20.2.19) 55, 153, 163, 177, 188, 204, 284
Littlejohn, Dorothy (Mrs Hedderwick) (cook) 13, 15, 17, 18, 22–3, 25–6, 32, 271, 276
Logan, Dr Dorothy (doctor, ? to 27.8.18) 156–7, 183
Loudon, Kate (administrator) 30–1, 49, 51, 56, 61, 85, 88, 90, 92, 93, 96, 122, 276
Louis IX 5–6
Lowe, Catherine (x-ray orderly, 22.8.18 to 31.12.18) 213

MacAlister, Marion Jamieson (sister, 29.7.18 to 16.12.18) 213
MacDougall, Dr Helen (Mrs Hendrie) 81, 89, 93, 94
McGregor (Mrs Hallam) (chauffeur) 123–5
McGregor, Jessie Leslie (sister, 28.7.16 to 18.11.17 and 2.3.18 to 30.12.18) 32, 202, 286

Mackay, Norah (clerk, 25.1.15 to 14.7.17) 19, 243, 281–2
Mackenzie, Geraldine (Mme Potez) (orderly, April 1916 to May 1917) 82–3
MacKnight, Jean (sister) 128, 285
McLeod, Helen (cook, 4.8.17 to ?) 98, 168
Mair, Miss Sarah Siddons (president, Scottish Federation of National Union of Women's Suffrage Societies) 9, 30, 39
Manoel, Dr Marie (25.10.17 to 21.1.19) 132–3, 204
Martin, Eveline C. (clerk) 281
Martindale, Dr Louisa 62–3
Martland, Dr Edith Marjorie (assistant surgeon, 7.16 to ?) 81, 154, 159, 194, 204, 253, 254, 258–9, 262–3
Meiklejohn, Dr Jean 48
Merrilees, Anna Louisa (auxiliary nurse) 115, 281
Miall-Smith, Dr Gladys Mary (Mrs Fry) (doctor, 26.6.18 to ?) 181–2
Michelet, Chef 4, 63, 95–8, 101, 122, 153, 190–1, 200
Middleton, Rachel (chauffeur) 281
Miller, Marjorie (orderly, later auxiliary nurse, 30.8.15 to 28.2.16 and 9.9.16 to 30.12.18) 45, 57, 112–113, 281
Minchin, Irma Eleanor (Mme Steinmann) (orderly, 17.10.18 to 30.12.18) 211, 247, 275, 278, 281
Moffat, Florence (orderly) 276
Monument 1, 140, 243–4
Moore, Evelyn Mercy (chauffeur, 5.5.18 to 6.11.18) 162, 278

Morgan, Dorothy Carey- (orderly) 122

Morris, Rose (sister) 286

Murray, Elizabeth Margaret (Mrs Galbraith) (chauffeur, 9.6.17 to 7.11.18) 163, 204

National Union of Women's Suffrage Societies (NUWSS) 8, 264

Navarro, Antonio de 3, 47, 96, 109–110, 229, 243

Neilson-Gray, Norah (orderly) 275, 276

Nicholson, Miss (Dr) Ruth 14, 71, 93, 133, 179, 200, 204, 215, 221, 238, 243, 247–8, 252, 255–6, 274

North Africans 94, 108, 110–111, 185–6, 188, 243

Nurses 127–8, 282–6 and *passim*

O'Rorke, Catherine (sister, 25.2.15 to 24.4.16 and 15.9.16 to 5.1.19) 204, 284–6

Orderlies 274–82, and *passim*

Owen, Mrs (administrator) 16, 41, 271

Parkinson, Dora (orderly) 141

Parties *see* Celebrations

Percival, A.M. (clerk) 280

Pétain, General Philippe 65, 100, 102, 118–18, 129, 150, 203

Peter, Mary Wilmot (Mme Campora) (auxiliary nurse) 106, 280

Pichon, M. (architect) 19–20, 67, 80

Poincaré, M. (president of France) 87

Potter, Dr Lena Mary 194–5, 248

Prance, Edith (chauffeur) 26–7, 238–9

Proctor, Evelyn Hope (orderly) 111, 141–8, 151–2, 195–6, 211–12, 216–17, 263, 276, 279

Ramsay-Smith, Madge (secretary/ administrator, 25.5.16 to 22.3.19) 115, 126, 136–7, 172, 179, 204, 207–9, 273–4

Raymond, Patricia (Mrs Lloyd) (orderly, 27.7.17 to 18.3.19) 170–1, 181

Red Cross *see* French Red Cross

Richardson, Dr Barbara 158

Richmond, Susan (Mrs Haydon) (orderly, 6.7.15 to 11.10.16) 57, 278

Robertson, Mrs A.M. (member of SWH committee) 68, 86–7, 88–97, 107–8, 112, 131–2, 153, 253–4

Rolt, Agnes Louisa (auxiliary nurse, 25.11.15 to 28.2.19) 130–1, 204, 280

Rose-Morris, Martha (sister) 261

Ross, Dr Winifred Margaret 14, 47, 71

Rousselle, M. l'Abbé *see* Curé

Royaumont, Abbey of *see* Abbey of Royaumont

Royaumont and Villers-Cotterets Association 46, 140, 183, 264, 284

Royaumont Monument *see* Monument

Russell, Mrs (Dr) (SWH committee) 59–61, 64, 136, 182, 190

Rutherford, Dr Margaret 59–61

Salway, Kitty (Mrs McIntosh) (orderly, 11.10.16 to 21.1.19) 159, 194, 204, 215

Savill, Dr (Mrs) Agnes 14, 48, 51–2, 71–2, 74, 77–8, 133, 135–6, 193–4, 198, 223, 224, 226, 227, 248–51, 261

Scottish Federation of Women's Suffrage Societies 8–10

Scottish Women's Hospitals (SWH) 7–11, 48, 189

Service de Santé, *see* French Red Cross

Senegalese 32, 58, 83, 91–2, 94, 107–110

Simms, Florence Beatrice (orderly, 1.12.17 to 28.8.18) 33, 177, 194, 279, 280

Simpson, Peternia M.B. (Mrs Gray) (cook, 12.10.17 to 22.6.18) 97, 98, 190–1

Sisters *see* Nurses

Smeal, Hilda Mary (chauffeur, 19.7.17 to 19.9.18) 170–1, 204, 277

Smieton, Maud Isolde (Lady Sanderson) (orderly, 4.7.16 to 22.3.19) 166–7, 194, 204, 224

Soissons canteen 129–31

Somme, Battle of the 65–6, 72–84

Spanish flu *see* Influenza

Spring Offensives, German (1918) 149–51, 158–81

Starr, Marjorie L. (Mrs Manson) (orderly) 6, 52–9, 64, 276, 277, 283

Statistics 70, 99, 156, 219–21, 228

Stein, Netta Hunter (orderly, 2.9.17 to 17.7.18) 216, 280

Stevenson, Doris (orderly) 183–9

Stoney, Edith Anne (x-ray) 138–40, 170–1, 172–3, 179–81, 194, 198, 204, 212–15, 224

Summerhayes, Grace (Dr Macrae) (orderly, 13.12.17 to 16.8.18) 33, 98, 107, 111, 146, 158, 177, 185–6, 192, 216, 224, 276, 277, 279, 280

Swanston, Mary (cook) 22, 25

Thom, Jean (Mrs Pierce) (sister, 21.2.17 to 5.12.18) 188

Tod, Isabel (matron, February 1915) 41–2

Tollitt, Florence (orderly, 1.6.15 to 24.7.18) 130–1, 162, 172, 204

Treatment 47, 62, 72, 104, 120–1, 133, 219–32

Uniforms 28–31, 84–5

Vêtements 43–4

Villers-Cotterets 133–8, 143–7, 151, 153, 155, 156–81, 186, 195, 207, 261

Walters, Dr Enid 132–3, 195

War, course of the 11–12, 35–6, 65–6, 117–19, 149–151

Warren, Christian Don (orderly) 278

Watt, Mabel (orderly) 278, 279

Weinberg, Professor 48, 225

Whitworth, Lucy M. (sister) 286

Williams, Mrs Crawshay- (later Mrs Alison) (clerk) 42

Williams, Janet (Mrs de Boutillier) (sister, 25.11.15 to 25.11.16) 32, 94–5, 107–8, 286

Wilson, Dr M.E. 33, 48, 71, 89, 92, 140
Winstanley, Maude (sister) 71, 122–3, 126, 135, 286
Woodall, Doris (orderly) 275

X-rays 20, 48, 51–2, 74–7, 89, 135–6, 138–9, 156, 170–1, 172, 180–1, 190, 193–4, 212–14, 251, 265

Yeats, Monica K.B. (chauffeur, 5.8.18 to 2.1.19) 205–7
Young, Marjorie (chauffeur, 5.10.15 to 1.7.17 and 3.11.18 to 23.3.19) 27–8, 123–4, 133